Not putting person in a box;
providing a box and seeing if they'll
jump in.

Core feature of each disorder

familiarity / comfortableness

Psychiatric Interviewing

The Art of Understanding

Shawn C. Shea, MD

Director, Diagnostic and Evaluation Center,
Associate Director of Residency Training, and
Assistant Professor of Psychiatry
Western Psychiatric Institute and Clinic
University of Pittsburgh
Pittsburgh, Pennsylvania

with illustrations by Meg Maloney

W. B. SAUNDERS COMPANY   1988
Harcourt Brace Jovanovich, Inc.

Philadelphia • London • Toronto • Montreal • Sydney • Tokyo

W. B. SAUNDERS COMPANY
Harcourt Brace Jovanovich, Inc.

West Washington Square
Philadelphia, PA 19105

Library of Congress Cataloging-in-Publication Data

Shea, Shawn C.
  Psychiatric interviewing.

  Includes index.
  1. Interviewing in psychiatry.   I. Title.
RC480.7.S54   1988   616.89   88-3155
ISBN 0-7216-1748-4

Editor: William Lamsback
Developmental Editor: Kathleen McCullough
Designer: W. B. Saunders Staff
Production Manager: Bill Preston
Manuscript Editor: W. B. Saunders Staff
Indexer: Dennis Dolan

Psychiatric Interviewing: The Art of Understanding. A Practical Guide for Psychiatrists, Psychologists, Social Workers, Nurses, Counselors, and Other Mental Health Professionals.

ISBN   0–7216–1748–4

Last digit is the print number: 9   8   7   6   5   4   3   2   1

To my father who showed me the door of creativity,
To my mother who urged me to open it,
And to Susan and Brenden who were waiting on the other side.

Preface

After all, there is nothing in the world as interesting as people, and one can never study them enough.

Vincent Van Gogh

The initial psychiatric interview is a creative act. It is a study of movement and change. It is unique. The circumstances, the environment, and the people involved can never be duplicated. Even if the interviewer and interviewee wanted to replicate their own interaction, they could not; for with each sentence their relationship has subtly changed. With each sentence they define a new phenomenon. This creativity is harnessed by two pivotal principles: (1) the patient must be powerfully engaged, and (2) a thorough and valid data base must be gathered in a limited amount of time. These two principles form the basis of the initial therapeutic encounter. They represent a complementary pair. When performed with sensitivity, thorough data gathering mirrors effective engagement.

Rapid advancements in the field of mental health have necessitated an evolution in the craft of assessment interviewing. In the past forty years an impressive array of new therapeutic interventions has emerged. These revolutionary advances include modalities such as tricyclic antidepressants, antipsychotic medications, behavior modification, family therapy, group therapy, and more sophisticated forms of dynamic and hypnotic psychotherapies, to name only a few.

The development of so many new tools has presented a startling challenge to the initial interviewer, especially when the interviewer is functioning as a triage agent or consultant who may never see the patient again. More specifically, in order to determine an effective treatment plan and disposition, the interviewer must gather an amount of information in fifty minutes which might have staggered an interviewer of forty years ago. At that time, one did not need to elicit the neurovegetative symptoms of depression, for tricyclic antidepressants did not exist. One did not have to carefully delineate the diagnosis of agoraphobia, because behavioral tools such as flooding were unavailable. It did not matter whether the interviewee had symptoms suggestive of mania, for lithium was a dream waiting to crystallize in John Cade's mind. In short, the therapeutic explosion has created an impressive need for more effective and thorough data gathering in the initial encounter.

The challenge of the interview currently revolves around the manner in which the initial interviewer collects critical data, while constantly attending to rapport. With each unique pairing of interviewer and interviewee this tension must be creatively resolved. A skilled interviewer is remarkably flexible. As has always been the case, the validity of the data depends directly upon the strength of the therapeutic engagement. In fact, if anything, the importance of the therapeutic alliance has increased over the years. In the long run, reliable diagnosis, effective treatment planning, treatment compliance, and family support of therapeutic intervention are all limited by a common factor: the therapist's ability to engage the patient. Consequently, the initial interview remains the foundation of all mental health interventions. This book focuses the attention on this craft that it rightfully deserves.

The text developed from my work as the medical director and instructor of interviewing at the Diagnostic and Evaluation Center (DEC) of the Western Psychiatric Institute and Clinic of the University of Pittsburgh. Our three-month interviewing program emphasizes didactic teaching, live interviewing, role playing, and direct feedback by fellow students, as well as videotaped and direct supervision. I felt a practical textbook, emphasizing the integration of engagement, diagnosis, and treatment planning, would be very helpful. To my surprise, I could not find such a book. Indeed, excellent books exist, but each tends to be primarily based upon a specific style of interviewing, such as the psychodynamic approach or the behavioral approach. *Psychiatric Interviewing: The Art of Understanding* attempts to fill this void, providing a synthesis of many perspectives, including various schools of psychiatry, psychology, and counseling.

More to the point, students seemed eager to read a book that integrated many different concerns, such as body language, engagement techniques, differential diagnosis by DSM-III-R criteria, treatment planning, and the internal structure of the interview. Students also repeatedly emphasized the usefulness of hearing the specific phrases and questions that different interviewers employed to explore distinct areas of information.

In the interviewing class (consisting of psychiatric residents, psychiatric nurses, psychology interns, social work interns, family practice residents, emergency room residents, and medical students), this practical exposure was accomplished by the experiential methods mentioned earlier. In this book, the same goal is approached by the generous use of sample questions, case vignettes, direct transcripts of actual interviews, and numerous mock interviews created to demonstrate specific teaching points. This textbook is a clinician's book, focusing directly upon the practical issues of sensitive interviewing.

As a field guide, this text reflects the concern of any professional asked to perform the initial interview. Therefore, it is primarily written with psychiatric residents, counselors, clinical psychologists, social workers, psychiatric nurses, and psychiatrists in mind. The format allows flexible use as a guide for individual study, a classroom textbook, and/or a seminar springboard. With regard to flexibility, the book may be read as a whole or in parts. Each chapter tends to function as a unit unto itself, thus allowing readers to pick and choose relevant material for their particular needs.

The book was also written to be a core textbook for medical and nursing students as they studied psychiatry. All physicians and nurses, no matter which field they choose as a specialty, must be able to effectively engage patients and determine whether major types of psychopathology are present and require treatment. All physicians and nurses should be adept at detecting critical processes such as suicidal ideation or the presence of psychosis. This text provides the groundwork for these critical skills. Moreover, many textbooks of psychiatry provide the facts but not the methods. Consequently medical students and nurses know what a major depression is but do not have any idea how to explore for it in an actual clinical setting. This book provides the practical bridge that can lead students from the classroom into practice. With regard to medical and nursing students the critical chapters for study are Chapters 1, 4, 5, 6, 7, and 8. The section on the mental status in Chapter 9 is also very useful for the students moving on to the clinical wards.

The text can also be used as a unique supplementary reading source in abnormal psychology, for it functions as a clinical reference point. It illustrates the human aspect of psychopathology, as evidenced by the interviewing experience. The interviewee appears as an individual, not a textbook label. In this regard Chapters 4, 5, 6, and 7 are most relevant.

Concerning structure, the book is organized into three sections: (I) Fundamentals of Interviewing, (II) The Interview and Psychopathology, and (III) Advanced Techniques of Interviewing.

In Part I, Fundamentals of Interviewing, the first two chapters center around core issues challenging the assessment interviewer, such as the structure and tasks of the interview, the validity and reliability of the data gathered, and basic types of resistance such as overly talkative patients or adamantly shut-down patients. In essence, these issues determine the nature of the interview itself. The understanding of how one should interview grows from an understanding of why one is interviewing.

The third chapter explores the fascinating world of body language, emphasizing the nonverbal dialogue that occurs throughout the interview process. It pays particular attention to the powerful impact of the clinician's own body language and paralanguage upon the interview process, influencing a diversity of factors such as patient engagement, validity of data, and the pacing of the interview itself.

The fourth chapter focuses upon treatment planning and the organization of clinical data. It also introduces the reader to a simplifying and practical approach to utilizing the DSM-III and DSM-III-R describing in detail the five diagnostic axes. Equally important approaches, such as the perspective of family systems and the patient's framework for meaning, are also explored in depth.

In Part II, The Interview and Psychopathology, the principles discussed earlier are viewed in the context of their application to three major areas of psychopathology: (1) affective disorders, (2) schizophrenia and psychotic process, and (3) personality disorders. A chapter is devoted to each of these areas. By intensively studying interviewing principles in these three circumscribed areas it is hoped that a variety of core principles will be delineated, which are generalizable to many other areas of psychopathology such as anxiety disorders and substance abuse. Thus, Chapters 5, 6, and 7 magnify the subtle nuances of the interviewing process, providing a more sophisticated understanding from which to develop one's own interviewing style.

To facilitate this exploration, Chapters 5 and 6 are split into two complementary sections. In the first section, interviewing techniques useful in the process of differential diagnosis by DSM-III and DSM-III-R criteria are examined in detail. These principles are explored through discussions of interviews based on actual case histories or hypothetical case histories created to enhance learning. In the second section, an attempt is made to understand the phenomenology of each pathological state, emphasizing the ramifications of these states on various systems pertinent to treatment planning in the initial interview itself.

Chapter 7 is devoted to personality disorders and emphasizes the need to understand not only diagnostic criteria but also the world view of the patients suffering from character psychopathology. A concerted effort is made to help the reader feel what it is like to be in the world as these patients experience their worlds. To this end, topics such as sensitively eliciting "difficult histories," including the sexual history and the drug and alcohol history, are examined in detail. Many other troublesome areas are discussed, such as performing a formal mental status and dealing with a tearful or angry patient.

In Part III, Advanced Techniques of Interviewing, the emphasis shifts to more sophisticated methods of analysis and interviewing. An entire chapter is devoted to the critical issue of evaluating suicidal and homicidal ideation. Besides examining the many pertinent risk factors through case histories, this chapter carefully explores many of the specific interviewing techniques useful in uncovering suicidal and homicidal ideation. The ninth chapter deals with shifting perspectives during the interview itself, as exemplified by looking at one's own emotional responses, fantasies, and countertransference. In the final chapter, the thorny issue of patient resistance is addressed directly, including both general principles and specific methods of handling awkward situations, which use actual patient questions as jumping-off points for discussion.

As this introduction draws to a close, I am reminded that if someone asked me to define the major goal of this book, I would be flooded with many possibilities. To begin with, it is not an attempt at an exhaustive study, which unfortunately can often transform into a study in exhaustion for the reader. Instead, I have attempted to produce a quick reading field guide that examines carefully many of the core practical and clinical issues surrounding the first clinical encounter. From this exploration I hope to achieve my major goal, the stimulation of intellectual excitement. Hopefully this excitement will entice readers to proceed upon their own ongoing exploration of this craft long after they have put this book down.

I would like to add that the style of interviewing described here represents only one of many effective styles. I do not present this style as "correct interviewing." Instead, I offer this material as an invitation to readers to develop their own styles, by borrowing some methods, discarding others, and creating new ones.

In closing, I want to say that interviewing has provided me with many fascinating moments. I believe we are studying a very special human interaction, one in which we are privileged to be participants. In the last analysis, interviewing is an ultimate art, a shared work of creativity, undertaken in the service of a person in need.

Please note that the names of all patients have been changed, and at times distinguishing characteristics or facts have been altered to further protect their identity.

Shawn C. Shea, M.D.

Acknowledgments

I would like to begin by expressing my deep gratitude to Thomas Detre, M.D., Director of Western Psychiatric Institute and Clinic, and David Kupfer, M.D., Chairman of the Department of Psychiatry at Western Psychiatric Institute and Clinic, for their enthusiastic support of the book. Both Dr. Detre and Dr. Kupfer have also given their strong support to my attempts to develop a training program dedicated to interviewing and to the development of an interviewing laboratory in which the interviewing process can be given the empirical study that it deserves. I would also like to thank the remaining administration of Western Psychiatric Institute and Clinic for their key support of our interviewing program, many of whom also provided invaluable feedback on the book, including Carol Anderson, Ph.D., George Board, Dr. PH, Richard Cohen, M.D., George Huber, J.D., Joan Kyes, M.S.N., Joaquim Puig-Antich, M.D., Jeffrey Romoff, M.Phil., Loren Roth, M.D., Duane Spiker, M.D., and Jack Wolford, M.D.

I would like to thank the following clinicians, each of whom reviewed various chapters from the book and whose comments were greatly appreciated, including Cleon Cornes, M.D., Peter Fabrega, M.D., Rohan Ganguli, M.D., Tom Horn, M.D., Stan Imber, Ph.D., Paul Pilkonis, Ph.D., and Grady Roberts, Ph.D. A warm thanks to Val Brown, Ph.D., and Mimi Brown, M.S.N., for both their constructive feedback and their delightful friendship. Thanks should also be given to Jeff Wilson, M.D., who allowed me to utilize various quotations he had discovered related to the phenomenology of psychotic process. The quotations greatly enhance Chapter Six.

I would like to give a special thanks to Richard Simons, M.D., a man I tracked down as he was racing to leave for the airport, after giving his keynote address at the Annual Meeting of the Association for Academic Psychiatry, who quickly agreed to review several chapters and proceeded to provide enthusiastic support. His willingness to help a young academician, whom he had never met before, represents a model of the academic spirit at its best.

I would like to also give a very special thanks to Juan Mezzich, M.D., Ph.D., who has served as my mentor over the years and without whom the book would never have developed. A special thanks is given in memory to the late Peter Henderson, M.D., whose dedication to training will always remain as a source of inspiration and whose support of my career and this book will never be forgotten.

As the author of a book dedicated to teaching, perhaps my strongest debt is to those who taught me. Many of them have already been mentioned, but I would also like to thank the following clinicians, whose compassion and excellence created a stimulating learning experience during my residency at Western Psychiatric Institute and Clinic: Anselm George, M.D., Carol Heape, R.N., M.S.N., Diane Holder, M.S.W., George Hsu, M.D., Tony Mannarino, Ph.D., Bob Marin, M.D., Swami Nathan, M.D., Elaine Portner, Ph.D., Al Rossi, M.D., Mike Shostack, M.D., Paul Soloff, M.D., Susan Stewart, M.S.W., Rick Tomb, M.D., Paul Weiss, M.D., Gerhard Werner, M.D., and Bob Wittig, M.D.

I would also like to thank my editor, Bill Lamsback, for his belief in the text and his efforts to achieve a book that would not only be enjoyable to read but a pleasure to the eyes. I would also like to thank Jack Farrell of the Marketing Department whose enthusiastic support for the book and creative ideas will hopefully ensure its success. I would also like to thank my secretary, Maria Antonich, for her patient help in preparing the text and correspondence associated with the book.

Before closing, a few more particularly important thanks are warranted. Working with Meg Maloney was a true treat. Her creativity and imagination, as well as her ability to bring our ideas to visual fruition, were a continuing source of excitement. I believe her illustrations bring a true feeling of awe and sensitivity to the written word.

I would like to thank all my students, from whom I am always learning and whose provocative questions provide a constant source of growth. A particular thanks to two former students, Barb McCann, Ph.D., and Scott Bohon, M.D., who have become my colleagues, working together with me towards a better understanding of the art of interviewing.

Ultimately a clinician and educator is only as good as the people with whom he works, who provide a constant source of creative ideas and emotional support. In this respect I would like to thank Karen Evanczuk, R.N., Anita Zeiders, M.S., and Patty McHugh, M.S.W., the clinical/administrative arm of the Diagnostic and Evaluation Center, for their continued support. And a special thanks to the staff nurses and telephone counselors of the Diagnostic and Evaluation Center; a more dedicated and talented staff cannot be found. They are a pleasure to work with, and it is with a great sense of gratitude that I have found a home in our work together.

A warm thanks also goes to my sister, Sandy, who showed me the beauty of teaching and to my brother, Chuck, who has always been a model in the art of compassion.

Finally, all my thanks goes to my wife, Susan, for her love, understanding, and support. She has believed in the book from the beginning, and her insight and editorial comments were invaluable in improving the text. Her help with word processing was also greatly appreciated.

Thanks again, to all.

Contents

1

Fundamentals of Interviewing

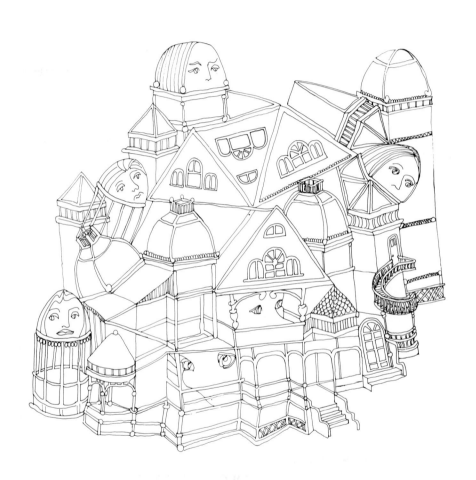

1

Interviewing: The Principles Behind the Art

When a doctor tells me that he adheres strictly to this or that method, I have my doubts about his therapeutic effect. . . . I treat every patient as individually as possible, because the solution of the problem is always an individual one . . .

Carl G. Jung, Memories, Dreams, Reflections

In the following pages, we will begin a study of the interviewing process. We will be examining the craft in which one human attempts the formidable task of understanding another human. By way of analogy, this task is not unlike exploring a darkened room in an old Victorian house, holding only a candle as a source of illumination. Occasionally, as one explores the shadows, a brisk wind may snuff the candle out and the room will grow less defined. But with patience, the explorer begins to see more clearly. The outlines of the family portraits and oil lamps become more distinct. In a similar fashion, the subtle characteristics of a patient begin gradually to emerge. This quiet uncovering is a process with which some clinicians appear to familiarize themselves more adeptly than others. It is as if these more perceptive clinicians had somehow known the layout of the room before entering it. And indeed, in some respects, they had.

Their a priori knowledge is the topic of this chapter. We will attempt to discern some of the underlying principles that determine whether an initial interview fails or succeeds. As Jung suggests in the epigraph to this chapter, these principles do not harden into rigid rules. Instead they represent flexible guidelines, providing structure to what at first appears structureless.

Perhaps a second analogy may be clarifying at this point. A recent book on nineteenth century art by Rosenblum and Janson provides some useful insight.[1] In it, the authors attempt to describe the many processes that lead to the creation of a work of art, including environmental influences, political concerns, and the goals and limitations of the artist. With each painting these historians appeared to question themselves vigorously concerning concepts such as color, composition, originality, perspective, and theme. In short, Rosenblum and Janson utilized a specific language of art consisting of concisely defined terms. This language provided them with the tools to conceptualize and communicate their understanding. Since the language was one understood by most artists, the concepts of Rosenblum and Janson could be widely discussed and debated.

The work of the art historian is not at all unlike our own; as clinicians, however, we are concerned with a living art. We can study the characteristics of this living art once we possess a language with which to conceptualize our interviewing styles. With this language, the principles that seem to provide an experienced clinician with a "map of the Victorian room" naturally evolve.

In this chapter we will begin to develop a language with which to describe the interviewing process. Towards this goal the chapter itself is divided into two parts: (1) an operational definition of interviewing and (2) a concrete conceptualization of the major goals of the interview. This foray into the language of interviewing will shed new light on familiar faces, providing a chance for the development of a more flexible and penetrating style of interviewing.

IN SEARCH OF A DEFINITION

There probably exists no better method for uncovering a definition of interviewing than by analyzing a brief piece of clinical dialogue. Even in a short excerpt, clarifying principles may begin to emerge.

The following dialogue was taken from a videotaped diagnostic interview. Of particular note is the fact that the supervisee was disturbed by a not uncommon problem faced by an interviewer, "the wandering patient." Specifically, the supervisee commented, "I couldn't really even get a picture of her major problem, because she took off on every subject that came to her mind." In this excerpt, the interviewer was attempting to discover whether the patient was suffering from the symptoms of a major depression. The patient, a middle-aged woman, had been describing some problems with her son, who was suffering from an attention deficit disorder.

> **Pt.:** . . . He's a behavior problem; maybe a phase he's going through. (Interviewer writes note.) He's exhibiting crying spells, which don't necessarily have a reason. The teacher is trying to interview him to see what exactly is

wrong with the child because he's tense and crying, which isn't like him; he's been a happy-go-lucky kid.

Clin.: Is he still kind of hyperactive?

Pt.: Oh yeah . . . now that we've lowered the medication he's a little bit better, but I was just mad at the doctor; you know, one of them should have explained it to me.

Clin.: I would think that must be very frustrating to you.

Pt.: It was.

Clin.: And how has this affected your mood?

Pt.: Ah . . . I have a husband who works shifts (interviewer takes note), and he wants to be in charge of everything. I had a job until last February, when I got laid off. I was working more than full time. My husband does not pitch in at all. I was working about 60 hours a week. He wouldn't lift a dish, which really gets to you.

Clin.: Uh huh; I'm sure.

Pt.: Especially when you're working Saturdays and Sundays and you start at 6:30 in the morning and don't get home 'til 8:00 at night.

Clin.: What kind of work?

Pt.: I was working in electronic assembly. I was an x-ray technician for ten years and then we decided to settle down and have a family. I was working at the hospital up in Terryhill. And, uh, he said, and I can see his point . . .

At first glance, one can quickly empathize with the interviewer's frustration, for indeed this patient is in no hurry to describe her mood or her depressive symptoms. Instead, when asked directly about her mood, she immediately darts down a side alley into a belittlement of her husband. She appears to wander from topic to topic. But with a second glance, an interesting observation emerges concerning the communication pattern between these two co-participants. It is unclear who is wandering more, the patient or the interviewer. It is as if the two had decided to take an evening stroll together, hand in hand.

Specifically, the interviewer had intended to explore for information concerning depression. But when the interviewer asked about mood, the patient chose to move tangentially. At this crucial point, where the patient left the desired topic, the interviewer left with her. Unintentionally the clinician may have immediately rewarded the patient for leaving the desired topic by taking notes. Her scribbling may have inadvertently told the patient to continue by suggesting that what the patient was saying was important enough for the clinician to jot down. The interviewer further rewarded the tangentiality of the patient by proffering an empathic statement, "Uh, huh; I'm sure." As if this were not enough, the clinician follows the patient down the alley by asking a question about the new topic.

Thus, both the patient and the clinician had an impact upon each other, their interface defining a dyadic system unconsciously committed to the perpetuation of a tangential interview.

This example illustrates the point that interviews define interactional processes, some of which facilitate communication and others of which inhibit communication. These processes are so distinctive that one can name them. For instance, the above process could be named "feeding the wanderer." If one is trying to uncover specific information within a set topic, then the process of feeding the wanderer represents a maladaptive technique. Curiously, if one were attempting to foster an atmosphere conducive to free association, the same technique might be beneficial. In either case, the interviewer can and should be consciously aware of this technique, implementing it when desirable and avoiding it when it would not be efficacious.

For example, in the next chapter we will discover that the interviewer may have been able, in the above dialogue, to lead this patient effectively into a less digressive mode of speech through the use of focusing statements. But the point of most immediacy to us concerns the hint provided by this excerpt as to the nature of the interviewing process itself, a definition of which is beginning to crystalize. This definition would be equally true for an assessment interview by a social worker or a television interview by a talk show host. The clinical definition reads as follows:

> An interview represents a verbal and nonverbal dialogue between two participants, whose behaviors affect each other's style of communication, resulting in specific patterns of interaction. In the interview one participant, who labels himself or herself as the "interviewer," attempts to achieve specific goals, while the other participant generally assumes the role of "answering the questions."

This definition emphasizes the interactional process of the interview. It also allows one to refine the definition depending upon the desired goals and the context of the interview. To make this definition more specific to the clinical assessment one has only to look for the goals particular to the clinical situation.

In a broad sense, these assessment goals are as follows:

1. To establish a sound engagement of the patient in a therapeutic alliance.

2. To collect a valid data base.

3. To develop an evolving and compassionate understanding of the patient.

4. To develop an assessment from which a tentative diagnosis can be made.

5. To develop an appropriate disposition and treatment plan.

6. To effect some decrease of anxiety in the patient.

Furthermore, the goals of the initial interview will vary depending upon the demands of the assessment situation, including issues such as time constraints and the interviewer's determination of what type of data seems clinically necessary in order to make an appropriate disposition. For instance, a crisis worker called into an extremely busy emergency room to interview a rape victim will clearly sculpt a different interview than an analyst asked to spend an hour or two with a well-educated patient requesting psychotherapy for chronic depression. In short, the needs of the clinical situation should determine the style of the interview but can do so only if the clinician remains willing to flexibly alter his or her approach.

In any case, the above consideration emphasizes one of the frequent challenges facing the initial interviewer, namely to gain a thorough and valid data base in a limited amount of time while sensitively engaging the patient. The shorter the time period provided, the more complex the task appears. To return to our Victorian room, it is as if a clinician were being asked to make an inventory of a darkened room in a restricted amount of time while being careful not to disturb the decor too much. No easy task, even for a master of parlor games. Perhaps this challenge reaches its most formidable peak when an interviewer or consultant is placed in the unenviable role of performing an intake assessment. From his or her assessment, frequently limited to about sixty minutes by the many time pressures present in a busy clinic, the interviewer must determine the treatment disposition of the patient.

I have chosen to focus upon this particularly challenging type of interview in this book, for the principles needed to perform it gracefully can be generalized to most other types of interviews, where more time may be available, resulting in a more leisurely pace. In short, the difficulties presented by the assessment interview provide tremendous opportunities for learning skills critical to understanding the core issue of most interviews, the delicate interplay between engagement and data gathering. Many of these same skills will ultimately also be of use in psychotherapy itself.

The discussion so far has provided an operational definition of an assessment interview. From this definition, a map of sorts can be formulated as shown in Figure 1.

This map, delineating the various goals of the assessment interview, begins with the engagement process, which, in many respects, determines whether the other goals will be successfully achieved. As engagement proceeds, the data gathering process unfolds, leading to a progressive understanding of the patient. This understanding of the

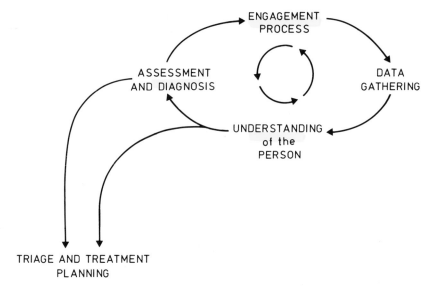

FIGURE 1. Map of the interviewing process.

patient as a unique person depends upon the clinician's ability to see the patient's view of the world and recognize the patient's fears, pains, and hopes. As the interview progresses, the clinician begins to formulate a clinical assessment, including a tentative differential diagnosis. From both the assessment of the patient's situation and an understanding of the patient as a person the clinician can formulate a treatment plan suited to the individual needs of the interviewee, while acknowledging the constraints placed upon treatment by the limitations of the mental health system itself.

These processes of engagement, data gathering, understanding, and assessment are in actuality parallel processes. The reverse arrows in the center of the map emphasize this fact, highlighting the clinician's need to attend to engagement activities throughout the first sixty minutes.

THE CREATION OF AN INTERVIEW: GOALS AND VARIATIONS

The Engagement Process

BLENDING AND EMPATHY

From the first moment they see, hear, smell, and touch each other, the clinician and the patient begin the engagement process. In this complex interplay they reflect their sensory information onto the slippery screen of their memories. From these comparisons, both the clinician and the patient attempt to determine where each will fit into the other's life. Even as simple a gesture as a handshake can lead to lasting impressions. The experienced clinician may note whether he or she encounters the iron fingers of a Hercules bent upon establishing control or the dampened palm of a Charlie Brown expecting imminent rejection.

Ironically, at this same moment, the patient will have begun his or her own mental status on the clinician. This process can be seen clearly in the patient who greets the clinician's outstretched hand not with a handshake but with a look of disdain. As the clinician responds to the patient's rejection of a simple social amenity, who can doubt that the patient will be gaining some hints about the psychological workings of the clinician. For example, one interviewer, perhaps with an obsessive need to "do things my way," may further extend his or her hand, testily adding, "Don't you want to shake?" Another clinician, perhaps jaded from overwork, may dryly comment, "Not in the mood for shaking today, are we?"

In either case, the patient has struck a rich vein from which to mine answers to questions such as the following: (1) Will this interviewer get angry with me?, (2) Will this interviewer make me do things I don't want to do? and (3) Am I safe here? This example hints at the complex and mutual activities affecting the engagement process, during which territorial issues are initially addressed.

Before proceeding it is important to define two terms, *engagement* and *blending*. Engagement refers to the ongoing development of a sense of safety and respect from which patients feel increasingly free to share their problems, while gaining an increased confidence in the clinician's potential to understand them. Blending represents the behavioral and emotional clues from the interview that suggest that this engagement process is proceeding effectively. Stated differently, the engagement process defines a set of activities, and the concept of blending provides a method of monitoring the effectiveness of these activities.

Not all writers emphasize the distinction between engagement and blending, but I feel it is an important one. Its significance lies in the fact that it does one little good to study engagement techniques if one does not develop a reliable method of measuring the effectiveness of these techniques in the interview itself. The concept of blending provides an avenue for active self-monitoring by the clinician. Problems in blending can alert the interviewer to the need to change interview strategies before serious damage to the clinician-patient alliance has developed.

One can assess blending by utilizing three complementary approaches: a subjective method, an objective method, and patient self-report. With regard to the subjective technique, an interviewer can learn what sensations he or she experiences when engagement is optimal — in essence, what a good interview feels like. Educators have suggested that once this internal and idiosyncratic feeling stage has been identified, the clinician can use it as a thermometer of sorts, to determine the intensity of blending at any given moment.[2]

Naturally, this subjective feeling will vary from interviewer to interviewer. Consequently it may help to examine some of the descriptions clinicians have related concerning this feeling state.

a. "To me good blending feels more like a conversation and a lot less like an interview or interrogation."

b. "I know blending has occurred when suddenly I realize during the interview that I'm actually talking with a person with real pain, not a case with imagined defenses."

c. "When the blending is good, I notice that I feel more relaxed, sometimes even giving off a sigh. Curiously I also feel more interested."

These descriptions suggest the personal uniqueness of the blending process. It is this personal uniqueness that allows the concept of blending to function as such a reliable and sensitive tool for monitoring the degree of engagement. If clinicians can train themselves to intermittently check the progress of blending, they will have discovered a window from which to study the unfolding engagement process. To this extent, the interview becomes less nebulous and more tangible. It evolves into something that can be modified.

This increased tangibility can be furthered by utilizing the second major avenue for monitoring the blending process, an objective look at the behavioral characteristics of the interview itself. The behavioral clues suggested by body language will be discussed in Chapter 3. In this chapter an examination of the timing and structural characteristics of the verbal exchange will be highlighted.

The issue facing the interviewer involves finding concrete behavioral cues, from the verbal exchange, that indicate the presence of good blending. Weins[3] and colleagues have provided some simple but fascinating methods of analyzing the temporal characteristics of speech by studying three major speech variables: duration of utterance (DOU), reaction time latency (RTL), and the percentage of interruptions. The DOU can be roughly equated with the length of time taken up by the interviewee's response following a question. The RTL represents the length of time it takes an interviewee to respond to a question. And the percentage of interruptions represents the tendency for the interviewee to cut the clinician off before a question has been finished. One can look at all of these variables in relation to the clinician's speech patterns as well.

With regard to blending, these variables offer a potentially more objective measure of effectiveness, for certain patterns of exchange may suggest weak blending. For instance, a guarded or suspicious patient often produces curt responses to questions (a short DOU), long pauses before answering (long RTL), and occasional cutoffs as the patient corrects the interviewer for inaccuracies in his or her statements. If an interviewer spots such a pattern emerging, it may be a clue to ineffective engagement.

Another example at the opposite end of a continuum concerns the hypomanic, histrionic, or anxious patient who tends to wander. These wandering patients frequently present with a long DOU, a very brief RTL, and may actually cut the interviewer off frequently. Interestingly the interviewer may find himself or herself reciprocating with cutoffs in a vain effort to get a word in edgewise.

Moreover, with histrionic, hypomanic, or manic patients, the blending is frequently marked by a peculiar superficial quality. With regard to spontaneity of speech these patient's open up inappropriately quickly, as opposed to the gradual increase in blending seen with most patients. Consequently, the observed blending possesses a one-sided and shallow quality, aptly called by one student "unipolar blending."

In the above two examples, we have seen that variations in basic patterns of verbal output, such as a DOU and RTL, can provide objective indications of the adequacy of the blending process. One might ask whether this objective technique offers any advantage over the subjective approach described previously. I believe it does. But one method does not appear more valuable than another; rather each method complements the other. For instance, not infrequently clinicians are duped into missing the psychopathology of histrionic or hypomanic patients.

One of the reasons this problem occurs is that the clinician feels at a subjective level that the blending is unusually good. Indeed, the clinician is fascinated by the patient's story. In actuality, the blending is artificially good, representing the unipolar blending just described. In fact, unipolar blending, if recognized by the clinician, could provide the clue that "something is wrong here." The patient's engaging style and subtle dramatics are misleading the clinician. If in this instance the clinician could step back to look at the DOU and RTL, the clinician might recognize the hallmarks of a unipolar blending and consequently evaluate the possible psychopathological causes of it. In this case the objective technique sidesteps the confusion created by judging the blending process solely by the subjective method.

The other advantage of paying attention to more concrete parameters such as DOU and RTL is the ability to use these criteria to judge the effectiveness of a specific technique employed by the clinician. If the clinician, for example, attempts to actively engage a patient who seems hesitant to talk, one of the earliest and most easily recognized markers of success will be an increase in DOU. Correspondingly, changes in the subjective feeling of increased blending may only appear later and may be less easily recognized.

A third method of determining the degree of blending consists of the patient's self-report. Occasionally, a patient will spontaneously tell an interviewer to what degree the interaction is enjoyable. More commonly, the interviewer may inquire, as the interview winds down, "What was it like talking with me today?" Oftentimes, because of a hesitancy to appear unappreciative or rude, patients will reply that everything was fine, even if it was not. On the other hand, patients may pointedly discuss specific concerns, which sometimes provides appropriate and constructive criticism.

In other instances, the patient's self-report may provide unexpected insights, especially when the self-report contradicts the subjective and objective methods of evaluating blending. For instance, I am reminded of a young man who appeared somewhat disinterested as we spoke. He talked softly and with little animation. As we proceeded, I felt awkward, as if this was going to be a bad mix of personalities. Though both the objective and subjective signs of blending suggested poor engagement, to my surprise, at the end of the interview he reported feeling very at home with me. He stated that he had enjoyed the interview, and he appeared sincere.

His diagnosis was paranoid schizophrenia in remission. It was a residual blunting of affect that was creating both an outward and an inward suggestion of poor blending; the engagement was not, in truth, weak. This disparity highlighted the type of miscommunication that this patient could easily convey to other people, an aloofness that was both disarming and misleading. Attention to blending by self-report greatly enhanced my understanding of the manner in which this patient embraces the world. It also suggested the possible utility of social skills training.

Thus, the clinician can benefit from learning to judge blending by the subjective, objective, and self-report approaches. With these three techniques in mind, the interview becomes at once less mystifying and more gratifying. The gratification stems from the realization that the interviewer can learn to creatively alter the interview process itself.

Once blending has been analyzed, the clinician possesses a concrete idea of the strength of the engagement process with any particular patient at any given moment. Weak engagement may imply that invalid data is more likely and compliance more problematic. Moreover, a weak engagement process suggests one of the following three conditions:

1. The interviewer's actions are actively disengaging the patient.
2. The interviewee's psychopathological processes or defenses are interfering with engagement.
3. A combination of the above.

If the clinician feels that the damaged blending can be attributed to the first condition, then the clinician can attempt to consciously alter his or her style of interaction. For instance, a paranoid patient may be put off by an extroverted style of interviewing. In such an instance, the clinician may decide to tone down the interview in an effort to ease the patient's fears.

If the weak blending can be ascribed to the second condition, then the clinician may be alerted to the types of psychopathology that could be blocking the blending, as with the histrionic process described earlier. Naturally, if the third condition is the issue, increased attention to both style of interaction and psychopathology can be brought into play.

At this point we have reviewed three methods of directly assessing blending that indirectly assess engagement itself. It is of value to reflect upon the map of the interviewing process delineated earlier. On this map, the interviewer begins with the engagement process for a good reason. The engagement process affects all subsequent goals of the interview.

More specifically, poor engagement raises significant doubts about the validity of the data base, for patients generally do not freely share with people they do not like. Moreover, without effective engagement, one will seldom gain knowledge of the private corners of the patient's room alluded to in our comparison of an interview with an exploration of a dark Victorian room. Hence, the clinician leaves with only a superficial understanding of the patient's pain. Furthermore, without valid data falling into place, the clinician's assessment and diagnosis are frequently in significant jeopardy. Finally, if the engagement process proceeds poorly, the patient may never return for a second appointment, casting the shadow of irrelevence over the work of the first interview.

Thus one is left with the realization that this somewhat nebulous concept of engagement appears to be the pivotal process upon which much of clinical practice turns. Fortunately, this process is not as mercurial as it first appears. Upon a more searching exploration specific principles for engagement emerge, including (a) the assessment of blending, (b) the effective conveyance of empathy, (c) the ability to foster a safe environment in which the patient can share, (d) the ability to appear genuine and natural to the patient, and (e) the ability to appear reassuringly competent. In the following pages we will attempt to get beyond the obvious meanings of these terms in an effort to recognize their practical applications. We shall begin with the term *empathy.*

Many clinicians assume that empathy is a simple concept. It is not. The large number of research papers devoted to its capture testifies to its elusiveness. Fortunately, over the years insights have been achieved that help to demystify empathy, a quality that all people feel they naturally possess but that in reality may be less ubiquitous than imagined. It seems only right to begin our story with Carl Rogers, who developed the field of client-centered counseling. He conceptualized empathy as the clinician's ability "to perceive the internal frame of reference of another with accuracy, and with the emotional components and meanings which pertain thereto, as if one were the other person, but without ever losing the 'as if' condition."[4] Stated more simply, empathy is the ability to accurately recognize the immediate emotional perspective of another person while maintaining one's own perspective.

As Rogers pointed out, there is an important distinction between empathy and identification, although they can overlap. In the latter process the clinician not only recognizes the emotional state of the other but also proceeds to feel it. The importance of this distinction lies in the fact that identification often marks the pathway towards such unrecognized therapeutic gremlins as burn out and unrecognized countertransference. The persistent appearance of strong feelings of identification may alert clinicians to the need to begin or return to their own therapy, for such identification can quickly destroy the therapeutic process.

One feels compelled to say a silent prayer for the poor patient with borderline features who meets a clinician who boldly proclaims, "I can feel your pain." Borderline patients have enough problems with identity diffusion without finding "silly putty" coating the edges of their clinician. Thus a simple but important lesson to be learned from the study of empathy is that most patients are not searching for a person who feels as they do; they are searching for someone who is trying to understand what they feel.

G. T. Barrett-Lennard sheds further light upon the concept of empathy by recognizing the fact that empathy is effective only if it involves both the interviewee and the interviewer.[5] He calls this shared response the "empathy cycle," a concept providing an excellent framework with which to study the practical application of empathy. Consequently we will look at each phase of this cycle in detail.

The empathy cycle consists of the following phases: (1) the patient expresses a feeling, (2) the clinician recognizes this feeling, (3) the clinician conveys recognition of the feeling to the patient, (4) the patient receives this conveyance of recognition, and (5) the patient provides feedback to the clinician that the recognition has been received.[5] With this cycle in mind, the empathic process begins to make significantly more sense. In fact, one can see that a breakdown in empathy can arise at each of these five stages.

In the first phase of the empathy cycle, in which the patient expresses a specific feeling, a variety of processes can disrupt empathy. For instance, both conscious and unconscious defenses may block the patient from expressing his or her actual emotions. A poignant example of this process is illustrated by the following dialogue, in which a mother of a mildly retarded seven-year-old discusses her son:

> **Clin.:** Tell me a little about John's behavior with other children.
> **Pt.:** Oh there is really little wrong there, he's really quite normal, just like the other kids. He doesn't like to play games very much or sports, but then he has a mind of his own, maybe someday he'll be a star golfer or skier.
> **Clin.:** You had mentioned something about his speech earlier.
> **Pt.:** Oh, hmm, you must be thinking of his lisp. Well I think we all went through that phase as children. In a few years it'll all work out. You know, I have trouble understanding most little kids when they talk, it's part of being a little person.

One feels the pathos of this situation, in which the mother's defenses of denial and rationalization prevent the expression of core feelings of pain. If the interviewer should attempt to make an empathic stagement such as, "It sounds like you're really going through a lot with John," I doubt the response would be positive. In this case the patient's own unconscious defenses have prevented the empathy cycle from spontaneously unfolding.

But phase one does not have a monopoly on the common breakdowns that prevent the establishment of an empathic contact. In phase two, the recognition of the patient's feeling, problems may arise if the clinician's perceptual or intuitive skills fall short, perhaps related to his or her own defenses or psychopathological undertow. In particular, interviewers need to be aware of the impact of their immediate emotional status upon their ability to empathize accurately. For example, a clinician who has recently experienced an unsettling session in supervision may have significant trouble attending to a patient's subtle clues of inner pain. At the other extreme, a recently divorced clinician could easily project his own feelings of betrayal onto a patient undergoing a trial separation, when, in fact, the patient is not experiencing such feelings at all. In both situations, the clinician's emotional state prevents an accurate perception of the interviewee's feelings.

In this light, it can be stated that interviewers have only themselves to serve as measuring instruments. The clinician has no microscope or CAT scan to provide insight. But like the sophisticated machine, interviewers can unintentionally bias their data. Before beginning an interview, it is often useful to check the bias of the instrument by pausing for a moment of reflection, asking what feelings are present before proceeding to meet the patient. Such a simple process may alert the clinician to potentially distorting factors such as feeling rushed, angry, sad, or simply weary. Once alerted to their biases, interviewers may hope to stand one step further away from invalid data.

The second phase of the empathy cycle also raises several interesting questions concerning the actual nature of intuition. Margulies and Havens[6,7] have emphasized two frames of mind that appear to be integral aspects of the empathic process. In the first place, the clinician must possess the ability to listen with an attitude of disciplined naivete, literally attempting to feel the world of the patient without seeking cause and effect, classification, or moral judgment. This receptive listening perspective was masterfully developed by the psychological school of phenomenology, which we shall discuss at greater length later in this chapter. But the bottom line can be simply stated: the clinician must learn to suspend analytic thought when such thought may be destructive to the engagement process.

The second frame of mind that Margulies discusses concerns the ability of the clinician to imagine the inner experiences of the patient by creatively projecting himself into the patient's world. He likens this ability to the poetic imagination of artists, emphasizing the ability to move actively into the patient's world, or "inscape," as this phenomenon has been called.[8] When done well, the clinician not only paints a picture of the patient's world, he or she enters it.

The ability to listen while suspending analysis and the ability to sensitively project what another person may be experiencing can be viewed as two skills from which intuition is born. They remain pivotal to effective clinical practice, typically reaching powerful proportions when clinicians achieve a high degree of blending.

Here we stumble upon a fascinating irony, for one of the characteristics of a gifted interviewer is the ability to know not only when to use these intuitive skills but when not to use them. Phrased slightly differently, a skilled clinician draws from both intuition and analysis. In a matter of a few minutes the skilled interviewer may juxtapose periods of intuitive listening with moments of analytic thought. Indeed, the two processes, in the hands of a seasoned clinician, tend to guide each other. For example, a clinician may intuitively sense a patient's extreme fear of a disintegration of the self. Besides immediately helping the clinician to blend with the patient, this intuitive feeling might prompt the clinician to later explore, in a diagnostic sense, whether the patient may represent a borderline personality or a narcissistic personality.

Similarly, an analytic process can lead a clinician to a higher level of empathy. For instance, a clinician may observe that as the interview proceeds, the patient avoids eye contact and becomes increasingly anxious. This analytical observation may prompt the clinician to be more empathically aware of the patient's feeling of being ill at ease. At such moments the clinician may gently ask, "I'm wondering what it has been like for you coming to see a psychiatrist?" Subsequently an empathic mode of listening may significantly help the patient to relieve his or her sense of guilt or embarassment. The important point remains that intuition and analysis are complements, not antagonists. Both skills are utilized frequently during the first encounter.

In the third phase of the cycle, the clinician's actual phrasing of the empathic statement, the complexities of human interaction further manifest themselves. Here is a phase in which some surprises may appear. One such unexpected twist arises from the fact that not all empathic statements work equally effectively with all patients. In order to understand why, this phase warrants close inspection.

One of the more puzzling aspects of empathic statements remains their uncanny ability to promptly disengage a small subset of patients, in short, to achieve the exact opposite of their intended use. One is reminded of the varying fashions in which people accept compliments in everyday situations. Some people take compliments well, while others take them poorly. Members of the latter group often become decidedly ill at ease following a sincere compliment, shrugging it off with "Thank you, but it's really nothing."

One manner of interpreting this peculiar phenomenon consists of viewing the compliment as pushing the recipient towards one of two uncomfortable states: (1) accepting a view of himself or herself that seems inaccurate or (2) feeling an emotional state (such as a pleasant sense of self-worth) that he or she does not want to experience, as may be seen in a person burdened by a chronically punitive superego. So it is with empathic statements, which backfire when they push people into interpersonal niches they do not wish to occupy.

The question is whether or not this situation can be avoided. To a large extent I think it can be. Preventing such undesirable repercussions represents one of those areas in which analytic thinking can be of considerable help. More specifically, one can categorize patients, with some degree of caution, into two types, those who are trusting and those who feel guarded. It is with the latter patient, the so-called guarded patient, that empathic statements most frequently display the nasty habit of disrupting the engagement process. The guarded quality of these patients may stem from a variety of sources, including a fear of the clinician, a long-standing character trait of suspiciousness, or frankly prepsychotic or psychotic paranoia.

Empathic statements made to guarded patients from whatever etiology frequently decrease the interpersonal distance between these patients and the clinician. This interpersonal intimacy is exactly what guarded or paranoid patients do not want. Stripped of their "buffer zones" by the well-intentioned clinician, these patients have only one option: to escape through retreat or attack. In short, guarded patients need "distance," a fact too frequently overlooked by interviewers.

So far we have delineated the concept that patients may respond to empathic overtures in different manners secondary to their degree of guardedness, ranging from a trusting bias to frank paranoia. Our understanding can be developed even more fully if we look at three of the characteristic qualities of empathic statements in general, for a change in these characteristics can affect the responses of guarded patients.

In this regard, empathic statements appear to vary along the following three axes: (1) the degree of implied certainty of the interviewee's feelings by the interviewer, (2) the degree of implied intimacy between the interviewer and the interviewee, and (3) the degree of intuited attribution made by the interviewer from statements offered by the interviewee. As one would expect, these axes overlap considerably. But, for purposes of acquiring a more sophisticated understanding, it will be worthwhile to look at them separately, their unique qualities offering the structural foundation from which to understand the impact of empathic statements in general. Along each of these axes one can move from *basic* to *complex empathic statements.*

To begin our inquiry let us speculate on the first axis, the degree of certainty implied by an empathic statement. Put simply, one considers to what degree the clinician implies that he or she knows exactly what the patient is experiencing. In basic statements, the interviewer expresses considerable uncertainty. In contrast, in complex empathic statements the interviewer conveys a high degree of certainty, as illustrated in the following dialogue, in which the patient, a poetic young man, has just suffered the cruelties of an unwanted divorce. This same man had lost his mother to leukemia when he was thirteen. Following the patient's statement, an example of both a basic and a complex response along the axis of implied certainty will be given.

Pt.: After my wife left, it was like a star exploded inward, everything seemed so empty . . . she seemed like a memory and my life began to fall apart. Very shortly afterwards I began feeling very depressed and very tearful.

Clin.: [Basic Empathic Statement] (said gently) It *sounds like* everything seemed to be collapsing around you.

or

> ***Clin.:*** [Complex Empathic Statement] (said gently) *You were feeling like everything was collapsing around you.*

As a general rule, basic empathic statements, which tend to possess a "sounds-like" quality, can be used effectively to enhance blending with *both* a trusting and a guarded patient. In the case of a trusting patient, the complex empathic statement may represent an even more effective device, for it may indicate to the patient a higher degree of seeing things through their eyes, in a phenomenological sense. On the other hand, complex empathic statements may disengage a guarded patient, as shown in the following:

> ***Pt.:*** I can't believe how cruel people can be. My ex-boss won't even talk with me, won't even give me a minute of his damn time. It hurts, yes it does. But at this point I've got a million problems and nobody to help me.
>
> ***Clin.:*** *You are feeling* very hurt.
>
> ***Pt.:*** How would you know what it feels like, have you ever been fired?
>
> ***Clin.:*** No, I can't say I have, but it surely must be a devastating process.
>
> ***Pt.:*** To some people perhaps (slight glare from patient).

In this passage, the clinician's attempt at a complex empathic statement with regard to certainty seems to have unsettled the paranoid patient, a verbal boomerang of sorts. Perhaps this backfire has its origins in the patient's desire for a private and hence safe world. More explicitly, this patient appears to dislike the process of being told what he is feeling or should be doing, for that world is his world, and trespassers are not encouraged.

This trespass has led to a rather awkward moment, in which the patient challenges the clinician's ability to understand him, which is not exactly the response desired by the interviewer, who suddenly finds himself dodging the cutting edge of a paranoid accusation.

One can speculate that if the clinician had used a simple empathic phrase such as, "It *sounds like* you have been feeling pretty hurt" instead of the complex phrase, "*You are* feeling hurt," that the interaction may have been less antagonistic.

The second axis of empathy concerns the degree to which the clinician's response implies emotional intimacy to the patient. It specifically evaluates the degree to which the clinician suggests that "I am or probably would be experiencing at this very moment the same emotion you are." In this sense, it implies a feeling of "our world" as opposed to "your world" and "my world," as seen below, using the patient discussed earlier as a model.

> **Pt.:** After my wife left, it was like a star exploded inward, everything seemed so empty . . . she seemed like a memory and my life began to fall apart. Very shortly afterwards I began feeling very depressed and very tearful.
>
> **Clin.:** [Basic Empathic Response] *To me it seems as if you may be* feeling a whole set of intensely painful emotions.
>
> or
>
> **Clin.:** [Complex Empathic Response] It hurts to lose someone like her.

Once again the basic empathic response will frequently foster the blending process with both trusting and guarded patients. Furthermore, with the guarded patient, the basic empathic response seems to provide ample distance or breathing room, a quality much in demand by guarded patients.

For a moment, let us focus upon the ramifications and potential advantages and disadvantages of complex empathic responses with regard to the axis of intimacy. With trusting patients, another example of a complex empathic statement begins with phrases such as "It is" or "There is." These phrases can sometimes be unusually effective for engagement purposes.[9] Such third-person singular impersonal phrases tend to suggest a shared experience to the patient, in the sense that the clinician acknowledges the validity of the patient's experience while simultaneously suggesting one would (or even has) experienced similar emotions. When well-timed, these phrases can shore up a faltering alliance. Of course the difficulty surfaces when complex statements are poorly timed, as with some paranoid patients. In such instances complex phrases can precipitate unwanted misunderstandings, as suggested by the following:

> **Pt.:** My husband is a strange man. You might call him evil. It's the "divorce game," him trying to drive me nuts so that he can divorce me.
>
> **Clin.:** How do you mean?
>
> **Pt.:** For about three months he's had them on me. I know they're watching, every night at 6 o'clock. I feel their presence. I think they use telescopes and maybe mind probes to see me, a terrible terrible position to be in.
>
> **Clin.:** *It is* frightening to be constantly watched by others.
>
> **Pt.:** Just what do you mean by that? How would you know what I'm feeling? (said testily)

Clin.: Well, in the situation you're describing I think it would be frightening.
Pt.: Frightening enough to make one lose their mind?
Clin.: Well . . . that's difficult to say, it's not . . .
Pt.: Its' *what* Dr. Jones? Frightening enough to make one crazy, well I'm not crazy Dr. Jones, no matter what you think, and trust me I'm not defenseless.

In this example, the clinician's complex empathic statement has suggested a shared intimacy that has been rudely rejected by the patient. In fact, for the patient, fleeing from a world studded with "mind probes," the clinician's unsolicited entry into her world seems most poorly timed. Indeed, the unintended invasiveness resulting from the phrasing has formed a paranoid rage of no small proportion, perhaps placing this patient near the edge of violence. Once again, with this type of paranoid process, it may have been wiser for the clinician to employ a basic empathic statement or perhaps no empathic statement at all. Along the third axis of empathy, we will once again see that the impact of empathic statements can vary depending upon the mental state of the patient.

The third axis, concerning the degree of implication of specific qualities to the patient, warrants considerable attention. Along this axis how much the clinician reads into the patient is compared with how much the clinician repeats back exactly what he or she has heard. The opposing ends of this spectrum appear in the following:

Pt.: After my wife left, it was like a star exploded inward, everything seemed so empty . . . she seemed like a memory and my life began to fall apart. Very shortly afterwards I began feeling very depressed and very tearful.
Clin.: [Basic Empathic Response] (said softly) It sounds as if your whole life began falling apart.
or
Clin.: [Complex Empathic Response] (said softly) It is very frightening to lose her so suddenly, so similar to the pain you felt when your mother died.

In the basic empathic response, the clinician, essentially employing the same wording as the patient, has truly mirrored back the patient's thoughts. No intuition is displayed here. Consequently there exists little chance that the statement will be perceived as inaccurate or too invasive by either a trusting or a guarded patient. Moreover, if said in a caring tone, this basic response can convey concern while demonstrating an attentive listening style. It may represent a rudimentary level of empathy, but it does convey caring when done well. This statement has significant limitations, for it does not particularly demonstrate great sensitivity or understanding by the clinician.

To the contrary, the complex response to a *trusting* patient may suggest to the patient that he or she is dealing with a keenly perceptive individual. For instance, in our example this sensitivity was suggested by the clinician's use of the term "frightening," a feeling never mentioned by the patient but nevertheless felt to be present by the clinician. When accurate, such empathic connections can be powerful indeed. Moreover, the second part of the clinician's response, suggesting a relationship of the current grief to an earlier mourning for the patient's mother, also represents an attribute made by the clinician to the patient that may suggest to the patient that he has found an understanding and insightful listener. The presence of such comments often characterizes the dialogue of an experienced clinician.

Once again, however, one must ask whether or not this complex empathic statement can get a clinician into trouble. Not surprisingly, the answer is "yes," especially with guarded patients. By way of example, paranoid process is often associated with an inordinate attention to details, demonstrated by an unexpected value on accuracy. This need for *accurate* understanding at all costs is bolstered by the paranoid fear that "no one understands what I'm really feeling." With these two processes in mind, one can easily imagine potential traps awaiting the clinician who unwittingly uses a complex empathic response with a paranoid patient, as displayed in what follows:

> *Pt.:* After my wife left, it was like a star exploded inward, everything seemed so empty . . . she seemed like a memory and my life began to fall apart. Very shortly afterwards I began feeling very depressed and very tearful.
>
> *Clin.:* It sounds terribly frightening to lose her so suddenly, so similar to the pain you felt when your mother died.
>
> *Pt.:* No . . . no, that's not right at all. My mother did not purposely abandon me. That's simply not true.
>
> *Clin.:* I did not mean that your mother purposely abandoned you, but rather that both people were unexpected losses.
>
> *Pt.:* I suppose . . . but they were very different. I never was afraid of my mother . . . they're really *very* different.

Needless to say, this attempt at empathic connection leaves something to be desired. The patient's attention to detail and fear of misunderstanding have obliterated the intended empathic message, leaving the clinician with a frustrating need to mollify a patient who has successfully twisted an empathic statement into an insult of sorts. At this point some relatively simple patterns are emerging, which can act as practical guidelines to effective phrasing of empathic statements.

1. In general, empathic statements represent extremely valuable methods for strengthening engagement. Consequently, the clinician will usually employ such statements intermittently throughout an interview.

2. The statements themselves vary in degree of implied certainty, intimacy, and attribution of qualities, which represent three axes of empathy.

3. Along these three axes, one can characterize empathic statements as either basic or complex.

4. Basic statements are generally useful with *both* trusting and guarded patients. Their weakness lies in the fact that they do not convey a particularly sensitive understanding to the patient, although they do demonstrate concern. Their strength lies in the fact that they seldom backfire.

5. With guarded patients it is frequently best to utilize basic empathic statements. At other times it is best to avoid empathic statements. If one attempts to use a more complex statement and discovers some evidence of resulting disengagement, then further complex statements should probably be avoided.

6. On the other hand, with trusting patients, interviewers frequently begin with basic statements and progress to more complex empathic statements, for such complex statements may prove more effective in producing a deepening sense of trust.

In our survey of the empathic axes we have uncovered an important principle of interviewing: empathic statements may disengage guarded or paranoid patients. This acute decrease in blending may show itself by a disavowal or correction of the empathic statement or by various nonverbal communications. Being aware of this principle can allow the clinician to consciously avoid the inappropriate use of empathy. But this principle provides another service to the clinician if looked at from the diagnostic perspective. If a clinician is in the midst of an interview and finds that the patient disengages when offered empathic statements, then the clinician should be aware that a hostile or paranoid process may be present, a process that may have been masked until that moment in the interview. Of course, not all patients who disavow empathic statements are guarded or paranoid. At times, patients who feel a need to appear strong will also refuse empathy. With such patients, it is often wise to emphasize their strengths as opposed to utilizing empathic statements.

At this juncture in our discussion of the third phase of the empathy cycle, the actual conveyance of empathy, three further variables determining the effectiveness of empathic statements warrant attention: frequency, timing, and length. With regard to frequency, no magic number exists. I do not think anyone can authoritatively state the number of optimal empathic comments per interview, for this number must surely vary for each paired interviewer and interviewee. On the other hand I would estimate that well-received clinicians frequently seem to scatter empathic statements throughout their interview, perhaps averaging one statement every five to twenty minutes. Moreover, it seems likely that one could either potentially overuse or underuse empathic statements. In the former case the clinician runs the risk of sounding superficially caring or paternalistic. In the latter case, the interviewer may be perceived to be as inscrutable as a sphinx, hardly an effective tool for ensuring a follow-up appointment.

This discussion of frequency naturally leads into the issue of timing. One underlying principle, perhaps the most important, remains the value of using at lease one or two empathic statements during the first five to ten minutes. Generally speaking, I would suspect that many patients often determine whether they like or dislike the clinician during these initial minutes, and their decision frequently rests upon whether the clinician seems accepting or not. Specifically, patients may fear that the clinician will not understand them or will think they are silly or weak. No better tool exists in the clinician's repertoire than an empathic statement for decisively allaying such fears. Although an easy maneuver, this technique can set the tone for an entire interview.

Of course, even with the best of intentions, empathic statements can miss their mark, as illustrated below:

> ***Pt.:*** Well I don't really think it's right for the university to be so upset with me for not paying back the loan. I mean it was seven years ago and I simply don't have the money. It really hurts me too.
>
> ***Clin.:*** It sure sounds like a difficult spot to be in, what with all those pressures and financial responsibilities. I bet it seems like you have no place to go, you know, sort of stranded, probably makes you feel like everyone is against you.
>
> ***Pt.:*** Uh-huh (painful pause)
>
> ***Clin.:*** What are you thinking of doing?

In this example the empathic statement has all the power of a two-page descriptive paragraph in an adventure story. It is far too long. In general, empathic comments display their engagement best when they are concise and unambiguous.

This example also points out one method of determining the effectiveness of any given empathic comment. Put succinctly, effective statements usually result in an increased verbal production by the patient. Shut-downs, as shown above, often follow an ineffective comment. Leston Havens describes this process elegantly:

A more exacting test of successful empathy is the extent to which our responses stimulate and deepen the other's narrative flow. Does the speaker stop or change subjects? Are the expressions of feeling increased or decreased? One of the moments of greatest clinician drama occurs when a strong empathic flow encounters a memory heretofore forbidden to consciousness or denied.[10]

There remains one last comment to make before leaving the discussion of the third phase of the cycle. Empathy is probably not primarily conveyed through empathic statements. Large amounts of empathy appear to be communicated through facial expressions, body language, tone of voice, and other "empathic noises," as Havens calls them.[10] These nonverbal elements will be given the attention they deserve in Chapter 3.

In the fourth phase of the empathy cycle, in which the patient receives the conveyed empathic statement, problems can also arise. Specifically, the patient's psychopathology may limit his or her ability to perceive empathy or even to understand language itself. Such a situation can occur with delirious patients or severely psychotic patients. In extreme cases, empathic statements can be malignantly transformed into an auditory illusion, perhaps becoming a derogatory statement or threatening insult.

Another case in point concerns manic patients who quite simply are sometimes too busy talking to even register an empathic statement. Indeed, at times, it is not clear whether they care if the clinician is being empathic or not. With these patients, attempts to empathize may actually be counterproductive, being in some respect contrary to what they most want at that moment, an audience.

In the fifth phase of the empathic cycle, in which the patient provides feedback to the clinician that the empathic statement was received, difficulties may once again surface. As before, the patient's psychopathology may prevent acknowledgment of the clinician's empathic communications. This is perhaps most poignantly demonstrated by the patient ravaged by a severe, regressive depression or a catatonic stupor. Such patients sometimes seem almost hollow, as if our words pass through them unheard and unanswered. But I think it is important not to be misled by this sensation, for these patients may very well be hearing and even responding to empathic statements despite their inability to convey their reception. Clinician statements such as, "I have no real way of knowing what you are feeling, but if you are feeling lonely or sad or want to talk, I will be available, just let me know", can be very important, perhaps even pivotal in providing a new bridge for communication, the first resonation in the empathy cycle.

Through this review of the empathy cycle, we have, it is hoped, moved from a cliché-like understanding of empathy towards a more sophisticated understanding of one of the most practical tools available to the initial interviewer. Furthermore, our discussion has indirectly led us to our next topic, the establishment in the interview of a feeling of safety.

THE INDUCEMENT OF A SAFE RELATIONSHIP

The patient's waiting room period before meeting his or her clinician may pass with an urgent slowness. It is frequently teeming with fears of rejection and with self-recrimination. It is often accompanied by ruminations such as, "Well, it's finally come to this, I'm so weak I need a shrink." As professionals we would like to think patients do not feel this way about us, but we should not kid ourselves. For most people (including most mental health professionals), it is genuinely upsetting to admit the need for help with a psychological problem. The sensitive handling of this anxiety represents one of the main tasks of the initial interviewer. In fact, if it is not handled well, there may not be a second interview.

In his insightful book *The Psychiatric Interview* Harry Stack Sullivan describes a novel idea he calls "the self system." This self system consists of "a vast system of processes, states of alertness, symbols, and signs of warnings," which protect us from a lowering of self-esteem as we meet new people.[11] This self system, consisting of both conscious and unconscious coping mechanisms, becomes activated in an effort to decrease the anxiety generated by fears of rejection. It is this self system that rises to a high pitch as a patient absent-mindedly turns the pages of a magazine in the waiting room.

Three ideas immediately come to mind. First, one of the primary goals of the clinician, in the initial interview, consists of attempting to decrease the patient's anxiety and hence the need for an extremely active self system. Second, the activation of the self system offers the clinician an excellent preview of the patient's defenses against interpersonal anxiety. Thus, the opening ten minutes of the interview provide an unexpected window into the workings of the patient's mental guard dogs, both healthy and rabid. And third, in most cases, the clinician's own self system is also aroused when the clinician meets a new patient. The interplay of these three processes lies at the very heart of the engagement process.

As we have seen, to some extent, the conveyance of empathy can significantly decrease the patient's need for an active self system, but other specific processes can also reassure the interviewee. In the 1950's and 1960's, Carl Rogers developed the concept of "unconditional positive regard," which he defines as follows: "The therapist communicates to his client a deep and genuine caring for him as a person with potentialities, a caring uncontaminated by evaluations of his thoughts, feelings, or behaviors." [12] It is a powerful statement. It is not unlike the suspension of analytic thought seen in the process of intuition.

Placed into the context of the initial interview, as opposed to ongoing therapy, unconditional positive regard translates as a suspension of moral opinion by the interviewer upon the interviewee. In short, the patient comes away with the feeling that the clinician is not going to pass judgment on him. In many cases, this safe feeling contrasts starkly with the patient's recent experience (and at times lifelong experience) of encountering a long string of raised eyebrows on the faces of friends, family members, and employers. It is up to the interviewer to not follow this parade of frowns.

In this regard, it becomes important for the clinician to work out the potentially disturbing feelings raised by emotionally charged issues such as divorce, religion, sexual preference, violence, rape, and abortion. No matter what the clinician's view of these activities, in the initial interview, the goal remains to show no judgment to the patient. Instead, the interviewer attempts to convey interest in finding out the significance of these ideas to the patient, recognizing the very wise statement of Armond Nicholi, Jr. that "whether the patient is young or old, neatly groomed or disheveled, outgoing or withdrawn, articulate, highly integrated or totally disintegrated, of high or low socioeconomic status, the skilled clinician realizes that the patient, as a fellow human being, is considerably more like himself than he is different . . ." [13]

Practically, one effective method of spotting potentially disruptive topics for oneself consists of monitoring interviews for those topics one consistently avoids. For instance, one interviewer may discover that he or she seldom knows anything about the religious beliefs of the patient, while another interviewer never asks about sexuality. Such gaps in data gathering may point to precisely those topics about which the interviewer has strong opinions. It is in these areas that conveying unconditional positive regard may be problematic.

It is not only controversial issues that can disrupt the conveyance of unconditional positive regard. In fact, as clinicians we may unwittingly sound like parents at the most unlikely times. In the following dialogue with a young man suffering from paranoid schizophrenia, this disconcerting process rears its head in a subtle form:

    Clin.:   Tell me more about what you've been doing since your last hospitalization.

    Pt.:   Things are going well. I'm getting along much better at

           home and I haven't needed all those drugs the doctor told
           me to take.

Clin.:   (pause, clinician looks up from clipboard) So you haven't
           been taking your medications like you're supposed to.

  Pt.:   No I just think they fog up my mind.

Clin.:   We'll need to talk about that a little later.

This clinician's choice of words has created an atomosphere potentially suggestive of a parent's reprimand. Indeed the interviewer's last statement sounds suspiciously like a threat to go to the principal's office.

As a contrast, in the following dialogue, a different approach yields a different interaction with significantly less activation of the patient's self system:

Clin.:   Tell me more about what you've been doing since your
           last hospitalization.

  Pt.:   Things are going well. I'm getting along much better at
           home and I haven't needed all those drugs the doctor told
           me to take.

Clin.:   What were some of the medications you were using?

  Pt.:   I think it was called Haldol and a little pill . . . Cogentin
           or something like that.

Clin.:   Tell me a little bit about what you felt like while you were
           on these medications.

  Pt.:   It was strange. I don't know which one was doing it, but I
           always felt doped up, like I was in a fog.

Clin.:   That sounds like an unpleasant side effect.

  Pt.:   Yes, it was.

This interviewer has successfully conveyed concern without a price tag of obedience. Ironically, later in the interview, I would suspect the latter clinician would be in a more favorable position to persuade the patient to try a neuroleptic again.

This discussion suggests another characteristic, nondefensiveness, that contributes to a feeling of safety for the patient. Patients are very quick to perceive defensiveness in an interviewer. Defensive posturing by the clinician may create in the interviewee the feeling that "I've got to watch what I say here." The following example illustrates a defensive position by the clinician, as a woman describes her anguish concerning her son's problems with schizophrenia:

Moth.:   I just don't know what to do with him. Nothing the
            doctors do ever helps. It's always the same. I don't think

they know what they are doing. They haven't tried mega-vitamin therapy and I hear that sometimes works miracles. I want you to try that treatment.

Clin.: Well, let's get something straight, these kinds of therapies are simply unproven and maybe unsafe. So we don't use those here.

Moth.: But some people claim they've been helped.

Clin.: Don't believe everything you read Mrs. Jones.

Here we see the paternalistic tone that can so readily destroy a patient's trust. The clinician's self system has been activated, resulting in a defensive, "educational" posture, which only serves to reciprocally activate the patient's own self system. This interaction might have been avoided with the following approach:

Moth.: . . . They haven't tried mega-vitamin therapy and I hear that sometimes works. I want you to try that treatment.

Clin.: It sounds like you've really gone through a lot of frustration Mrs. Jones. In a little while we'll talk about the pros and cons of different treatments, including mega-vitamin therapy, but first I want to hear more about your son so that I have a better understanding of exactly what we are dealing with here.

Moth.: Sure. It's long and complicated. But it all started about three years ago . . .

Our discussion of the principles behind the development of a safe alliance began with the words of Harry Stack Sullivan. Sullivan also provided an important note upon which to close our discussion. One of the contributing factors to the development of an overactive self system is the not so maladaptive fear that strangers may harbor ulterior motives. In short, a patient may fear that he or she is going to be used, or even abused.

It is hoped that conscious abuse of a patient is a rarity in our field, but less sinister abuse may enter the picture unconsciously. Clinicians may have ulterior motives of which they have little if any awareness. For example, a clinician may depend upon a patient for the gratification of the clinician's need to feel liked or important. If the patient feels that the clinician needs something from them, such as respect, caring, or fondness, the relationship is no longer a safe one. Once again the patient is faced with watching what he or she says, from the fear that professional help will be withdrawn if certain needs are not satisfied.

Sullivan stated this principle elegantly.

He [the clinician] is an expert having expert knowledge of interpersonal relations, personality problems, and so on; he has no traffic in the satisfactions which may come from interpersonal relations, and he does not pursue prestige or standing in the eyes of his clients, or at the expense of his clients. In accordance with this definition, the psychiatrist is quite obviously uninterested in what the patient might have to offer, temporarily or permanently, as a companion, and quite resistant to any support by the patient for his prestige, importance, and so on. It is only if the psychiatrist is very clearly aware of this taboo, as it were, on trafficking in the ordinary commodities of interpersonal relations, that many suspicious people discover that they can deal with him and can actually communicate to him their problems with other people.[14]

Besides offering a safe relationship, the initial interviewer also actively engages the patient in a positive fashion, utilizing those gestures and words that suggest to the patient that future interaction will be enjoyable and rewarding, as seen in our next topic.

CLINICIAN GENUINENESS

The term "genuineness" has been described by a variety of researchers.[15,16] As was the case with empathy, genuineness appears to be a nebulous term at first glance. Once again, an operative definition provides clarification. One can state that "being genuine" occurs when the following is present:

The behavioral characteristics of the clinician suggest to the patient that the clinician is feeling at ease both with himself and with the patient. It is frequently marked by three characteristics in the clinician: (1) responsiveness, (2) spontaneity, and (3) consistency.

Perhaps there exists no better arena for examining these characteristics of clinician genuineness than looking at the reactions of a clinician to patient humor.

When faced with humor some clinicians display a curious sense of awkwardness, as if humor should not be allowed during an interview. In essence these clinicians "run-over" the moment of humor. Rather than responding with a smile or a chuckle, they maintain a somber expression.

This rather extreme form of nonresponsiveness can produce an immediate increase in patient anxiety, not unlike the discomfort many of us have had the misfortune of experiencing in a social setting when one of our jokes is followed by an absence of laughter. Ironically, such clinicians may argue that their nonresponsiveness represents professionalism, but it seems odd that professional behavior should result in increased patient anxiety during the early stages of an interview. Moreover, this same lack of clinician responsiveness may be uniformly provided in response to a variety of patient affects, including tearfulness, anger, and fear, all in the name of professionalism.

Many patients balk at such pseudoprofessionalism, preferring a clinician who interacts with a gentle responsiveness. In the final analysis, the mark of a true professional seems to be his or her lack of a need to feign professionalism. Such clinicians quickly and easily appear at ease with both their body language and their reactivity. They are attentively relaxed. Moreover, they bring to the inteview a sense of appropriate spontaneity, the second characteristic of genuine interaction as described in our definition.

This spontaneity does not exist as a license for sharing whatever comes to mind. To the contrary, a skilled clinician consistently assesses the potential impact of all statements but also possesses the ability to share some spontaneous feelings if they are deemed appropriate for the patient. This spontaneous quality often demonstrates itself in characteristics such as a well-timed sense of humor, a flexible method of structuring the interview, and a nondefensive attitude towards questions voiced by the patient.

As just mentioned, one must be careful about the degree of responsiveness and spontaneity one displays. Both too much and too little can present problems. For instance, a bouyant interviewer can intimidate certain patients, while a wooden interviewer may frighten them. In the latter regard, if the frightened patient feels too uncomfortable with the clinician to share suicidal ideation, then the unresponsive interviewer may truly regret the need to present a wooden attitude. The clinician needs to nurture a flexible style. The degree of spontaneity and responsiveness will probably vary from patient to patient and with the clinical setting.

In this regard, the myth of "professional blandness" may have evolved from a misinterpretation of the psychoanalytic concept of presenting a neutral screen, upon which the patient could project his or her transference. This neutral screen concept does not represent a dictum for unresponsiveness. In the first place, an expressionless presentation hardly represents a neutral stance, as Ryle[17] has commented, for such a bland reaction typically suggests that the nonresponder dislikes the other participant. This supposed "neutral stance" is, in actuality, potentially very disengaging. Moreover, rather than providing a blank screen, it seems to bias the patient towards negative transference.

Even if one adhered to this neutral stance theory for therapeutic application, and few talented analysts I have met do so in a strict sense, it does not necessarily follow that the neutral stance is effective for assessment interviewing. Indeed, as we have seen, one of the major goals of the initial interview remains the development of a powerful blending, which will, it is hoped, lead to both powerful compliance and a second appointment. A wooden interview hardly lends itself to the facilitation of engagement.

It seems timely to examine consistency, the third element commonly characterizing a genuine interaction. Gerard Egan has emphasized the importance of consistency as demonstrated by the clinician's willingness to explore the patient's world in a shared manner, while respecting the patient's present limitations and defenses. More specifically, the clinician avoids discordant actions such as appearing warmly responsive in part of the interview and cooly distant later. Nor does the clinician suddenly become confrontative, as demonstrated by Counselor A in the following example provided by Egan.[18]

> **Client.:** I want to know what you really think of me.
>
> **Counselor A.:** I think you're lazy and that you would like things to get better if that could happen by magic.
>
> **Counselor B.:** Frankly, I don't find a great deal of value in such direct evaluation, but I think it's good to talk about this directly. Maybe we can take a look at what's happening between you and me.

The response of Counselor B demonstrates a willingness to share exploration, including a foray into the developing interviewer-interviewee relationship.

Together, the traits of appropriate responsiveness, spontaneity, and consistency coalesce to create an appealing milieu for the sharing of problems. When adroitly blended, these three traits of genuineness convey a sense of emotional balance in the clinician, a balance that suggests a possible source of help to the person in need.

In the following dialogue, these traits as well as a sense of nondefensiveness are elegantly displayed in a situation in which a therapist could easily have swallowed his or her foot. In this interaction, the clinician, a physician, had determined from the preceding conversation that the patient was pleasant and well-integrated but very anxious. Consequently, the interviewer felt that humor could be safely employed.

> **Clin.:** What has it been like coming down to the emergency room today?
>
> **Pt.:** Unsettling, to say the least. I feel very awkward here, sort of like I'm vulnerable. To be honest, I've had some horrible experiences with doctors, I don't like them.

Clin.:   I see, well, they scare the hell out of me too (smiles, indicating the humor in his comment).

Pt.:   (chuckle) I thought you were a doctor.

Clin.:   I am (pause, smiles) that's what's so scary.

Pt.:   (smiles and laughs)

Clin.:   Tell me a little more about some of your unpleasant experiences with doctors because I want to make sure I'm not doing anything that is upsetting you or frightening you. I don't want that to happen.

Pt.:   Well, that's very nice to hear. My last doctor didn't give a hoot about what I said and he only spoke in huge words.

In this example, the clinician has skillfully transformed a potentially "loaded moment" into a shared resolution through humor. If patients realize that avenues for discussing their needs and complaints are open, they frequently feel less frightened. The presence of pathways for "filing complaints" paradoxically often decreases the need for their use.

This excerpt also illustrates the common finding that experienced interviewers frequently appear to enjoy the process of interviewing itself. Experienced clinicians feel at home in the interviewing process, their own self systems purring quietly. It is this sense of natural balance in the clinician that remains one of the most powerful of engagement tools. This balance is complemented by the next trait to be discussed, yet another important tool in the engagement process.

CLINICIAN EXPERTISE

In order to explain the concept of clinician expertise most effectively, it may be best to temporarily view the interviewing process solely from the patient's perspective. To the patient, certain questions are of paramont importance. The answer to one of these questions in particular holds unusually powerful significance, perhaps even determining the degree of final compliance. It is a logical question. It is a natural question. And it can be paraphrased simply as follows: "Can this person help me?"

To ignore the reality that the patient is attempting to answer this question can lead to serious problems in engagement. To begin with, the act of hanging out our shingles as mental health professionals suggests that we have something to offer to patients for which they are exchanging money, time, and trust. On a basic level, they are generally expecting to find a good listener, albeit a "paid ear" of sorts. But at a deeper level, they are also expecting something else, something more. They are expecting to find an expert, a term I find mildly threatening, for it comes preseasoned with more than a pinch of pride. One feels hesitant to declare oneself an expert in so vast a field as human behavior, feelings, and psychophysiology.

But the term becomes more palatable, and indeed appropriate, if one keeps in mind two of the principles behind it. First, being an expert does not mean that one has all the answers or, for that matter, can necessarily provide relief. And second, being an expert does suggest that we have been rigorously schooled in an effort to consolidate a body of knowledge found useful in our field. It is the presence of this body of knowledge that may most successfully answer the patient's pressing question, "Can this person help me?"

In this regard, it is also useful to remember that in an anthropological sense, the initial clinician is fulfilling the role of a healer, and whether one is a shaman or a social worker, as a healer one is expected to possess knowledge not commonly available to the patient. From the above discussions, it should be apparent that at both a personal and a societal level, the clinician's expertise as perceived by the patient is critical to the engagement process.

The next logical question is, "How does one convey expertise effectively during an initial interview?" The answer lies primarily not in what we tell the patient but in what we ask the patient. It is the quality of our questions, not the quantity of our words, that generally convinces a patient that the clinician knows something that might help.

Questions, like empathic statements, can be categorized along a number of continua, including: (1) open-ended versus closed-ended, (2) probing versus nonprobing, (3) fact-finding versus opinion-finding, and (4) structured versus unstructured. Questions along the full range of these continua can be clinically useful, and all can be surprisingly ineffective as well. Their effectiveness or ineffectiveness seems to depend upon their timing as well as the appropriateness of the type of question for the task of the interviewer at any specific moment.

In the next chapter a great deal of time will be spent discussing the flexible use of questions at different phases of the interview. But at this point, I want to focus on an especially useful question, a type of question that can unobtrusively yet effectively convey expertise to the patient, the fact-oriented question.

By a fact-oriented question, I am referring to questions concerned with the concrete realities of the patient's situation, symptoms, and problems. Questions such as, "Are you having any problem falling asleep?" or "Has your appetite changed?" represent typical examples of fact-oriented questions. Frequently fact-oriented questions concern diagnostic issues, and they are generally closed-ended in nature.

Some initial interviewers shy away from fact-oriented questions, because they believe that such questions are generally disengaging. In this regard I agree that they can be disengaging when used at the wrong moments, too frequently, or in check-list fashion. And an interviewer should learn to avoid these pitfalls. But when asked sensitively, fact-oriented questions are powerful engagement tools, which also yield large amounts of valuable information for triage decisions.

To illustrate the point, let us look at the mid-phase of an initial interview with a woman in her late twenties. Rather than just going with the patient, the interviewer begins a more structured effort to tease out the symptoms upsetting this patient in an effort to arrive at a useful diagnosis.

> *Pt.:* I am terribly frightened about going back for my masters, I mean, is it worth it? . . . When I think about it, I get all uptight.
>
> *Clin.:* How do you mean?
>
> *Pt.:* I start to fret and worry. I feel extremely tense and wound up like a crazy alarm clock, ready to explode.
>
> *Clin.:* Over the course of any given day, say over the last month, how much of your day do you spend worrying like that?
>
> *Pt.:* Oh, I'd say at least seventy per cent, sometimes almost the whole day.
>
> *Clin.:* (said gently) Sounds miserable.
>
> *Pt.:* It really is, and the bad part is, I can't stop it.
>
> *Clin.:* Sounds like you find it difficult to relax.
>
> *Pt.:* Oh my god Yes! Even when I come home I feel like I've got to do something, something needs to be done and if I don't do it I'm a bad person. It's strange.
>
> *Clin.:* People develop a lot of tensions during the day, especially in a job like yours. I'm wondering if you find yourself having muscle aches, trembling sensations, or eye twitches related to your tension.
>
> *Pt.:* Funny you should ask. You may have noticed, but my left eye twitches when I'm tense, drives me nuts.
>
> *Clin.:* How long has that been going on?
>
> *Pt.:* I've had it . . . let's see . . . maybe five or six years but ever since deciding on grad school it's been really much worse.
>
> *Clin.:* How do you mean?
>
> *Pt.:* I look like a "mad winker" (patient and clinician chuckle). It really can be embarrasing.
>
> *Clin.:* I'm sure it can be. (warmly chuckles again) Tell me, have you noticed any other evidence of tension in your body, other than the twitching?
>
> *Pt.:* I've had a lot of diarrhea lately, I don't know if that's

related or not and I also have been feeling flashes of feeling real hot, makes me think of my mother and menopause, but I've had those kinds of flashes off and on for years.

Clin.: With these hot flashes do you notice any change in your pulse rate or breathing rate?

Pt.: No, I can't say I have.

Clin.: Have you ever found yourself suddenly having an abrupt episode of being extremely anxious, all at once?

Pt.: No . . . let me think, . . . not really.

Clin.: When you say "not really," what have you experienced?

Pt.: About a week ago I really got upset about Bob, but I wasn't really anxious, I was mad.

Clin.: What about periods where you suddenly became very frightened, perhaps of dying, without any apparent reason?

Pt.: No, that I can clearly say I've never had.

Clin.: Any periods where you suddenly found yourself panicking and perhaps short of breath or noticing tingling sensations in your fingers or around your mouth?

Pt.: No, I don't get that either.

Clin.: What about your concentration?

Pt.: Now that's shot. I can't concentrate at all. I've particularly noticed that when doing the books at work. Math comes simple to me and usually I fly through that stuff, but over the past two months I feel really frazzled. It takes forever.

Clin.: Earlier you mentioned the relationship of these feelings to your fears about grad school. What are some of the connections you see?

Pt.: Well, in the first place, I don't think I can do it. I mean I'm smart, at least I think I'm reasonably intelligent, but I don't know about the discipline I'd need. I think that worries me most.

Clin.: What else worries you?

Pt.: What would happen to Bob and me, I mean, when would I see him? I don't know, maybe never . . .

I have used a rather lengthy example because I want to emphasize the usefulness of sensitively utilized fact-oriented questions. In this excerpt, their gentle structuring, while clearly providing answers to diagnostic questions concerning anxiety disorders, may have also helped to convey a variety of important metacommunications to the patient, such as the following:

1. This interviewer is obviously interested in finding out exactly what symptoms and experiences I have been feeling.

2. This interviewer must have worked with similar problems before because the questions asked hit upon a lot of the feelings I have had.

3. This interviewer seems to be thorough and is actively exploring many different issues.

In short, all of these metacommunications serve to increase the patient's confidence in the clinician's expertise and ultimately in the clinician's potential to provide help. Good friends can provide sensitive listening, but only good clinicians can provide both sensitive listening and knowledgeable questioning.

It is also informative to see the frequent peppering of this fact-oriented dialogue with unstructured questions and basic empathic comments. In fact, it looks as if the interviewer was about to leave structured questioning in order to pursue a region of open-ended inquiries into psychodynamic issues. Once again the art lies in a flexible attitude, a suiting of the most effective form of questioning to the task at hand.

It is interesting to note that an interviewer who gets stuck on the idea of open-ended questioning throughout the entire initial interview potentially robs himself or herself of the chance to be perceived not only as a good listener but also as a skilled caregiver. In addition, it goes without saying that the clinician limited to an open-ended approach may also come away with an inadequate data base for triage purposes. The use of fact-oriented questions in the above example has provided a sound exploration of the symptoms of a generalized anxiety disorder and a panic disorder by DSM-III-R criteria. The treatment may vary for these two disorders, especially if the questioning around panic episodes had uncovered entities such as agoraphobia or a simple phobia, in which case specific treatment modalities are available.

In a last note concerning clinician expertise, we can see the complementary functions of all the factors discussed so far under the rubric of engagement. Indeed, the ability to blend effectively with a patient is mirrored by the clinician's ability to blend a variety of techniques, such as (a) the skilled use of empathic statements, (b) the creation of a safe environment, (c) the ability to convey genuineness through spontaneity, responsiveness, and consistency, and (d) the conveyance of a reassuring knowledge base. These four attributes lay the groundwork for quickly establishing an effective therapeutic alliance.

At this point we have completed our exploration of the engagement process, the first goal in our map of the interview. The reader will recall that the next way station concerns the process of effective data gathering.

The Subtleties of Collecting a Data Base

In many respects the major goal of the initial interview remains the elicitation of information. At first glance, this process sounds simple enough, perhaps too simple. Earlier we had likened the initial interview to a person exploring an old Victorian room with only a candle in hand, the limited light source representing an exterior hindrance to the endeavor at hand. But a weak light source does not represent the only barrier to a familiarization with the antique furniture scattered about, for the method of exploration employed can provide internal barriers to the effectiveness of gathering an accurate picture of the room. For instance, one explorer may walk about with his hands only held at shoulder level, hence missing all the curios lying upon a well-varnished table. A second explorer may underuse her sense of hearing, thus ignoring the presence of a clock tucked away in a quiet niche beside Sarah Bernhardt's portrait. A third explorer may be afraid of dark corners, thus never spotting the elaborately carved chess set hidden away in the shadows. Thus, it is not only a matter of gathering data, it is a question of realizing that one alters the data base by the very act of gathering the data. For these reasons it is of benefit to explore the issues of validity and reliability, for both of these factors can be altered by the idiosyncratic traits of each clinician's style.

VALIDITY

Statisticians discuss a variety of forms of validity, including content validity, empirical validity, and construct validity. To discuss all three of these concepts remains beyond the scope of our study, however. Instead, we will look at an admittedly simplified concept of validity, which nevertheless sheds considerable light on its clinical application. In a clinical sense, validity can be formulated as a question, "Are we actually eliciting the information we are trying to elicit?" From a slightly different perspective, the issue of validity can be conceptualized as the question, "Is the data base accurate?"

Clearly, because of psychological defenses, predispositions for deceit, fading memories, and actual cognitive deficits (as seen in dementia), patients may not provide accurate histories. For instance, a patient suffering from schizophrenia, and who wants to return to work quickly, may not readily tell the interviewer about the persistence of auditory hallucinations. On the other hand, a different patient, not suffering from schizophrenia but actively seeking disability, may tell the clinician about a plethora of tormenting yet nonexistent voices.

Along these lines, it is important for the interviewer to be alert for signs that the patient harbors a hidden agenda, such as needing a mental health professional to appear in court or to provide illicit drugs. For instance, in an emergency room setting, it is not uncommon for people with imminent court appearances to seem unusually interested in hospital admission, for hospitalization may represent a clever and logical excuse for missing the court date. In such cases, the tip-off is often the spontaneous request for admission from a patient who is typically noncompliant and indeed antagonistic towards health care. This example stands as one of many instances in which the patient may be actively distorting information. But it is frequently not the patient's resistances or deceits that alter validity. It may be the clinician who stands in the way of accurate information.

To focus on this issue, we will look at a concept known as "the behavioral incident," which was developed by Pascal and Jenkins and presented in an imminently useful fashion by Pascal in his book *The Practical Art of Diagnostic Interviewing.*[19] The basic concept can be delineated as follows.

When a clinician is particularly concerned about gaining accurate information, it is often best to ask the patient to describe specific historical details as opposed to asking them their opinions about these details. Once a patient is asked to make an opinion, the validity of the data becomes more suspect, since the clinician does not know how accurate the patient's perceptions may be.

All sorts of resistances may predispose a patient to distort information. For instance, if the clinician wants to determine whether a patient dates frequently, a patient may respond to a question such as "Do you date fairly regularly?" with a simple "yes," for the patient may be embarrassed to relate a sparse dating pattern. To sidestep this problem, the clinician could specifically ask about the frequency of dates over the past several years and ultimately the past several months. If the clinician finds only several dates spanning five or six months, then the clinician will have discovered a lack of dating activity without necessarily embarrassing the patient. As Pascal states, in general, it is best for clinicians to make their own judgment based upon the details of the story itself, for it seems unwise to assume that patients can objectively describe matters that have strong subjective implications.

Pascal calls the discrete historical behaviors elicited "behavioral incidents" and suggests that interviewers frequently collect invalid data by not asking for such concrete information, an extremely useful principle worthy of clarification.

Let us assume that an interviewer is interested in accurately determining the amount of open affection shared between a woman and her husband. We will look at two hypothetical dialogues with the same woman but with different interviewers. In excerpt one, the interviewer asks primarily for the patient's opinions, a process that yields invalid data. In excerpt two, the sensitive search for behavioral incidents provides a different story.

Interview One

Pt.: Basically I've been very busy, what with the kids and my mother getting sick.

Clin.: Do you feel happy with your husband's support?

Pt.: Yes . . . yes he's been fairly good about it all.

Clin.: Is he very affectionate?

Pt.: (pause) Uh huh, affectionate enough.

Clin.: Have there been any financial strains?

Pt.: No, not really. Although the past several months have been a little tight, what with decreased benefits and a new school year starting.

Interview Two

Pt.: Basically I've been very busy, what with the kids and my mother getting sick.

Clin.: What kinds of things does your husband do to support you?

Pt.: Well, he's been a little less demanding, he doesn't get upset if the dirty dishes stack up a little longer or a shirt is a little wrinkled.

Clin.: When he comes home from work, what is his typical routine?

Pt.: That's pretty simple. He'll walk in the door, I usually don't see him come in and he goes straight back to his room to change clothes.

Clin.: And then?

Pt.: Well, let's see, I usually knock on the door and let him know dinner will be ready.

Clin.: Do you go in and talk with him then?

Pt.: No, I go straight back, oh I usually peek in and say hello, but I have to get back to the stove.

Clin.: During the course of the night, is he the type of man who likes to hug, or does he prefer to keep a little more to himself?

> **Pt.:** Well, let me see, he really doesn't hug a lot. No I can't say he does.
>
> **Clin.:** Do you remember the last time he hugged you?
>
> **Pt.:** I honestly can't remember (patient's affect is becoming more sad).
>
> **Clin.:** You look a little sad. Has it been some time since the two of you felt close?
>
> **Pt.:** (patient looks at interviewer and pauses with a little sigh) I think the last time he hugged me was about six months ago near Christmas, I remember because I was so pleased by it. It's rare for him to touch me like that anymore. (pause) It didn't used to be this way . . . (breaks into tears).

Clearly, the second interviewer seems to have uncovered a different and more valid story than the first one. Through the gentle use of behavioral incidents, the second clinician has gathered evidence that problems exist in the marriage, a situation the first interviewer missed.

The apparent loss of validity caused by the first interviewer's reliance on patient opinion, as opposed to behavioral incident, can be seen in many areas, ranging from simple questions such as "Do you have problems falling asleep? to more critical questions such as "Do you ever want to kill yourself?" Consequently, the usefulness of listening for behavioral incidents when seeking valid data speaks for itself. There remain a few points worth mentioning, however. First, this form of questioning can be time consuming, and in initial triage interviews the clinician will probably utilize it judiciously in areas in which the clinician deems validity to be of particular importance. Second, the idea of a behavioral incident does not mean that patient opinions are not to be sought. Quite to the contrary, the patient's perspective often yields revealing insights into various dynamic issues. The point is not that one should avoid patient opinions but rather that one should not rely solely on them. In short, different styles of questioning tend to yield differing degrees of validity.

RELIABILITY

With the advent of the concept of reliability, a new factor awaits the self-attentive interviewer. In a statistical sense, reliability can be defined as follows:

> Reliability is an indication of the extent to which a measure contains variable errors; that is, *errors* that differed from

individual to individual using any one measuring instrument, and that varied from time to time for a given individual measured twice by the same instrument. For example, if one measures the length of a given object in two points of time with the same instrument — say, a ruler — and gets slightly different results, the instrument contains variable errors.[20]

One can translate the above concept into practical interviewing terms by remembering that our own interviewing style functions as our measuring instrument. The question then becomes: Does our way of asking questions change from individual to individual and, if so, do we bias patients towards certain answers?

This issue of interviewer reliability can be framed within two problem areas, although many other areas also exist: (1) the interviewer changes his or her style of asking a question and is not aware of the impact of this change and (2) the interviewer has good reliability but unfortunately reliably evokes invalid information. We will briefly examine each of these potential pitfalls.

Specific clinical settings predispose to the problem of inadvertently changing styles. This issue appears to frequently shadow the presence of countertransference and/or emotional strains in the clinician. For example, if an interviewer feels pushed for time or begins to dislike an interviewee, subtle changes in interviewing style frequently emerge. For instance, the interviewer may cut off the patient's responses or actually cast a disarming scowl. In other instances in which a clinician may have gently requested a pleasant patient to explain a vague response further, the same clinician might ask for no further clarification from a sarcastic patient, resulting in a shortened interview.

In any case, such changes in style can significantly decrease the reliability of the interviewing instrument, with subsequent deficits in the validity of the data. All clinicians will experience such negative emotions. There is nothing innately wrong with these feelings as long as their potential impact is considered. Indeed, at times an awareness of such emotions may provide us with clues to the inner workings of both the clinician and the patient.

The second area of concern focuses on the knotty issue that I shall loosely label as being "reliably invalid." In brief, one wonders whether interviewers can develop habits that consistently increase the risk of obtaining invalid data. Actually we have already seen an example of this process, for an interviewer who never uses behavioral incidents is probably reliably invalid. Furthermore, as normal human beings, most of us have developed other rather clever ways of not hearing what we do not want to hear. Such ingenious devices may get us through some touch-and-go dinners with in-laws, but if unchecked, these habits may cause problems during a clinical interview. In a more precise fashion, I am describing processes such as cajoling desirable answers from patients through choices of words and tone of voice.

Interviewers may not want to hear positive responses to questions concerning sensitive topics such as suicidal ideation, homicidal ideation, child abuse, or even the emergence of certain target symptoms such as depression. The hesitancy to uncover positive replies to such questions probably results from the fact that such responses may demand increased time from the clinician or legal action or even generate fear or a sense of failure in the clinician. Consequently, clinicians may unconsciously develop methods of decreasing the risk of a positive reply by beginning their questions with a negative (e.g., not), as follows:

a. You don't really feel more depressed, do you?
b. You're not feeling any chest pain today, are you?
c. You're not having thoughts of hurting yourself, are you?
d. (Said to your mother or father-in-law) You're not really thinking of spending the whole week here, are you?

An unusually sophisticated clinician will reinforce the negative bias by adding a subtle shake of the head from side to side. In essence, this negative approach to asking for a yes or no answer strongly biases the patient to say no. The reason for this negative bias most likely relates to the fact that the patient feels a need to please the clinician with a negative response. This biasing remains one of the most common errors I see during supervision. It represents a particular nemesis when employed around issues of high sensitivity such as sexuality or lethality, areas in which patients are hesitant to share positive answers to begin with and clinicians are occasionally afraid to hear them.

Another reliably invalid type of questioning consists of habitually asking multiple questions disguised as a single query, as demonstrated below:

> ***Pt.:*** I just don't feel the same, there's no question about that. Even my weekends seem bland.
>
> ***Clin.:*** When did you begin to feel depressed, to feel like life was not worth living?
>
> ***Pt.:*** Probably back around May. Everything seemed to be collapsing back then, near our anniversary.

In this excerpt the clinician has unwittingly set up a confusing situation. He or she does not know if the patient's depression *or* the patient's hopelessness began back in May. It is possible, even probable, that the patient's depression began much earlier than the deep sense of hopelessness. Only further questioning could clarify this issue that resulted from the multiple question. In addition, multiple questions are frequently employed during a review of physical systems, such as:

Clin.: Are you having any problem with your eyes, ears, heart or stomach?
Pt.: No.
Clin.: Have you noticed any coughing, constipation, diarrhea, headache, backache, or change in bowel habits?
Pt.: No, I don't think so.

Although time constraints may necessitate such multiple questions, it remains important to realize that such questions may be confusing to patients. Only one of the words may stick out in their minds, and such confusion can cause considerable problems with validity.

For supervision purposes, errors in validity and reliability can be conveniently labeled as type A or type B errors. Type A errors consist of all errors associated with the verbal content of the clinician's speech, including omission of behavioral incidents, lack of persistent probing when a patient seems to falter, negative questions, and multiple questions. Type B errors relate to nonverbal biasing elements, such as the shaking of the head from side to side while asking a question and many others, which will be discussed in Chapter 3.

Towards an Understanding of the Patient

As the clinician integrates the processes of engagement and data gathering, a curious phenomenon emerges. Gradually, the clinician begins to gain an understanding of the world through another person's eyes. This process does not happen suddenly or dramatically. Instead, like the imperceptible clearing of a mist, the clinician's conceptualization of the patient's perspective crystallizes. To return to our analogy of the Victorian room, the nooks and crannies of the environment gradually become more familiar. As interviewers we are no longer strangers. In the concluding section of this chapter, we will look at three areas that may enrich our ability to understand the patient, and perhaps ultimately our ability to offer compassion. These three areas are (1) interpersonal dynamics, (2) parataxic distortion, and (3) phenomenological perspective.

THE INTERPERSONAL PERSPECTIVE

It seems naive to assume a simple causative agent for most examples of human anxiety. For instance, future research will probably unmask many physiologic as well as psychosocial precipitants to anxiety. In this section we will focus upon some of the interpersonal forces at work in the creation of anxiety as it unfolds in an initial interview. Much of the following discussion is borrowed directly from the work of John Whitehorn[21] and Harry Stack Sullivan,[11] both pivotal explorers of interpersonal psychology.

To begin our discussion, the following question is worth considering as the interview proceeds, "How does this patient feel that he or she is viewed by others?" In many instances, the answers to this question will provide clues to the patient's immediate presence in our office. Guilt, shame, inadequacy, and fear of failure, these concerns are the stuff of neurosis. Many of the paralyzing defenses developed by people are erected to deflect such painful feelings. Whitehorn cogently expressed this idea, "Even in deadly warfare one's greatest apprehension is not of death but of being maimed or of failing in one's duty, and that, in large part, because one dreads the reactions of other persons.[22] This is not to downplay the fear of death but rather to emphasize the fear of life.

In another sense, developmentally speaking, the child appears to incorporate its sense of self-worth through a synthesis of perceived parental and family attitudes towards it. Indeed, persons demonstrating poorly developed personality states, such as the borderline personality and the narcissistic personality, have frequently evolved from chaotic childhoods. These developmental issues highlight the importance of interpersonal issues in the birth and feeding of unpleasant affects such as anxiety and depression. An actress has told me, "I can play any role once I understand what the character feels guilty about."

With regard to the art of understanding in the initial interview, these concerns suggest the utility of a sensitive search for answers to the questions discussed earlier. In particular, certain questions concerning the adolescent years may help open the interpersonal door a bit, such as:

a. What were some of your teachers like?
b. Tell me a little bit about the kids in your neighborhood where you grew up.
c. What was it like for you to walk home from school or go on the bus?
d. Which of your brothers or sisters are you most like?
e. Who do you think is the happiest in your family?
f. Who do you admire most in your family?

g. What do you think are some of your parents' concerns for you?
h. What was gym class like for you?
i. What was report card day like for you?

Most likely this list could be endless, but these questions represent samples of pathways into interpersonal affect related to past and perhaps current symptomatology. Of course, besides these reflections on the past, the interviewer will also pay heed to the patient's immediate concerns about spouse, family members, friends, bosses, and fellow employees.

Of even more immediate concern to the interviewer is the generalization of the patient's interpersonal fears to the interview itself. As mentioned earlier, the patient's self system may be activated by the perceived threat of rejection or disapproval from the interviewer. Whitehorn once again crystallizes the idea, "The patient's attitudes are not likely to appear at first, in answer to prepared questions, but later, in reaction to what he feels is the interviewer's response to his statements." [22] In this regard the clinician may be aptly rewarded by reflecting upon the following two queries: (1) How is this particular patient trying to come across to me? and (2) Why does he or she feel a need to present himself or herself in this fashion?

Some patients may feel that either the clinician or their friends feel they must be weak or "nuts" to be "seeing a shrink." This anxiety can seriously hamper engagement and may be partially alleviated by allowing some ventilation later in the interview with questions such as "What has it been like for you to come to see a mental health professional?" Such a question may provide reassuring feelings of interpersonal safety for the patient, for they realize the clinician is aware of the all too human anxieties associated with admitting a need for help.

Another possible method of gaining insight into interpersonal issues stems from asking patients to describe their attitudes towards others. As Whitehorn states, "A fruitful field of study lies in a consideration of his sentiments or prejudices, that is, his attitudes toward father, mother, siblings and other significant others, toward church and state, toward his home town and toward secret societies, antisemitism, Socialism, Fascism, and other 'isms'. In the discussion of such matters, the patient reveals more clearly than in response to direct questions the character of his ideals and the way in which he has come to dramatize his role in life." [22]

During an interview with an adolescent boy of about fourteen, the wisdom of this approach became apparent to me. The boy was suffering from a severe depression and seemed reluctant to talk about himself, but to my surprise he was not reluctant to talk about others. The request, "Tell me about some of the things you would change at school," led to a long and revealing discussion of complex social issues such as his school's policy towards racial integration and his own contempt for prejudice. Clearly this was not a boy interested only in the next football game or party. His detailed analysis suggested a person preoccupied with powerful moral concerns, which, when on overtime, could transform into harsh superego admonishings. His was a tense world, dotted with rights and wrongs, creating an intrapsychic field of land mines.

This boy's interview also raises another pertinent issue, "Can an interviewer probe too much or too quickly?" Generally speaking, when questioning is done sensitively, it infrequently goes too far. But the trick lies in being attuned to the degree of interpersonal guilt generated by the patient's responses. If the questions generate too much guilt, the initial interviewer may find that an impressively thorough data base has been developed but that there is no patient present with whom to discuss this data base at the second appointment.

To avoid this problem, the clinician keeps an eye open for signs of embarrassment or shame in the patient, perhaps indicated by an averted gaze or a hesitant first step into speech. This awareness is coupled with a common sense attitude towards which subject areas typically produce anxiety. When present, these signs may suggest the presence of potentially disengaging guilt, at which point the clinician may opt to reduce the tension by gently asking questions such as, "What has it been like for you to share such complicated material today?"

Asked calmly and sincerely, such questions demonstrate Rogers' unconditional positive regard while allowing patients to ventilate fears of clinician rejection, discovering to their surprise that such rejection is not imminent. The clinician can further decrease tension by positively reinforcing the patient's courage for sharing delicate material with phrases such as, "You've done an excellent job of sharing difficult material. It's really helping me to understand what you've been experiencing."

A combination of these techniques was useful in allaying the intense interpersonal anxieties generated in a man of about thirty who had presented for an initial assessment. Ostensibly requesting self-assertiveness training, he eventually related a striking list of paraphilias, including voyeurism, exhibitionism, and frotteurism (rubbing one's genitals against people in crowded public places). As he spoke, eye contact vanished, while his hands picked at one another. Near the end of the session, the dialogue evolved roughly as follows:

Clin.:   John, I've been wondering what it has been like for you to share this material? You look like you're feeling a little upset.

Pt.:   It's been very unsettling. I have never shared this stuff with anybody, it's so weird, . . . uh . . . uh . . . I, I feel ashamed every time I meet someone new, afraid of . . . what they might think.

Clin.: What have you been afraid I might be thinking?

Pt.: Oh that I'm really sick or disgusting.

Clin.: Has there been anything I've done or said that has conveyed that to you?

Pt.: (pause) No, no, I can't say there has been.

Clin.: Good, because I have a feeling there is only one person in this room who feels you are sick or disgusting, and that person isn't me.

Pt.: (patient nods head and smiles gently) That could be. (patient visibly releases)

Clin.: Why don't we try to find out more about why these unwanted behaviors developed so that we can look at potential ways of changing them. It's important we can talk about them openly and you've done an excellent job so far.

Pt.: Oh, that sounds real good to me.

Clin.: Tell me what you were feeling the last time you exposed yourself.

Pt.: I had had a bad day, I was really angry at a sales clerk . . .

John went on to be successfully treated using cognitive/behavioral techniques. The above interaction had helped him to dismantle a powerful projection, a projection that threatened to disrupt the therapy before it even began.

Thus as clinicians we need to consider carefully the impact of our probings, recognizing that certain patients may not be ready to discuss certain issues, while others might actually benefit from our exploration. At these moments, during the initial assessment, we must rely upon our ever-growing experience to guide us, keeping in mind a most relevant statement made by a wizened monk in the novel *The Name of the Rose* by Umberto Eco: "Because learning does not consist only of knowing what we must or we can do, but also of knowing what we could do and perhaps should not do."[23]

PARATAXIC DISTORTION

So far we have been examining the generation of interpersonal perceptions primarily via conscious or preconscious processes. If it could be so simple! Unfortunately, the patient's developing image of the clinician and, for that matter, the clinician's developing image of the patient are colored by unconscious processes. Unbeknownst to the clinician, he or she may resemble a family member of the patient or an ex-spouse or fill a stereotype of a concrete prejudice. As Sullivan put it, "The *real* characteristics of the other fellow at that time may be of negligible importance to the interpersonal situation. This we call parataxic distortion."[24]

This distorting process can affect both the patient and/or the clinician and sometimes both parties. In actuality, parataxic distortion may evolve from the early seeding of both transference and counter-transference; as such, its formation and resolution may play a pivotal role in subsequent therapy. But, in the initial interview such unde-tected early distortions may beleaguer an already fragile alliance.

Fortunately, such intense parataxic distortion is atypical. But when it does occur, it generally displays itself either through unusually poor blending or by atypically high levels of anxiety in the patient, perhaps even frank antagonism. This weakening of the blending pro-cess represents one more area in which monitoring of the blending process can provide important clues to the engagement process. Once such weak blending is recognized, the clinician can begin repair work. The first step in the repair process consists of questioning whether one's own actions are somehow disengaging the patient. At times these self-defeating behaviors may be related to countertransference issues with the patient (parataxic distortion on the part of the clinician).

If free of such process, the clinician can then legitimately wonder whether parataxic distortion is at work in the patient's mind. If such distortion is suggested, an open exploration may decrease the growing resistance. For instance, the clinician can ask, "I'm wondering what you're feeling as we are talking," or "I sense you are feeling a little displeased with the interview so far, and I'm wondering what's going on?"

This type of nondefensive statement may seem to defuse the situ-ation, for it brings hostile feelings into the open where they can at least be approached. Moreover, the clinician should not be afraid to uncover specific feelings of ill will, such as, "I find you very controlling," be-cause these feelings can be tapped for clues of dynamic significance with questions such as, "When are some times you've felt similar feelings in the past?" Once again the emphasis rests upon allowing the patient to openly express his or her view of the world, in this case, of the interview itself. This emphasis upon understanding the patient's view of the world provides the focus for our last topic in this chapter.

PHENOMENOLOGICAL INQUIRY

We now have a moment to re-examine the process of blending. At times, blending can be improved by utilizing a style of questioning that can lead directly to a clearer understanding of the patient. This style has its roots in the fields of existentialism and phenomenological psychology to which the book, *Existence,* by R. May,[25] remains an excellent introduction. While employing a more phenomenological style, the clinician attempts to see the world as the person experiences it, to literally see the world through the patient's eyes, to understand the phenomenon of being that person.

The emphasis rests upon what Medard Boss called "Daseinsanalysis," a German word translatable as "analysis of being-in-the-world."[26] In short, the clinician attempts to know what it *would* be like and what it *is* like to be the person sitting across from himself. To this end, it is often useful to emphasize the world of the senses by asking specifically about what the patient is seeing, hearing, feeling, smelling, or tasting. From this sensate inquiry, doors may open into the patient's feelings, attitudes, and thoughts. To borrow a phrase from Aldous Huxley and William Blake, it is "through the doors of perception" that one may enter a patient's unique way of being, the patient's inner home. Indeed, this home may be turbulent, beautiful, or terrifying, but once experienced, the clinician's understanding cannot help but be clearer.

Moreover, such sensitive questioning can convey to the patient that the clinician remains interested in the patient as a person not merely as a new case. In this regard, in the first interview the clinician may decide to include brief (sometimes not so brief) forays into the phenomenology of the patient. These dialogues may be similar to the following one involving an overweight woman, reflecting a string of suicidal gestures in her eyes:

> **Pt.:** I guess I was just sick of everything . . . everything . . . so I wanted to get away, to be by myself away from everybody who can hurt me. So I went into my room and shut off the light. I lit a few candles and I sat there.
>
> **Clin.:** What were you looking at as you sat there?
>
> **Pt.:** Nothing really . . . occasionally I watched the candle light flickering, it made the shadows of the vase dance around on the wall.
>
> **Clin.:** Do you remember anything else that caught your eye?
>
> **Pt.:** Uh huh, I remember looking at my high school prom picture.
>
> **Clin.:** And?
>
> **Pt.:** I thought how cruel it was the way relations have to break up. The person in that picture meant nothing to me now, and I don't think I really meant anything to him ever (patient sighs).
>
> **Clin.:** What else are you feeling in the room?

Pt.:   Lonely and empty. I just wanted to crawl up into a tiny ball like a cocoon.

Clin.:   What does the world feel like to you in your cocoon?

Pt.:   It feels distant, dark, and numb. I feel, feel sort of blank, but I also am angry. I'm angry at my mother for never really caring, for putting me in the cocoon in the first place. I don't ever remember her hugging me (begins crying gently). I remember going away for the summer once to stay with my grandparents. And at the train station I felt very frightened and sad. I kept wondering what my mother would do when she said good bye, would she hug me or kiss me, and for how long? And you know what she did? She did nothing. She said good-bye.

Clin.:   That must have hurt.

Pt.:   It really did, it really hurt . . . (perks up) But that's the way it's always been.

Clin.:   Do you expect people to hurt you?

Pt.:   . . . Yes, yes I do, maybe I'm growing accustomed to it, maybe I even like it.

Clin.:   Going back to that night in the room with the candle flickering, did you have any thoughts of wanting to hurt yourself?

Pt.:   Yes, I did. As I sat there it all seemed sort of silly, so I began thinking about taking some pills. I'd stored up some Valium.

Clin.:   What thoughts went through your mind?

From this dialogue the clinician can begin to feel the resounding hollowness of this patient's world, the intensity of her pain. One gains a sense of her neediness and her latent expectation of rejection, an expectation that may very well create the very bitterness that seeds actual antagonistic behavior from others put off by the patient's hostility. In any case the patient seems somehow more "real." Moreover, this phenomenological excursion has provided many hints for the clinician of potentially productive regions of future exploration, another example of intuition guiding further analysis. Indeed one wonders if this hollow world represents one petal in the abated flower we call a borderline personality.

This excerpt began with an active investigation of the room with the patient, moving into associations generated by this phenomenological exploration. Sometimes the patient will share associations experienced at the time being discussed, while at other times new associations stirred by recounting the experience may surface. In either case, rich material may become accessible to the clinician. Phenomenological inquiries are not necessarily based on questions dealing with the five senses. Frequently the patient's experience of the world is entered by questions exploring attitudes, opinions, recollections, and by an immediate sharing of feelings as they arise within the clinician/patient dyad.

Before leaving this excerpt a quick perusal reveals an interesting twist. The clinician has switched tenses from past tense to present tense with the phrase, "What else are you feeling in the room?" Such a switch sometimes facilitates a regression in the patient to a point at which images become more real and less memory. This type of maneuver can unlock repressed memories and emotions, as witnessed here by the unexpected emergence of anger directed towards a parent figure perceived as cool and distant. Naturally, if one feels the patient cannot tolerate such a regression, as in an unstable patient or a psychotic patient, one would not utilize such a technique. In conclusion, phenomenological inquiry provides one more powerful method by which understanding may be increased.

Concluding Statements

In this chapter we have attempted to develop a practical language through which we can study the interviewing process. We began with an operative definition and proceeded to study various aspects of that definition, including the engagement process, the ramifications of data collection such as validity and reliability, and, finally, the subtleties of understanding another person's pains.

It is hoped this new language offers us a chance to explore effectively our own styles of interviewing, while greatly increasing the opportunity to learn from observing others. This language of the interview has revealed the fact that interviewing is an art, and like the art historian mentioned in the introduction, one can discuss this craft precisely and concretely. Indeed the language we have uncovered, utilizing words such as engagement, blending, behavioral incidents, and parataxic distortion, provides us with the map of the interviewing process discussed earlier. The interior of our Victorian room now appears considerably less foreboding.

At this point, we have developed a language with which to begin our study of the interviewing process. But this language is incomplete, for an exploration of the interplay between clinician and patient represents a pressing matter not yet fully examined. It is this interaction that creates the structure of the interview. This structure provides the passageway to clinical effectiveness.

References

1. Rosenblum, R., and Janson, H. W.: *19th Century Art*. New York, Harry N. Abrams Inc., 1984.
2. Ward, N. G., and Stein, G.: Reducing emotional distance: A new method to teaching interviewing skills. *Journal of Medical Education* 50:605–614, 1975.
3. Wiens, A. N.: The assessment interview. In *Clinical Methods in Psychology,* edited by Irving Weiner. New York, John Wiley and Sons, 1976.
4. Barrett-Lennard, G. T.: The empathy cycle: Refinement of a nuclear concept. *Journal of Counseling Psychology* 28:2, 91–100, 1981.
5. Barrett-Lennard, G. T., 1981, p. 94.
6. Margulies, A.: Toward empathy: The uses of wonder. *American Journal of Psychiatry* 141(9):1025–1033, 1984.
7. Margulies, A., and Havens, L.: The initial encounter: What to do first. *American Journal of Psychiatry* 138(4):421–428, 1981.
8. Margulies, A., 1984, p. 1031.
9. Havens, L.: Exploration in the uses of language in psychotherapy: Simple empathic statements. *Psychiatry* 41:430, 1978.
10. Havens, L., 1978, p. 338.
11. Sullivan, H. S.: *The Psychiatric Interview.* New York, W. W. Norton and Company, 1970.
12. Egan, G.: *The Skilled Helper: A Model for Systematic Helping and Interpersonal Relating.* Monterey, California, Brooks/Cole Publishing Company, 1975, p. 97.
13. Nicholi, A. M., Jr.: The Therapist-Patient Relationship. From *The Harvard Guide to Modern Psychiatry,* edited by A. M. Nicholi, Jr. Cambridge, The Belknap Press of Harvard University Press, 1978.
14. Sullivan, H. S., 1970, p. 12.
15. Rogers, C. R., and Traux, C. B.: The therapeutic conditions antecedent to change: A theoretical view. From *The Therapeutic Relationship and Its Impact,* edited by Carl Rogers. Madison, The University of Wisconsin Press, 1967, pp. 97–108.
16. Egan, G., 1975, p. 90.
17. Ryle, A.: *Psychotherapy: A Cognitive Integration of Theory and Practice.* New York, Grune and Stratton, 1982, p. 103.
18. Egan, G., 1975, p. 93.
19. Pascal, G. R.: *The Practical Art of Diagnostic Interviewing.* Homewood, Illinois, Dow Jones-Irwin, 1983.
20. Nachmias, D., and Nachmias, C.: *Research Methods in the Social Sciences.* New York, St. Martin's Press, 1976.
21. Whitehorn, J. C.: Guide to interviewing and clinical personality study. *Archives of Neurology and Psychiatry* 52:197–216, 1944.
22. Whitehorn, J. C., 1944, pp. 197–216.
23. Eco, U.: *The Name of the Rose.* San Diego, Harcourt Brace Jovanovich, Publishers, 1983.
24. Sullivan, H. S., 1970, p. 25.
25. May, R. (ed.): *Existence.* New York, Simon and Schuster, 1958.
26. Hall, C. S., and Lindzey, G.: *Theories of Personality.* Third edition. New York, John Wiley and Sons, 1978, p. 320.

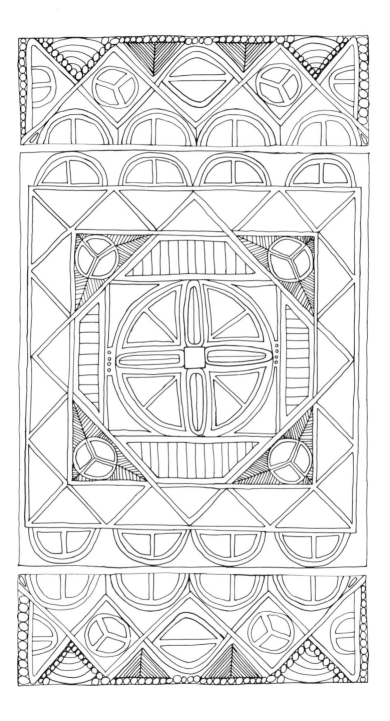

2

The Dynamic Structure of the Interview

Insecurity and uncertainty are everywhere. If you don't let it become part of your flow, you will always be resisting and fighting. . . . If the ground here suddenly shakes and trembles, can you give with it and still maintain your center? If you can become fluid and open even when you are standing still, then this fluidness and openness makes you able to respond to changes.[1]

Al Chung-liang Huang, Embrace Tiger, Return to Mountain

The clinical interview manifests as a relationship. As with all relationships, it undergoes a continuous process of change, evolving like a delicate landscape by a Chinese artist or the movements of a T'ai Chi Master like Al Chung-liang Huang. It will change as the needs and the fears of the two participants evolve. This metamorphosis occurs whether either participant wants it to occur or not. The clinician must choose whether to move with these changes gracefully or struggle against them.

In this chapter we will examine one method of conceptualizing the structure of the interview. This conceptualization focuses upon the naturally occurring phases of the interview. By uncovering the structure of the interview, clinicians can develop methods of utilizing the natural flow of the interview to their benefit.

The five phases of the interview are as follows: (1) the introduction, (2) the opening, (3) the body, (4) the closing, and (5) the termination. Categorizing the stages of the interview in this fashion is somewhat artificial, but this separation temporarily provides an avenue for a more sophisticated study. In reality, like the movement of a Chinese martial arts practitioner, these stages merge with one another, a process at least partially determined by the pathways chosen by the clinician. Appreciating that the clinician has a choice creates both a more efficient interview and a more exciting one. The ability to consciously guide the interview is one of the differences between a good clinician

55

and an outstanding one. It lies at the core of what has been called the art of interviewing.

THE INTRODUCTION: PHASE ONE

The introduction begins when the clinician and the patient first see one another. It ends when the clinician feels comfortable enough to begin an inquiry into the reasons the patient has sought help. When done well, it lasts a minute or two. When done poorly, it hardly occurs at all, or worse yet, the clinician regrets having been a part of it. The introduction represents one of the most important phases of the interview, for patients will frequently have formed their initial impression of the clinician by its end. This initial impression, whether justified or not, may help determine the remaining course of the interview and perhaps even of therapy itself.

The goal of the interviewer during the introduction remains relatively simple: engage the patient by decreasing the patient's anxiety. Employing one of Sullivan's terms mentioned earlier, we can state the goal as follows: the clinician attempts to decrease the patient's need for an overactive self system. In a similar vein, the goal of the patient is also relatively easy: "to find out what is going on here," for many patients are encountering a mental health professional for the first time.

The patient's need to understand the process tends to be rather intense, for it is rooted in some of the following basic fears:

1. Who is this clinician?
2. Is he or she competent?
3. Is this person understanding?
4. What does he or she already know about me?
5. Whose side is this clinician on?
6. How long will this assessment take?
7. Am I going to be hurt?
8. Do I have any control in this matter? (Am I going to be "mind-raped"? as one patient described her initial fear.)

Not all patients are dealing with all these fears, but most patients are probably coping with a good number of them either consciously or unconsciously. The goal of the clinician and the goal of the patient are really the same at this moment in the interview, in short, to help the patient to feel more at ease. To achieve this more comfortable state of affairs, the clinician may want to answer some of these questions either directly or indirectly. If done sensitively, the patient's initial anxiety should begin to decrease and the interview begin to move.

There exists no correct method of handling these fears. Consequently, each clinician needs to determine a comfortable style of addressing these issues in his or her own fashion. Below I shall give two examples. The first example is the work of an inexperienced clinician. The second dialogue demonstrates one method that addresses the issues more smoothly.

[The clinician enters brusquely, shaking the patient's hand very firmly. The clinician does not smile.]

Clin.: Well John, my name is Dr. James, I'll be conducting the interview. I understand you have some problems. Tell me about them.

Pt.: Let me see, I'm not really sure where to begin.

Clin.: Why don't you start at the beginning. I understand you've been acting a little odd.

Pt.: Who told you that?

Clin.: Your wife, but that's neither here nor there, I need to know when it all began.

It is hard not to chuckle at this exchange, for the interviewer has successfully aroused almost all of the anxieties mentioned earlier. Even such word choices as "I'll be conducting the interview" suggest that the patient should expect no control here, although the clinician's overpowering handshake may have already served as a premonition of this fact.

The following dialogue represents a more satisfying solution to the demands of the situation.

[The patient knocks. The clinician says "Come in." The patient enters the room. The clinician smiles warmly and spontaneously. He walks over to the patient at a normal pace and shakes the patient's hand with a gentle firmness.]

Clin.: Hello, my name is Dr. James. I'm one of the senior psychiatrists at the clinic here. Why don't we sit over here. By the way, if you like, I can hang your coat up (gestures toward wall).

Pt.: Thank you (patient passes coat and sits down).

Clin.: Did you have any trouble finding a parking space?

Pt.: No, not really, It's not that bad at this time of the day.

Clin.: Good. Sometimes people have some problems with it . . . Why don't we begin by my giving you some idea of what to expect today.

Pt.: That sounds good to me.

Clin.: First of all, do you like to be called Mr. Fenner or William or Bill?

> *Pt.:* I don't like the name William. "Bill" would be just fine.
>
> *Clin.:* Good. Your wife had called earlier . . . were you aware she had called ahead?
>
> *Pt.:* Well, sort of. She said she would, and I told her to go ahead. I didn't know if she had or not.
>
> *Clin.:* Let me summarize my impression from her call. She certainly seems concerned and a little confused about what you've been thinking and feeling recently. She seems to feel that you may be somewhat depressed. What I'd like to do is begin by hearing from you and getting your perspectives on what, if anything, has been going on. Perhaps we could start with your telling me a little about how you see things at this point.
>
> *Pt.:* It takes a second to get in gear here . . . well . . . let's see . . . In the first place, I must admit I've been feeling sort of down, not depressed mind you, but down.
>
> *Clin.:* Uh-huh.
>
> *Pt.:* Things have been going poorly at work. My boss left and he was replaced by a, let me just say, someone more difficult to get along with. The end result has been that I'm not enjoying my work like I used to.
>
> *Clin.:* And where is it you work?
>
> *Pt.:* Down at the lumber company.
>
> *Clin.:* Go on. (Said gently.)
>
> *Pt.:* Well, about three weeks ago I did something I've never done in all my twenty years of work (pause) (clinician waits) I called in sick without actually being sick.
>
> *Clin.:* Uh-huh.
>
> *Pt.:* It's really unusual for me to do that.
>
> *Clin.:* O.K.

In this introduction, which has imperceptibly moved into the opening phase, the clinician has smoothly addressed many of the potential resistances mentioned earlier. In particular, a large element of respect has been conveyed to the patient by the simple gesture of offering to hang up the patient's coat and by asking the patient whether he had been aware of the call from his wife. The clinician also clearly appears to be on no one's side, emphasizing the desire to hear the patient's opinions and even stating that the issue of a problem with the patient has not been determined yet by the comment, "and getting your perspectives on what, if anything, has been going on."

Anthony Storr points out that the situation may be slightly different if the patient has been referred by a fellow professional. In these cases, Storr adds a nice touch, as follows:

Clin.: I've read your notes and I have some idea of your background and your present trouble, but I would be grateful if you would go over some of it again. I know that you have told it all before to various people, and that it must be very tedious for you to repeat it, but I find it difficult to remember details from notes made by other people. I understand that your present trouble is depression. . . . Could we start there? What is your kind of depression really like?[1]

In this example Storr conveys respect and concern, essentially acknowledging that he, too, might find repeating the story again somewhat difficult. The last statement also indicates the clinician's desire to understand the patient as a unique individual, not just a case. Some clinicians also prefer to end the introduction by asking, "Before we go on, do you have any questions?" Such a question once again conveys a sense of respect, while checking for possible resistances.

Going back to our own example of an effective introduction, we find that the clinician has also managed to give a sense of control to the patient with phrases such as, "Perhaps we could start with your telling me a little about how you see things at this point."

The clinician also asked the patient how he would like to be addressed. One can find many vehemently written pages both for and against using a patient's first name. I shall not add many pages to this debate, because I think the intensity of the debate has led to overstated arguments on both sides.

I, personally, feel that one should not assume a first name basis without asking first. Some patients may find a first name threatening or a "put down," especially if the patient is a young adult or much older than the clinician. Consequently, when first greeting a patient I always use his or her last name.

On the other hand, the ability to use the patient's first name can be a powerful asset in engagement. When used sparingly and with good timing, it can effectively help patients share difficult material. In a cultural sense, first names are generally used by people who care about us and are privy to our private thoughts.

Consequently, I have found it both satisfying and rewarding to simply ask the patient how he or she would like to be addressed. This question accomplishes several tasks:

1. It conveys respect.
2. It gives the patient direct control over an important ego issue (some patients do not like to be called by last names and others do not like to be called by first names.)

3. One may learn a significant amount concerning the dynamics of the patient as revealed by the patient's preference.

For instance, very strong opinions voiced by the patient may represent the presence of character pathology or defensive posturing, thus offering the clinician immediate grist for the mill. A patient developing grandiose thinking as part of a manic episode may adamantly insist on being called "Dr. Jones." At the other extreme, patients with regressive tendencies may sheepishly smile while stating, "Please just call me Jim." With experience one can begin to discern the sense of self-identity implied by the patient's response to this simple question. Indeed, one wonders what dynamic issues may lie beneath ambivalent responses such as, "It doesn't really matter, you can call me Jim, Jack, or Jimmy."

There are some exceptions to the above guidelines. If the clinician knows beforehand that the patient has a history of paranoia, it may be advisable to use the last name throughout the interview, for such "distance" may be more comfortable for the paranoid patient. Patients who are much older than the clinician may prefer to be addressed by the last name. In the opposite direction, children and early adolescents generally should be addressed by first name from the start. In these cases, though, it is often useful to ask the child which first name to use. For instance, the family may call the child "Johnny," yet the child would prefer being called "John." Such a simple show of respect can go a long way towards ensuring a powerful engagement.

I should add that with regard to addressing the patient, I have yet to find any problem arising in either the initial interview or subsequent psychotherapy using the above approach. In the end, the reader must decide, from his or her own experience, what feels most comfortable.

In familiarizing the patient with the ensuing interview process, some clinicians go one step further than illustrated above. They specifically describe for the patient what to expect, depending upon the goals of the interview. After the clinician and patient have introduced themselves, the dialogue may proceed as follows:

Clin.: Perhaps it would be of value to describe what we'll be doing today.

Pt.: I would really appreciate that.

Clin.: Of course, first, I'd like to get an idea of what some of your concerns are and what types of stresses you're coping with. I'll try to get a clear idea of your symptoms with an idea of seeing how we may be able to help you. Later in the interview, I'll try to get a better idea of what has been happening by asking some background questions about your family, your health, your schooling, and any pre-

vious symptoms you've had. I find that getting an understanding of your background can really help me understand your current problem better. Do you have any
questions?

Pt.: Not really, no . . . not really.

Clin.: Then let's begin by looking at what brought you here
today.

Pt.: (Sigh) I'll tell you, it's a long story.

Clin.: I have big ears (smiles).

Pt.: (Chuckles) Well, it has to do with some problems with my
wife and me. It began about two months after our first
child, Jenny . . .

The purpose of a more extended description of the process is
twofold. First, it is hoped that the patient's fear of the unknown will be
decreased. Second, the description of the process serves as an educational ploy, subtly alerting the patient to the fact that large amounts of
data will be covered. This may allow the clinician to structure the
ensuing interview more effectively and with less resistance. It also
provides one method for smoothly switching gears later with transitions such as, "As I mentioned earlier, I'd like to learn a little more
about your family. How many children do you have besides Jenny?" At
the end of this interaction, the clinician also demonstrated the use of
well-timed humor to break the anxiety of the first meeting.

Before moving on, one final point may be of value. As with all the
other aspects of interviewing we have discussed so far, the format of
the introduction varies from patient to patient. In some instances in
which the patient is extremely psychotic, the patient may quickly cut
short the introduction. In such instances, it is wise to follow the patient's lead, for clearly such patients have a need to tell their story
quickly. It would be inappropriate to adhere rigidly to the typical
format of the introduction with such patients. The format is a guide,
not a rule.

In any case, the previous statements serve as a foundation for an
exploration of the introduction. When performed well, this phase can
provide the beginnings of a powerful blending, for patients truly appreciate the sense of acceptance created by a sensitive clinician. In the
next phase the patient does most of the talking while the clinician
listens attentively.

THE OPENING: PHASE TWO

With the clinician's first inquiry into the patient's immediate
state of affairs, the opening phase begins. It ends when the clinician

begins to focus his or her questions on specific topics deemed important by the clinician, after listening to the patient nondirectively. If the interview is only thirty minutes, the opening phase may only last about five minutes. In hour-long diagnostic interviews the opening phase often lasts about five to eight minutes.

Coupled with the introductory phase, the opening phase probably represents the most critical area for establishing patient rapport. If the end of the introduction marked the formation of the patient's initial impression of the clinician, the end of the opening phase represents the solidification or rejection of that impression. For the most part, patients have determined by the end of the opening whether they basically like or dislike the interviewer. These patient opinions are not irrevocably etched in stone, but it would take a rather large chisel to change them. In many instances when patients abandon therapy after two or three sessions, their disapproval may have been planted in the opening ten minutes of the first interview.

The patient has two primary goals during the opening phase: (1) to determine whether it is "okay" to share personal matters with this particular clinician and (2) to determine which personal matters to share. A third major goal of the patient also surfaces, namely "to tell my story right, so that the clinician understands me." Despite a well-handled introduction, the patient's self system will usually be activated during this phase, for it is here that self-exposure begins.

With these ideas in mind, one of the complementary goals of the interviewer becomes apparent: the engagement process begun in the introduction must be secured during the opening. The durability and elasticity of this engagement bonding, to a large degree, determine the depth of probing and the degree of structuring that the patient will tolerate in the subsequent phases of the interview. It is at this time that many of the engagement skills discussed in Chapter 1 meet their greatest challenge and yield their highest reward.

The approach to the opening phase generally proceeds along the following lines. Once the clinician has ended his or her introduction, an open-ended question is used to turn the interview over to the patient on a verbal level. Frequently used openings include the following:

a. Tell me a little about what brought you here today.

b. Perhaps you can begin by letting me know what some of your concerns have been recently.

c. To start with, tell me a little about what has been happening in the past couple of weeks.

d. What are some of the stresses you have been coping with recently?

Such open-ended questions or statements provide the patient with a chance to begin talking at a comfortable point. Broadly speaking, the goals are to decrease the patient's anxiety while beginning to uncover the patient's viewpoint. Both of these goals are generally met by giving the patient plenty of room to wander during the opening phase.

During this facilitating opening phase, one hopes to begin to see outward signs of good blending, such as the patient's assumption of a more relaxed body posture and a reasonably long duration of utterance (DOU) by the patient following the clinician's questions.

This facilitation can be nurtured by the use of phrases such as "Go on," "And then what happened," and frequent short conveyances of the clinician's interest such as "Uh-huh." Generally it appears useful to employ at least one or two simple empathic statements during the opening phase, for such phrases frequently circumvent the patient's fear of imminent rejection.

The opening phase bears a characteristic that distinguishes it from other phases of the interview. In sharp contrast to the introduction, in the opening phase the clinician speaks very little. To the contrary, there exists a strong emphasis upon open-ended questions or open-ended statements in an effort to get the patient talking. In an uncomplicated opening phase, roughly 30–70% of the clinician's questions or statements will be open-ended. During an assessment interview, the opening phase will probably represent the least verbally active phase for the clinician, for in the subsequent body of the interview, clinicians tend to increase the frequency of their questions as they attempt to clarify diagnostic and triage questions.

With regard to this open-ended emphasis, two frequent problems are encountered: (1) premature structuring of the interview before the patient has begun to relax and (2) the too frequent use of close-ended questions. Both of these tendencies remove control of the interview from the patient, a policy that only serves to heighten the patient's interpersonal anxiety. Perhaps equally important, these activities represent an increased amount of clinician speech, and at this early stage of the interview a direct correlation can be drawn between clinician confusion and the amount of time the clinician spends with his or her mouth open. In short, the opening phase is a time for reflection, not action.

Before proceeding, it is worth noting that some clinicians like to employ a bridge between the introduction and the opening. This bridge consists of a brief series of demographic questions that function to provide a cursory background while not intimidating the patient. The clinician may state, "As we get started I'd like to ask a few background questions that can help give me some perspective. For instance, how old are you, Mr. Jones?" Further questions may concern the place of residence, occupation, or a description of the patient's family. Following these questions, the clinician may proceed with the opening as described above. Once again, the emphasis remains upon effective and rapid engagement.

But active engagement techniques are not the only activities of the clinician during the opening phase. Much of the activity cannot be seen, for it is mental in nature. More specifically, the opening phase represents an intensely productive assessment period for the clinician. During these initial minutes, the clinician scours the interpersonal countryside in search of clues that may lead to the most effective engagement techniques for this particular patient. Simultaneously, the clinician determines the best manner in which to structure the body of the interview itself. In short, the clinician develops a tentative game plan, in the sense that a strategy for the interview will be developed, hand-tailored to the needs of the patient.

This early assessment process, which may be significantly revised as the interview proceeds, represents a mental "scouting period." This scouting period actually encompasses both the introduction phase, already discussed, and the opening phase. But since the main work of the scouting period occurs during the opening phase, it seems most appropriate to explore its intricacies at this time.

In the scouting period, encompassing the first five to ten minutes of the interview, the clinician receives a rare opportunity to assess four vital areas: (1) the patient's conscious view of his or her problems, as well as the patient's conscious agenda for the interview itself (e.g., What does the patient want from the interview?), (2) the patient's mental status, which can influence the type of interview the clinician feels would be most clinically effective for this particular patient, (3) the clinician's conceptualization of the patient's problems as well as the clinician's view of the patient's *unconscious* agenda for the interview (e.g., What in reality, does this patient desire from this interview?), and (4) an evaluation of the interview process itself.

Through an understanding of these four variables, the clinician can begin the delicate matter of matching the patient's agenda with his or her own agenda. If these agenda cannot be resolved, the resulting interview may prove to be relatively unproductive. It is interesting to note, just as Lazare[2] states that outpatient psychotherapy has a contractual nature, in a sense each interview shares this contractual element. The contract can be either implicit or explicit. But it always occurs. Indeed, interviews break down when the participants cannot agree to shared goals. Many of these communication breakdowns result when the clinician does not recognize the goals of the patient, or worse yet, knows the goals but does not acknowledge them.

The four analytic tasks of the scouting period are creatively coupled with the intuitive skills of the clinician. Armed with this interplay between analysis and intuition, the clinician quickly begins a "knowing" of the patient. In an attempt to sharpen the analytic skills of the scouting phase, the following acronym PACE is useful in reminding the clinician of the goals of this phase:

*P*atient's perspectives and conscious agenda.
*A*ssessment of the patient's mental status.
*C*linician's perspective of the patient's problems and the patient's unconscious agenda.
*E*valuation of the interview itself.

An ability to make these assessments quickly and accurately often signifies the presence of a skilled clinician. To develop this ability, one must first understand its utility.

Patient's Perspectives and Conscious Agenda

Each patient brings a unique set of perceptions and opinions to the initial interview. Two patient perspectives appear to be particularly crucial in determining whether contractual agreement will occur: (1) the patient's concept of what is wrong and (2) the patient's expectations of the interview or the interviewer. Many resistances to the interview process arise when these parameters are not understood by the clinician. On the other hand, if the interviewer is aware of these concerns, some resistances may be diminished, worked through, or perhaps even nipped in the bud.

To illustrate this aspect of the scouting period it may be useful to look at a short piece of dialogue. We will picture a man in his mid-thirties, who has scheduled an appointment at the strong urges of his wife. He nervously looks about the office, as if anticipating the appearance of a Grand Inquisitor. He has a small mustache and a nervous nose. Early in the scouting period the following interaction develops:

Clin.: Tell me a little bit about some of the reasons you came here today.

Pt.: It is very difficult to say. I don't know what Jane thinks is happening, but I'm not nuts. It's all got something to do with my chemistry, of that I'm sure. Somehow or other I'm a little speeded up.

Clin.: In what sense do you feel you're speeded up?

Pt.: I'm feeling excitable, ready to roll, very creative, but maybe a little too juiced up. That's why I think it's biologic, not mental. I've been doing some reading about physical fitness and its impact on emotions and I think I've got some understanding of what the hell is going on here.

The art inherent in the scouting period consists of listening not only to what the patient says but also to what the patient implies. A careful delineation of this patient's opening dialogue may yield some pertinent information.

His opening gambit, "It is very difficult to say," suggests a fear of being misunderstood by the interviewer. This phrase is followed by the statement, "I don't know what Jane thinks is happening, but I'm not nuts." Paradoxically, the patient reveals that he does know what his wife thinks yet he feels that she has labeled him as "nuts." The connection with his fear of being misunderstood seems clearer. More specifically, he may be worried that the clinician will immediately view him as irrational. He probably also fears that the clinician will not value his opinions. These opinions he openly shares with the phrase, "It's all got something to do with my chemistry, of that I'm sure."

With this last statement, he offers an explanation for his problem on one level but also provides two more important pieces of information: (1) At some plane of awareness, he recognizes a problem, and (2) he has a need to not view the problem as psychological. With the subsequent phrase, "Somehow or other, I'm a little speeded up," he further describes his perception of the problem. In the next question, the clinician demonstrates a desire to understand the patient's world by requesting a more phenomenological description of his stated symptom. The patient's reply once again confirms his immediate need to conceptualize the problem in physical terms, betraying his fear that the "clinician-inquisitor" will not share this perspective. Of course, the patient's insistence on a physical cause may represent an example of a person who "doth protest too much." Even the patient may subconsciously fear a psychological problem.

Although short in length, this excerpt provides a variety of pertinent clues for engagement. At one level, some unconscious agenda and needs have been delineated, but such unconscious needs will be discussed later. At this point, we are interested in the patient's conscious views of his problem. These can be summarized as follows:

1. The problem is physiologic, not psychologic.
2. A conscious desire to discuss his own view during the hour.
3. A conscious desire to convince the clinician of his view.

The next question arises, what can be done with this information? First, one can easily imagine what not to do, as would be exemplified by the clinician's proceeding with questions such as, "Perhaps you can start by telling me about some of your stresses with your son, since your wife seems to feel these stresses are at the root of your problem," or "Physiology may play a part here, but first let's look at the real problem." Such blundering inquiries must represent the clinician's hidden masochistic needs, for the clinician is adamantly refusing to explore the patient's world through the patient's eyes. A reciprocal desire by the patient not to accommodate the clinician's agenda should not be unexpected. In contrast, let us look at a possible line of questioning that attempts to move with these needs while ultimately joining both agenda:

Pt.: I'm feeling excitable, ready to roll, very creative, but maybe a little too juiced up. That's why I think it's biologic, not mental. I've been doing some reading about physical fitness and its impact on emotions and I think I've got some understanding of what is going on here.

Clin.: Oh, what kinds of things have you come up with?

Pt.: Well, some people have found that running and jogging can release substances in the brain called endorphins that help people feel good. I'm thinking that maybe that is why I'm speeded up.

Clin.: Hmm, that's interesting, how frequently do you run?

Pt.: About three miles every day, sometimes up to five miles.

Clin.: It sounds like you must be in pretty good shape. How did you get interested in physical fitness to begin with?

Pt.: I guess you could say it runs in the family, no pun intended (patient and clinician smile). My father was a jock and my two brothers both went to college on football scholarships.

Clin.: Tell me a little bit about them.

Pt.: Oh, they are both high-powered people, both very successful, (pause) more successful than me, but I do O.K. John is a corporate lawyer in Dallas and Jack is a physician.

As opposed to a denial of the patient's overt needs, this interviewer has implicitly acknowledged them. For example, the clinician picks up on the patient's hint, ". . . and I think I've got some understanding of what is going on here," by asking what the patient has discovered, thus allowing the patient to discuss his view openly. One of the most useful techniques with which to increase blending consists of asking patients for their opinions. These questions frequently open up patients, for most people have a need to be heard.

This particular choice of topics by the interviewer has also reinforced the issue of physiology, which symbolizes an area in which this patient feels safe. By moving with this patient's needs, the conversation transforms itself gracefully into an exploration of family relations.

This example stands merely as an illustration. Patient needs and perspectives change with each individual. But certain conscious patient agenda items are fairly common, and the interviewer may want to listen attentively for their presence. The following list includes some of the more common needs:

1. Somebody to listen to their story (e.g., "I've got to get this off my chest.")
2. Somebody to give them medications.
3. Somebody to "discover secrets" such as suicidal intent or a history of incest, which the patient has been afraid to share previously.
4. Somebody to confirm that they are sane.
5. Somebody to confirm that they are not sane.
6. Somebody to "tell me what's happening to me."

Naturally, some of these agenda items may or may not be compatible with the goals of the clinician. In particular, problems arise when patients' agenda may not originate from a sincere motivation for help, as with the following more manipulative needs:

1. A desire for illicit drugs.
2. A desire to be hospitalized secondary to a need for shelter.
3. A desire to have the clinician help them in a legal hassle by proving the patient is "seeing a therapist."
4. A desire to appear insane for legal purposes.
5. A desire to have the clinician confirm that the patient's regular therapist is "all wrong."
6. A desire simply to get a relative "off their back" by "seeing a specialist."
7. A desire for the clinician to tell relatives and friends that there is "nothing wrong with them."

All of these conscious agenda items can realistically lead to significant areas of resistance during the initial interview. Surprisingly, when one of these items is suspected by the interviewer, it may surface with the simple question, "At this point in our talk, it might help both of us to clarify what we want to accomplish today. I'm wondering what you were hoping might be done today." Some clinicians find this type of question to be routinely useful during the opening phase. In a literal sense, one can agree to a contract of shared goals for the first hour.

In any case, an attentive assessment of the patient's perspectives and conscious agenda provides valuable information during the scouting period. The usefulness of this information can be increased when it is added to a keen observation of the patient's behavior and appearance. A talented clinician develops the type of sensitivity to details that a good Agatha Christie detective like Miss Marple would admire. This quick-witted ability to observe leads to the second letter in the acronym PACE.

Assessment of the Patient's Mental Status

Much can be learned from a single glance if the glance has years of experience behind it. Although the formal mental status examination will generally occur in the body of the interview, during the scouting period a quick and informal assessment of mental status can provide invaluable information. In particular, the clinician searches for mental status clues that suggest a need for changing the strategy of the interview itself.

These clues are of three major types: (1) clues suggesting possible diagnoses and, hence, suggesting future areas for more extensive exploration, (2) clues suggesting significant resistances in the patient that need to be addressed, and (3) clues indicating that rather radical changes in the interview format may be needed. In a later chapter, we will look at the mental status in more detail, but for now we will briefly survey these three topics as they pertain to the scouting period.

With regard to diagnostic clues, one of the more interesting findings revolves about the issue of psychosis. If a patient presents with a smoldering psychotic process, it is not unusual for subtle signs to be present during the scouting period. Such subtle signs may include processes such as an infrequent loosening of associations, a slightly inappropriate affect, or an over-riding intensity to the patient's feelings and affects. The presence of such clues may suggest that questions dealing with psychosis may yield a rich harvest later in the interview.

Concerning the second area, evidence of resistance, the scouting period remains of vital importance. If strong resistance is present, it generally becomes necessary to work through this resistance, if possible, before proceeding into the main body of data gathering. Unresolved resistance may leave the clinician with an unresolved data base, for invalid data often lies in its wake.

To this end, the clinician keeps a wary eye out for behavioral evidence suggesting unspoken resistance. As discussed earlier, interpersonal anxiety is to be expected, but unusually high anxiety states may indicate intense fears of rejection, embarrassment, or ridicule. If the clinician suspects the presence of these fears, the following, said gently, may bring the resistance to the surface, where it can be dealt with more effectively, "It's somewhat anxiety provoking to be interviewed. I'm wondering what types of things you may be concerned or worried about as we are talking here today." Of course, other clues of resistance may be more direct, such as vague answers, an irritated or hostile affect, or no answer at all.

With regard to the third area, the discovery of a need to significantly change the structure of the interview, the issue of disruptive psychopathology rears its head. The question becomes whether a given patient can tolerate a standard initial interview. This question, frequently relevant to the emergency room setting, focuses directly upon the patient's immediate impulse control. A good clinician becomes facile at recognizing the situation in which the best interview may be a short one.

For instance, the clinician may happen upon a patient whose thinking has become laced with delusional ideation. The patient may be furiously pacing about the waiting room, shaking a fist at voices heard only in the private world of a psychotic nightmare. When questioning begins, this type of patient may rapidly escalate towards violence.

As such a rapid escalation begins to unfold, the clinician may decide to alter the strategy of the interview drastically, including its length. This type of agitated behavior may also suggest the wisdom of interrupting the interview briefly in order to alert the charge nurse of the possibility of impending violence. In any case, during the scouting period, mental status observations provide valuable clues as to which directions to take in the interview. These mental status observations may also provide clues related to the third letter of the acronym PACE.

Clinician's Perspective of the Patient's Problems and the Patient's Unconscious Agenda

A significant chasm may separate the patient's perspective from the clinician's perspective. For example, a patient may feel that the central problem consists of a vicious harassment devised by the F.B.I. The clinician may view this patient's problem as the development of a paranoid delusion. In other instances, the clinician and the patient may share similar views concerning the nature of the problem but differ upon its etiology. Fortunately, at times, both the clinician and the patient may share similar conceptualizations.

The clinician needs to begin a clinical and diagnostic formulation early in the interview, for this tentative formulation may help determine the basic strategy of the interview itself. By way of illustration, the clinician may be interviewing an elderly male brought by his family because, "he can't take care of himself anymore." During the scouting period, the clinician may notice thought disorganization, thought blocking, and an apparent memory deficit. Normally, the cognitive mental status exam is brief and generally appears late in the body of the interview. But in this instance, the clinician may decide that a determination should be made of the severity of this patient's cognitive deficit early in the interviewing process. Moreover, with this type of patient the cognitive exam may be lengthened in an effort to explore the degree of cognitive deficit.

If severe memory deficits are recognized, then little can be gained by a lengthy and tiring inquiry with the patient about the course of his illness. Instead, this time may be more profitably spent with members of the patient's family, for they may provide a more reliable history. Once again, the clinician moves flexibly, adjusting to the needs of the clinical situation. But such a creative change in strategy can only follow in the footsteps of a conscious awareness of the patient's condition by the clinician.

Of equal importance, the clinician will want to make a determination of the patient's unconscious agenda. It is worth emphasizing repeatedly that much of the art of interviewing consists not of analyzing what the patient said but speculating on what was not said and why it was not said. In a similar vein, patients often "half mention" issues, and the clinician needs to uncover what has been left partially clad. In particular, the issue of unconscious agenda remains one of the major tasks of the scouting period.

The unconscious agenda includes those drives of which the patient may be partially or totally unaware. These needs, frequently arising from core psychological pains, may represent the most telling reasons the patient has come for help and/or may also cause significant resistance to the task of the initial assessment. An example will help to clarify this concept.

In this illustration the patient is a young male about thirty years of age. His speech has a pressured quality, as if his words need to escape his mouth. He has been brought by his father, who threatened to commit him, after the patient squirted his father with tear gas during a family squabble.

> **Clin.:** Tell me some more about what brought you here today.
> **Pt.:** (Patient looks away disdainfully.) I'll tell you what brought me here today ... No! Before I tell you that, let me reassure you that I'm not crazy! My father's crazy, yeah, crazy, a real nut. . . . I'm an important person with important business, I don't have time to waste and I don't belong here, my father belongs here, you should see him, let's wrap this thing up here quickly.
> **Clin.:** Perhaps we could (patient interrupts).
> **Pt.:** I need an ashtray, you got a light?

Clin.: Yes, I do (clinician offers matches and places an ashtray near the patient).

Pt.: Look, I need to be out of here by four o'clock . . . the bottom line, the goal line is that there is nothing wrong with me that a little peace and quiet won't help, too many people do all the talking and no one listens. I'm a man whose time is worth big bucks, here, look at this (patient shows clinician business card).

Clin.: Let me take a closer look at that (inspects card). I see you are a vice president, no wonder your time is valuable. Perhaps we should start to get to the point.

Pt.: No kidding, that's a good idea. I think you and I could work this thing out logically. We are both professionals, so professional to professional is the way to work this out. There is a big misunderstanding here. He's got it all wrong, I didn't want to squirt him in the face but he attacked me, he needed a lesson, a whopper, something to put him in his place, always talking, always telling me what to do. That's the way he's always been and I'm sick of it.

Clin.: Tell me more about the misunderstanding, the way you see it, and take as much time as you need.

Pt.: The way I see it, no one appreciates me. I just started a mail order business with my fiancee, she is wonderful, she understands. It's a dog eat dog world out there and the old man doesn't give a damn, he lives in the age of horse-hoofs, the Stone Age.

Clin.: What are some of the specific stresses you are handling right now?

Pt.: Financial strain, paying the rent, getting ready for the wedding, this, that, and the other.

Clin.: Sounds like a lot of bills to pay.

Pt.: You're darn right. The trouble is my landlord is a jerk. All he thinks about is money and payments. I've been a good tenant, and he has no right to throw me out.

Clin.: When is he threatening to throw you out?

Pt.: Two weeks from now, the man's got a lot of nerve. To think I used to say nice things about him.

Clin.: How have all these pressures affected your sleep?

Pt.: I don't need much sleep, I get along with very little sleep because I'm energized.

Clin.: What time do you go to sleep roughly?

Pt.: Well, that varies. Usually around twelve or one o'clock, but recently I've been staying up later to do my work.

Clin.: And what kinds of things do you do when you stay up?

In this vignette, one can see the subtle maneuverings of the opening phase. The art lies in the interviewer's ability to recognize the unstated needs of the patient, while subsequently attending to some of these same needs. The passage warrants a closer look.

On a conscious level, the patient's agenda includes items such as convincing the clinician that nothing is wrong, convincing the clinician that the patient's father is wrong, and making a quick exit subsequent to an equally quick interview. But it is the unconscious agenda that yields the most fertile engagement secrets.

Two of these unstated needs could be described as follows:

1. The need to appear important, possibly related to an underlying fear of inferiority.
2. The need to be in control, perhaps generated by the impending threat of an involuntary commitment, which would represent a total loss of control.

The first need, the need for praise, manifests itself early in the dialogue. For instance, the patient immediately raises himself by putting down his father, "the nut," and the interviewer with a disdainful look. These defiant steps, indicative of a frightened ego, are quickly followed by a blunt request for praise, "I'm an important person who has important business." Later we hear, "I'm a man whose time is worth big bucks," at which point he proceeds to display his business card.

It is at this point that the clinician plays a gentle gambit. Specifically, he goes out of his way to provide the much needed praise. The clinician does not merely glance at the offered business card, he calmly admires it. Indeed, it is this quiet admiration that represents the real and immediate business of this interview, for with its presence the engagement process can begin to unfold. This quiet praise is furthered by a simple but elegantly effective acknowledgment of the patient's importance, "I see you are a vice president, no wonder your time is valuable." At last, the patient's self system receives a chance to relax. Someone has seen his worth. Defenses, such as pressured speech and accusation, may become less necessary.

Further acknowledgment of the patient's importance resides in the clinician's recognition of the patient's stated time needs, "Perhaps we should start to get to the point." With this apparently appeasing statement, the clinician, in reality, is beginning to structure the interview. In a relatively short time this patient will be providing diagnostic information related to mania instead of demanding a shorter interaction.

The second hidden need, the need for control, begins with a subtle redirecting of the clinician's attention by the patient, ". . . my father belongs here, you should see him . . ." and ends with a not so subtle directive, ". . . let's wrap this thing up here quickly."

The patient continues to control the interview by interrupting the clinician's question by stating a demand, "I need an ashtray. . . ." It is not so hard to imagine that someone close to involuntary commitment would feel threatened, for he is in reality threatened with an imprisonment of sorts. Fortunately, the interviewer recognizes this need and focuses attention on helping this patient regain some semblance of self-determination. This release of control in the service of gaining control is accomplished by the phrase, "Tell me more about the misunderstanding, the way you see it, and take as much time as you need." This conveyance of control is gently bolstered by suggesting that the patient has been appropriately managing at least some aspects of his life as implied by the wording, "What are some of the specific stresses you are handling right now?" How different this phrase must sound compared with a similar content message, "What problems are unsettling you right now," a phrase that would have ignored the patient's need to feel confident.

This dialogue represents only one of numberless interactions. It is not the specific words that are important here. It is the underlying principle of listening for the hidden needs that warrants emphasis. It is this third assessment of the scouting period, the search for the pains that drive the patient, that opens the door to engagement. Understanding this aspect of the scouting period is akin to understanding resistance itself, but that topic awaits future discussion. Presently, the fourth assessment, the fourth letter in the acronym PAC*E*, deserves attention.

Evaluation of the Interview Itself

Interviews, like the people creating them, tend to develop personalities of a sort. The personality of the interview appears to be determined by the quality and quantity of the communication evolving between the participants. Ideally, a clinician would like to become a co-participant in an interview characterized by a patient who produces relatively large amounts of pertinent and valid information, while easily focusing on issues raised by the clinician. This ideal patient would become increasingly at ease as the interview proceeded, becoming the proverbial open book. Within minutes, an adequate level of blending would be achieved, the patient and clinician working together towards unified goals. Someday, I would like to be a participant in such an interview.

In reality, ideal interviews are hard to find. Fortunately, good interviews are not. One of the keys to developing consistently productive interviews remains the ability to spot bad interviews before they become painful lessons in frustration. By consciously evaluating the interview process, the clinician opens the door to control and flexibility. Phrased more accurately, once the clinician has determined the personality of the interview, the clinician may gain control by adaptively altering technique. To this end, during the scouting period, the clinician needs to attempt a conscious assessment of the progress of the interview. If pleased with its nascent development, then similar strategies may be continued. If displeased, new options may be entertained.

The interviewer should be on the lookout for a variety of less productive patterns in communication, three of which are the shutdown interview, the wandering interview, and the rehearsed interview. All three of these interview types can lead to serious problems with engagement and data gathering. All three, once spotted, warrant a change in strategy (see Table 1).

THE SHUT-DOWN INTERVIEW

In the shut-down interview, the patient displays a short duration of utterance, a long response time latency, and usually a variety of body language clues indicating that things are not going well. In particular, eye contact is often poor. I am reminded of a patient I observed during supervision who sat morosely, her legs propped up on a stool, her own crossed arms representing the main objects of interest to her eyes. As if to place appropriate exclamation points in her nonverbal communication, she yawned with impeccable timing. She represented the ideal persona of a shut-down in communication.

But shut-down interviews are not the creation of the patient alone. As emphasized earlier, all interviews represent interaction. In this respect, the action of the patient described above suggests the possibility that the interview will become a shut-down interview. But for this process to unfold fully, the interviewer must feed it.

This feeding occurs when the interviewer fosters the shut-down pattern by utilizing a low ratio of open-ended to closed-ended questions. These closed-ended questions tend to decrease patient spontaneity and, hence, hinder the blending process. This tendency becomes further entrenched when the interviewer uses a high proportion of focusing statements and other structuring techniques. It may be even further entrenched if the clinician tends to utilize facilitating maneuvers poorly, such as head nodding, empathic statements, and an encouraging tone of voice.

During shut-down interviews, it is not uncommon for clinicians to

TABLE 1. Interview Typologies

Interview Type	Characteristics of Patient			Characteristics of Interviewer		
	Duration of Utterance (D.O.U.)	Response Time Latency (R.T.L.)	Natural Body Language such as Eye Contact	Ratio of Open-ended Questions to Close-ended Questions	Focusing Statements	Facilitating Maneuvers, Empathic Statements
Shut Down Interview	↓	↑	↓	↓	↑	↓
Wandering Interview	↑	↓	↑	↑	↓	↑
Rehearsed Interview	↑	↓	↕	↕	↓	↑

KEY: ↑ = increased; ↓ = decreased; ↕ = either increased or decreased.

feel frustration, which often manifests itself in a sharpness to the tone of voice and a distinct lack of empathic communication. Ironically, such action merely fosters the further development of the shut-down process itself. Thus, the dyadic nature of the interview surfaces once again.

If the interviewer spots the characteristics in the patient that may lead to a shut-down in communications, certain steps may be taken to reverse the process. This issue of practical interview management brings us directly to the topic of open-ended questioning.

The concept of an open-ended question appears at first glance as so self-explanatory that it warrants little discussion. But one could not be more mistaken. In actual practice, the open-ended question is frequently not utilized effectively. Moreover, numerous references to the technique in both research literature and interviewing texts tend to disagree with each other about the definition of open-endedness and about which questions are open versus closed.[3-18] The following approach clarifies these discrepancies and provides a practical approach to the application of open-ended techniques in shut-down interviews.

Open-ended Verbalizations. Both questions and statements can be classified as open-ended or closed. For example, the statement, "Tell me something about your old high-school girlfriend" is significantly more open-ended than the question, "Did you have a high-school girlfriend?" Any question or statement can be classified along the continuum of openness. Three variables seem to influence where a verbalization sits on this continuum: (1) the degree with which the verbalization tends to produce spontaneous and lengthy responses, (2) the degree with which the verbalization does not limit the patient's answer set, and (3) the degree with which the verbalization opens up a moderately shut-down interviewee.

At this juncture let us examine the continuum of openness more closely. In general, verbalizations can, by referring to the above variables, be classified into one of three broad categories, open-ended verbalizations, closed-ended verbalizations, and variable verbalizations, which lie somewhere between the two poles. In the following discussion these three categories will be defined and examples of each type given.

By definition, open-ended verbalizations are difficult to answer with one word or a short phrase even if the interviewee is moderately guarded or resistant. It is extremely difficult to respond to open-ended verbalizations with a simple "yes" or "no." Moreover, questions that provide or imply possible answers, ask for specific items, places, dates, numbers, or names are closed-ended, for they limit the patient's freedom of choice. Broadly speaking, with patients in whom the blending is high, open-ended verbalizations tend to produce relatively large quantities of speech.

Open-ended verbalizations appear in one of two forms, open-ended questions or gentle commands. A classic example of an open-ended question would look as follows, "What would you do if your wife decided to leave you?" (See Table 2 for further examples.) This question does not guide the patient towards any specific answer nor can it easily be tersely answered. It invites the patient to share personal experience.

We have already seen one example of a gentle command. They consist of statements such as, "Tell me something about your old high-school girlfriend," which direct the patient to speak but do not limit the potential answer. Gentle commands begin with words such as "Tell me . . ." or "Describe for me . . . ." They are stated with a gentle tone of voice while expressing a genuine interest. A series of such gentle commands or a mixture of these statements with open-ended questions frequently increases the blending and spontaneity of even the most shut-down interaction. Generally speaking, gentle commands represent one of the most powerful tools available to the clinician for opening up resistant patients.

Closed-ended Verbalizations. At the other end of the openness continuum one encounters closed-ended verbalizations. With closed-ended techniques it is extremely easy for a moderately shut-down patient to answer with one word, a short phrase, or a simple "yes" or "no." Even in instances in which the blending is high, these techniques may tend to decrease interviewee response length. Indeed, as we shall see shortly, closed-ended inquiries are frequently useful in focusing wandering patients.

Closed-ended verbalizations come in two types, closed-ended questions and closed-ended statements (see Table 2). Closed-ended questions are frequently of a yes/no format such as, "Did you seek therapy at the time of the accident?" or ask for specific details as with, "Which hospital were you at in 1982?" Although frequently hunting for facts, they may also seek out opinions and emotions as seen with, "Do you think your husband is hard working?"

Closed-ended statements do not suggest that any response is expected from the patient and frequently are of an explanatory or educational slant as with, "We will begin by looking at some of your symptoms."

Variable Verbalizations. Thus far we have examined both open and closed techniques, but what should we make of a question such as, "Can you tell me something about your first date?" This

TABLE 2. Degree of Openness Continuum

Verbalization	Example
OPEN-ENDED	
1. Open-ended questions	1. What are your plans for the future? 2. How will you approach your father? 3. What are some of your thoughts about the marriage?
2. Gentle commands	1. Tell me something about your brother. 2. Describe her initial reaction to me. 3. Share with me some of your hopes about the marriage.
VARIABLE	
1. Swing questions	1. Can you describe your feelings? 2. Can you tell me a little about your boss? 3. Can you say anything about the marriage?
2. Qualitative questions	1. How's your appetite? 2. How's your job going? 3. How's your mood been?
3. Statements of inquiry	1. You have never smoked marijuana? 2. You say you were fifth in your class? 3. So you left the marriage after three years?
4. Empathic statements	1. It sounds like a troubling time for you. 2. It's difficult to end a marriage after ten years. 3. It looks like you're feeling very sad.
5. Facilitory statements	1. Uh-huh. 2. Go on. 3. I see.
CLOSED-ENDED	
1. Closed-ended questions	1. Do you think your son will pass? 2. Are you feeling happy, sad, or angry? 3. What medication is he taking?
2. Closed-ended statements	1. Please sit over there. 2. I read the letter Dr. Smith wrote. 3. Anxiety can be helped with behavioral therapies.

question seems to lie somewhere in between, for it is open-ended in the sense of suggesting no specific answer set but also appears closed-ended, for it can be easily brushed aside with a short phrase such as, "not much to say." This type of question, "the swing question" represents one of five variable verbalizations. Variable verbalizations represent a middle ground with regard to openness, for they tend to vary in the responses they create depending upon the degree of blending. When blending is high, these types of questions often result in the production of large amounts of spontaneous speech. But when blending is low and the patient is resistant, the very same questions can be easily answered tersely. And therein lies their danger for the clinician, for these questions are tickets towards monologue when used in a shut-down interview. Consequently, we will examine the five variable verbalizations, swing questions, qualitative questions, statements of inquiry, empathic statements, and facilitory statements, more closely.

Swing questions are characterized by the quality of asking the patient whether he or she wants to answer. They often begin with phrases such as, "Would you tell me . . ." or "Can you describe . . ." (see Table 2). The impact of such questions literally swings from open to closed depending upon the degree of blending present. When blending is high, a patient may merrily chatter away following such a question. But when a patient feels resistant, these questions can be curtly answered with statements such as, "not really," "don't feel like it," or simply "no". Consequently, as mentioned above, they should not be used in a shut-down interview.

A second type of variable verbalization is the qualitative question, with which the clinician inquires about the quality of the state of the patient, his symptoms, or his relations and activities. They frequently begin with the words, "How is your . . .?" Qualitative questions such as, "How's your relationship with your son?" have the potential to produce a significant elaboration if the blending is high. But, as was the case with swing questions, a resistant patient could easily answer tersely with a phrase such as, "Just fine." Operationally speaking, if a question begins with the word "how" and can be answered by the single word "fine," then it is by definition a qualitative question.

The third type of variable verbalization, the statement of inquiry, is represented by a complete sentence followed by a question mark. Unlike closed-ended statements, they are intended to stimulate a response from the patient as seen with, "You were working at the factory right after college?" or "You're viewed as the black sheep in the family?" The tone of voice of the clinician has a lot to do with the transformation of these statements into questions. The clinician's tone of voice can also move these statements from a gentle probing to a blunt confrontation. Statements of inquiry tend to perform one of several functions: clarification, summarization, confrontation, or interpretation by reflecting the patient's words back to them so that the patient can hear the implication of what was just said. As with the two previous variable verbalizations, statements of inquiry can be easily shut-down by resistant patients, whereas in situations of high blending these statements may function as springboards for further patient elaboration.

It should also be noted that leading questions frequently take the form of statements of inquiry. If a clinician uses statements of inquiry too frequently or at the wrong moment, then errors in validity may result. Statements of inquiry that are leading in nature often begin with the word "so," as seen with "So, you began drinking even in junior high?"

The final two types of variable verbalizations, empathic statements and facilitory statements, can be usefully discussed together, for they generally tend to open patients up, but with guarded or hostile patients they may backfire, as discussed in Chapter 1. By definition, empathic statements are attempts to convey to clients that one is gaining an understanding of their feelings and perceptions of the world (see Figure 2). Facilitory statements include the wide range of single utterances or short phrases used to signal that the clinician is carefully listening such as, "Uh-huh" and, "Go on." Although these facilitory phrases tend to urge the patient towards more speech, looked at on an individual basis they are not as powerfully open as a gentle command or an open-ended question. With hostile patients they may even backfire. I recall one instance in the emergency room, when an intoxicated alcoholic began angrily aping both my facilitory statements and my head nodding, saying, "Yeah, you're a shrink all right, yeah, you're a shrink." Several minutes later he attacked a safety officer.

Unlocking Shut-down Interviews. Now that we have surveyed the types of questions along the continuum of openness, it is of value to look at a frequent problem encountered with shut-down patients. Specifically, variable verbalizations such as swing questions and statements of inquiry tend to become a habit. And as an interview becomes more shut-down, maladaptive habits have a tendency to return, just when they are least useful. As the patient grunts out short answers and begins to appear aggravated, the natural tendency is to ask questions even faster. These questions are frequently of a swing nature, almost asked apologetically. Closed-ended questions also seem to appear more frequently, probably because they are easier to formulate than open-ended questions. The unpleasant result may be as follows:

Clin.: How long were you in prison? (closed question)
Pt.: (Looking somewhat disgusted) Two years.
Clin.: Was it a bad experience? (closed question)
Pt.: What do you think? (said sarcastically)
Clin.: Were the guards tough? (closed question)
Pt.: Yeah.
Clin.: Did they get on your nerves? (closed question)
Pt.: Yeah.
Clin.: Did you get time for exercise? (closed question)
Pt.: Sometimes.
Clin.: Pretty bad food, I bet. (empathic statement)
Pt.: Yeah.
Clin.: Did you get very lonely there? (closed question)
Pt.: Yep.
Clin.: Could you tell me a little about what that felt like? (swing question)
Pt.: Not much to tell you.
Clin.: Well, I, uh, was it tough being away from your wife? (closed question)
Pt.: Sort of.
Clin.: Would you be able to tell me how she felt about it? (swing question)
Pt.: Don't really know.
Clin.: Can you tell me if she still loves you? (swing question)
Pt.: Don't really know that either.
Clin.: What do you think? (open-ended question)
Pt.: I think she might.
Clin.: How's the communication between you two? (qualitative question)
Pt.: Just dandy.
Clin.: How do you mean? (open-ended question)
Pt.: I mean she still writes and visits.
Clin.: Ah, how often does she visit? (closed question)
Pt.: About twice a year.
Clin.: When is that? (closed question)
Pt.: Take a guess . . . around Christmas and on my birthday.

The only person probably less comfortable than the patient is the clinician. Indeed, here is a classic shut-down interview moving into a spiral of silence. It illustrates several errors that are frequently made by clinicians. In the latter half, one sees the use of swing questions, under the mistaken thought that they are open-ended. The result proves otherwise. Then one sees the use of two true open-ended questions, "What do you think?" and "How do you mean?" But, two open-ended questions are too few. For the open-ended effect to really take hold, the clinician generally needs to ask a series of open-ended questions or use a series of gentle commands, not just a couple. In fact, following the first couple of open-ended questions, the patient's responses will probably still be brief. But after five or six open-ended questions in a row, many patients will start to yield to the awkwardness of not responding appropriately. The above exchange also illustrates how easily other variable verbalizations such as qualitative questions can be shut-down by resistant patients.

In the following example, we will see the course the previous dialogue might have taken if handled differently:

    Clin.: How long were you in prison? (closed question)
      Pt.: (Looking somewhat disgusted) Two years.
    Clin.: Huh ... Some people hate being in prison and others find it less upsetting. What did you do to keep yourself busy? (open-ended question)
      Pt.: Sports and cards, sports and cards, but it grows old real fast.
    Clin.: I really don't know much about what a prison is like; tell me something about it. (gentle command)
      Pt.: Let me put it this way. You wouldn't last a day (patient smiles). Yeah, they'd get you fast.
    Clin.: Tell me what it's really like in there. (gentle command)
      Pt.: Well, it's boring, day after day of the same shit. And time goes much slower. Everything, everything changes for you, man. Eating dinner is something to do, a movie is a scene, man. And you become a "con" man, not a jerk-off.
    Clin.: How do you mean, a "con." (open-ended question)
      Pt.: A "con" is no one's fool. We don't come on to the guards or anyone. You can't survive unless you watch out for yourself.

This clinician is cleverly engaging the patient by utilizing open-ended questions and gentle commands. In particular, the clinician has avoided the pitfall of utilizing swing questions and other variable verbalizations, which could function in a closed role, as evidenced in the earlier example. This clinician also wisely went into an area in which the patient felt comfortable and, indeed, could "instruct" the clinician.

The following list reviews the techniques we have discussed for working through a shut-down interview and suggests as well a few more tips:

1. Employ large numbers of combinations of open-ended questions and gentle commands in a series. Too frequently interviewers ask one or two open-ended questions followed by a close-ended question or a variable verbalization, which can immediately defeat the gains made by the open-ended approach.

2. Follow up any topic that the patient gives the slightest hint that he or she wants to discuss (i.e., any topic on which the patient shows an increasing duration of utterance, even for a brief period of time).

3. Avoid, in general, difficult or sensitive topics such as lethality, drugs and alcohol abuse, and sexual history.

4. Pick topics that gather general background information such as, "Tell me a little bit about the neighborhood you live in?" or "What are the people like where you work?" Or choose topics about which the patient has strong opinions as with, "What are some of the things your boss does that seem unfair?"

5. Avoid initiating questions with phrases such as, "Can you tell me . . ." or "Would you tell me. . . ." Such swing questions are easily answered with silence or frowns. Instead, it is frequently best to use gentle commands to instruct the patient to answer.

6. Increase attempts at eye contact, while increasing the reinforcement of verbal output with head nodding, empathic sounds, and phrases such as, "Go on," except with hostile patients, with whom a less frequent use of such techniques may be advisable.

7. Avoid long pauses before asking the next question. Long pauses are effective techniques for eliciting information from reasonably well-engaged patients who stop their flow because of their desire to avoid a topic. On the other hand, long pauses in shut-down patients frequently create further resistance and resentment. Effective use of long pauses depends upon effective timing and good common sense.

It should also be kept in mind that the above techniques are generally applicable not only in shut-down interviews but also during the opening phase of any interview. In contrast, in interviews with good blending, patients may spontaneously talk about a variety of painful and/or sensitive areas fairly early. In even sharper contrast, the first principle outlined above is specific to shut-down interviews. In naturally evolving interviews, open-ended techniques are interwoven with statements of inquiry and closed-ended questions, both of which serve to clarify issues and demonstrate the clinician's interest. Thus it is uncommon in interviews with good initial blending to employ long strings of open-ended techniques, and only about 30 to 70 per cent of verbalizations in the opening phase are open.

This list offers some of the guiding principles with which to approach stalled interviews. Most importantly, a concentrated effort should be made to increase patient output before proceeding with information gathering. If these techniques do not work, then a more deep-rooted resistance may have formed. Approaches to resolving such deep-rooted resistances will be discussed in Chapter 10. Another method of approaching shut-down interviews is to address the underlying resistance almost immediately. This technique is also discussed in Chapter 10. The most telling point remains that the presence of a shut-down interview indicates a need for an active change in interviewing style. These changes frequently and rapidly result in a more fruitful dialogue.

As with any interview, one must work flexibly and creatively with the individual patient. In some instances of a shut-down interview, the above techniques may actually hinder progress. In particular, some patients, whose thinking is grossly disorganized, secondary to either psychotic process or interpersonal anxiety, may respond poorly to open-ended questions or gentle imperatives. These techniques force these patients to conceptualize at a level at which they may not be capable, further increasing anxiety.

In these instances, very structured and concrete questions may help the patient with organization. In this effort, the clinician may employ a higher number of closed-ended questions and statements of inquiry. With experience one quickly learns which technique works best with which type of patient.

In a similar vein, some adolescents and adults need to "warm up" with a higher ratio of closed-ended questions, for these tend to be less probing and can be more quickly answered. Two other types of questions merit attention. At first glance they seem like classic open-ended techniques and they are open-ended, but they tend to perplex patients and should be avoided in shut-down interviews.

The first problematic question begins with the word "why" such as, "Why did you stop going to your classes?" As Alfred Benjamin has cogently discussed, questions beginning with "why" frequently sound judgmental and break the feeling of unconditional positive regard, especially if the tone of voice is even mildly harsh.[19] They also seem to suggest that there exists one answer to the question, and it may be difficult for the patient to sort through all the confounding factors to produce the single right answer. Instead of beginning with "why" one can rephrase the question in one of several ways, such as, "What were some of the things going through your mind when you decided that it would be best to leave school?" or "What were the pros and cons of leaving school when you made your decision?"

The second troublesome question that tends to hinder dialogue in a shut-down interview may represent the all-time stereotypical "shrink question," and it reads something like this, "What are you feeling as we talk?" In actuality, it is both uncommon and difficult for most people to be aware of their inner feelings. Thus in shut-down interviews this type of question is particularly good at producing looks of consternation on patients' faces. Avoid it. It may be of use later in therapy or with patients with whom the blending is high, but not in shut-down interviews. By the way, children and adolescents, in particular, find this question puzzling.

FOCUSING THE WANDERING INTERVIEW

At this point we have spent a large amount of time discussing methods of working through a shut-down interview, for this type of interaction is both common and frustrating. At the other end of the continuum, one may be unfortunate enough to become a participant in a wandering interview. We met this entity at the very beginning of the book. As we saw then, in the wandering interview, the patient displays a tendency toward mildly tangential and circumstantial thought, their serpentine meanderings swallow the interviewer's train of questioning in a cloud of spicy irrelevancies. The patient's loquaciousness is often characterized by a mild pressure to their speech, resulting in a long duration of utterance, almost tempting the interviewer not to ask questions, for each question creates a new verbal leak. The response time latency (RTL) is short, and eye contact is often good.

A variant of the wandering interview, "the loquacious interview," occurs when the patient demonstrates pressured speech but does not stray off the topic. In fact, at times the patient becomes lost in a mass of related details. The characteristics described above represent the attributes of a patient that predispose the patient towards the development of a wandering interview. But once again, a true wandering interview remains the joint creation of both the patient and the clinician. Clinicians foster the wandering by asking open-ended questions and not utilizing focusing statements. In short, as the patient extends his or her hand, the clinician accepts it. And the rambling walk begins.

Frequently clinicians unwittingly further their own demise by employing many facilitory gestures and sounds, which only serve to reward the patient's abundant flow of speech. Note-taking can also serve to reward this process, functioning as a metacommunication such as "What you just said is important, keep going." Interviewers can learn to quiet all of these facilitory activities in the service of closing off a runaway interview, if the clinician is aware of them in the first place.

The patient's contribution to the wandering interview has many etiologies. Such an interpersonal style may accompany histrionic personality structure or indicate the earliest stages of a mania. Or this style may represent something much less serious, as seen with a patient who is simply anxious. In any case, several principles may be of value in transforming such an interview into a more productive exchange. While moving out of the scouting phase, begin to help the patient structure his or her answers as follows:

a. Gently increase the ratio of close-ended questions to open-ended ones.

b. Avoid reinforcing the wandering pattern by excessive head nodding or paralanguage cues to "go on." This process was referred to earlier as "feeding the wanderer."

c. Begin with a gentle structuring by immediately returning to the topic of the question that led to the tangential thought.

d. If the wandering continues, become progressively more structured with statements such as, "For a moment, let's focus on what your mood was like back then."

e. With further wandering, one can further increase the focusing with statements such as, "This is such an important area I would like to focus on it alone for a few minutes."

f. If the above techniques fail, one can simply tell the patient what is needed, "We have a limited amount of time. Consequently, I'm going to focus on some of the very important areas you mentioned in an effort to understand more clearly. It's important for us to focus on one topic at a time."

g. Another approach consists of addressing the resistance itself, "I have noticed that when I ask questions we quickly seem to wander off the subject. What do you think may be going on"?

h. Finally, one can become very structured, "Because of time, we need to focus directly on the last two weeks of your mood. It will be important not to wander on to other topics because learning specifically about your mood is so important for our understanding. In fact, if we wander off, you'll notice that I'll bring us back to the last two weeks. Is that all right with you? . . . Let's start with your sleep. Over the past two weeks how long has it been taking you to fall asleep?"

Generally speaking, unless the patient has some serious underlying psychopathology, such as a manic process, the first several techniques will decrease the wandering process.

At times it may also be necessary to literally cut a patient off in mid-sentence. This technique is fairly forceful and consequently should only be utilized after less aggressive focusing techniques have failed. Frequently cut-offs are less disengaging if piggybacked onto empathic statements as shown below:

Clin.: Exactly how depressed have you been feeling?
Pt.: Well, let's see, in the past several months a lot has been

> happening to me, you know, what with the move and everything. I was very upset by my mother's nagging and the bills are really mounting, much as they did when I was living with Aunt Louise. Fortunately, I'm not quite as bad off as with Aunt Louise because . . .

Clin.: (clinician cuts off patient) It really sounds like you've been through a lot, and how has all this affected your mood in the past two weeks?

Pt.: Oh, I've been feeling very depressed.

Clin.: Have you cried or felt like crying?

In this example the cut-off included an empathic statement, which provided a softening touch without decreasing the effectiveness of the cut-off. Another method of effectively using a cut-off is to include a comment acknowledging the importance of what the patient is saying such as, "So much of what you are saying is important that we need to focus a bit to ensure we get the most important points. Exactly what has your mood been like over the past two weeks?" Once again the patient was cut off in mid-stream, but the opening line acknowledges the importance of what the patient is saying while focusing the conversation.

I would like to emphasize that the recognition of a wandering interview occurs during the scouting period, but the attempt to transform this process actually occurs somewhere in the body of the interview. This point warrants emphasis because one of the major deterrants to focusing a patient effectively is the attempt to focus too early. Ironically, such premature focusing can leave the patient and the clinician in a duel for control. In such a duel, both participants may go home wounded, for the patient responds by talking even more profusely. The main point remains: facilitate first, structure second.

A second major factor in successfully focusing a patient lies in the effective use of paralanguage and body language during the structuring process. The art is not so much in the choice of words but in the method of presentation. For instance, if said with a concerned tone of voice, a phrase such as, "Let's look again at what your mood was like over the past two weeks," will seldom be interpreted as a structuring ploy. On the other hand, the same phrase said harshly or in frustration may quickly disengage a timid patient.

At present, it may be valuable to examine an interviewer successfully working with a persistent wanderer. The interviewer recognized the wandering pattern during the scouting period and, consequently, began to structure as the scouting period ended and the body of the interview began.

Clin.: Tell me what your sleep has been like. (gentle command)

Pt.: My sleep, now that's a good question. Nobody in my family has ever been a sound sleeper. I remember my father always talking about his restless nights. Same way with Uncle Harry, although, personally, I think Uncle Harry was a drunk. They say drunks, I shouldn't call him that (patient giggles), have really bad sleep.

Clin.: How has your sleep been over the past two weeks? (qualitative question)

Pt.: Pretty bad, more wound up, what with all the worries on my mind. I'm really upset about my decrease in pay. I don't think my boss should have cut my salary.

Clin.: It sounds like you've had a lot of worries. How many hours do you think it takes you to fall asleep? (closed question)

Pt.: Oh, maybe two or three.

Clin.: Once you're asleep, do you stay asleep the whole night or do you tend to wake up occasionally? (closed question)

Pt.: No, no, once I'm out, I'm really out, just like the night after my chem final. I was so tired I literally slept like a log, but fortunately I was alert enough to pack up for home, although I don't know why I should want to go home, why . . .

Clin.: Before talking about home, let us get an even clearer picture of how your sleep has been affected. For instance, over the past two weeks have you been awakening earlier than usual for yourself? (closed question)

Pt.: No, I can't say that I have.

Clin.: Do you sleep at all during the day? (closed question)

Pt.: No, once I'm up, I'm really up.

Clin.: How has your energy been recently? (qualitative question)

Pt.: Up and down, mostly down. I guess I'm not as interested in things as I used to be.

Clin.: How do you mean? (open-ended question)

Pt.: Well, I used to be into jazz dance and ballet. On Wednesday nights I did aerobics. My sister, Jane, had gotten me into aerobics, she was always a super athlete.

Clin.: What about your own interest in things like dance now, has it increased or decreased? (closed question)

Pt.: Definitely decreased. I'm finding it harder and harder to enjoy all my hobbies. I'm even having a hard time reading . . .

In this illustration, the clinician has begun structuring this interview without disengaging the patient. This toning down of a wound-up wanderer was accomplished using a variety of techniques, including focusing statements, closed-ended questions, and even interrupting the patient with a cut-off statement at one point. Note that variable verbalizations, such as qualitative questions, though more effective than open-ended questions at focusing the patient, are not as effective as closed-ended questions in this regard. Consequently, when focusing, it is best to stick with closed-ended questions most of the time. The art lies in focusing while sensitively monitoring the blending.

Even when using a patient cut-off, the clinician maintained blending by conveying the importance of gaining a clear picture of exactly what the patient had been experiencing. Moreover, the clinician also emphasized the importance of what the patient was discussing by implying that the topic would be examined later in the interview. Both of these goals were accomplished with a single phrase, "Before talking about home, let us get a clearer picture of how your sleep has been affected." Even the use of the pronoun "us" helps to convey to the patient a shared goal and task.

Not surprisingly, working with a wandering patient is one of the most frequent problems for which clinicians request supervision, probably because we are often hesitant to structure, anticipating a rebuff from the patient. This hesitancy prevents us from learning how to structure effectively. In a sense, a wandering interview reminds one of an unchecked nuclear reaction; its ultimate result is a chaotic and sparse understanding of the patient. On the other hand, the ability to structure the flow of the interview offers the clinician a method of controlling the reaction, much as nuclear fission is controlled in a reactor.

Later, in the body of the interview, the clinician may find good reasons to unleash the reaction again while exploring the patient's dynamics or feelings. The important point remains that the clinician can modify the interview process in either direction, depending upon what the goals of the interview are at the moment.

To end this discussion of the wandering interview, it is of value to list some of the most common errors clinicians commit while handling a wandering patient:

1. Continuing to "feed the wanderer" instead of beginning to structure gently as one enters the main body of the interview.

2. Being afraid to focus or interrupt the patient. When done effectively focusing statements are generally well tolerated by patients.

3. Structuring too early. During the scouting period one generally lets the patient go wherever the patient wants to go. The interview, at

this stage, is highly unstructured. This facilitation period allows one to increase blending, while letting the clinician assess the various areas of PACE, as mentioned earlier.

4. Focusing too bluntly before trying more subtle approaches. It is best to begin with subtle focusing techniques, increasing the firmness as needed.

Breaking Through the Rehearsed Interview

At this point, it seems pertinent to examine briefly another problematical style of interview, keeping in mind that many other styles exist and that many interviews represent mixtures of these three styles. This third type can be labeled as "the rehearsed interview." It commonly appears when working with a chronic mental health patient who "knows the system." In this process, patients tell a story that may even bore the patient himself or herself, for it has been told so often. The history seems pat and simple, and therein lies the problem.

Both the patient and the clinician can be lulled into a joint acceptance of half truths. No person's life history or history of their present illness is simple. To get at the appropriate facts, both the patient and the clinician need motivation and involvement. Without these features, the validity and thoroughness of the data base may be seriously jeopardized.

To do something about the rehearsed interview one must first recognize it. It frequently announces itself with early diagnostic statements by the patient and a quick and unsolicited review of the history of the present illness. Sometimes patients will reel off a list of symptoms pertinent to the disorder with which the patient wants to present. These monologues frequently result in a long DOU and a short RTL. Eye contact varies depending upon the situation. It is generally good, but if the patient is feeling guilt or covering something up, eye contact may be poor.

On the interpersonal level, the patient may be quick to tell his or her side, while dismantling opposing views before the clinician can even think of them. This last phenomenon also illustrates that the rehearsed interview does not always arise from indifference. Quite the opposite, rehearsed interviews may grow from the patient's need to control the interview. The clinician colludes with a rehearsed interview by focusing poorly or by providing an abundance of facilitation activities, as seen in the wandering interview. A rehearsed interview can be unfortunately fed by the use of open-ended, variable, or closed-ended verbalizations, for any question that tracks with the patient can reinforce the direction of the interview.

The following brief vignette conveys a feeling for such an interview:

> *Clin.:* Tell me what brings you here today?
>
> *Pt.:* Well, I got out of St. Joseph's hospital two months ago. After I got out, I moved to a new catchment area, so I need new doctors. I've been feeling a little edgy and need to be on lithium. You see I'm manic depressive.
>
> *Clin.:* I see.
>
> *Pt.:* Now, I'm not having racing thoughts or problems sleeping and my energy is just fine. You'll probably be hearing from my sister and don't listen to a word she says. She over-reacts and she doesn't understand this disease. Other than my edginess everything is fine.

The problem here is the validity of this data. All angles are being covered so quickly that one can feel hedged in by the patient's story, almost as if one should not ask any more questions. To break this mechanical storytelling a variety of methods can be used.

One of the methods consists of disrupting the flow of patient opinion by asking for behavioral incidents, as discussed in Chapter 1. This type of behavioral questioning serves the dual purpose of forcing the patient to reflect, while also helping the clinician to gain a more effective data base.

A second method consists of interrupting the twice-told tale by getting the patient to discuss areas that require new conceptualization and/or bring the patient face to face with affectively charged topics.

For instance, later in the above interview, perhaps as the clinician was leaving the scouting phase, the patient could be led into more immediate material as follows:

> *Clin.:* You mentioned your sister several times, tell me a little bit about her.
>
> *Pt.:* She's sort of a jerk and I'll tell you one thing, I want her to keep her nose out of my affairs.
>
> *Clin.:* What has she been doing recently that has been so upsetting?
>
> *Pt.:* She's been mouthing off, getting me in trouble.
>
> *Clin.:* What sort of ways?
>
> *Pt.:* She got me into the hospital, when I didn't want to go. I didn't need to be in there, but she called the cops and the next thing I know, I'm committed. She claims I'm a danger to her children. I would say the greatest danger to her children is their mother.

In this instance, the patient has been led away from his rehearsed story, through the gate of affect. With this side trip, important information that may not have been intended for psychiatric ears has surfaced, namely the patient was recently committed involuntarily. Perhaps things are not as cut and dry as the patient wanted the clinician to believe.

At this juncture, we have concluded our survey of the various assessments that occur during the scouting period as summarized by the acronym PACE. This rapid assessment occurs during the first two phases of the interview, the introduction and the opening.

It is hoped the above information explains why a large amount of time has been devoted to the scouting period. Its importance would be hard to exaggerate, for in it the first hints of understanding are born in the clinician. The interviewer may have intuited some of the core pains and needs of the patient. Aware of these issues, the clinician is now prepared to enter the patient's world more fully. If the scouting period is done effectively, the clinician will generally be asked to enter the patient's world as an invited guest, and there will be no need for a "break in." The question now becomes an issue of finding the most effective means to gather the needed clinical information efficiently while powerfully engaging the patient.

THE BODY OF THE INTERVIEW: PHASE THREE

The chapter began with a quotation concerning the ability to move flexibly, as seen with a martial artist, and it can be as directly applied to the clinician's movements in the scouting period. It seems only appropriate to look at another Eastern quotation, from Chang Chung-Yuan, which concerns the ability to make flexible transitions gracefully, for a sense of timing and naturalness represents the essence of our approach in the body of the interview:

It was said that Wang Hsia's [a Chinese painter] brush sometimes waves and sometimes sweeps. The color of his ink is sometimes light and sometimes dark. Following the splotches of the ink he shapes them into mountains, rocks, clouds, and water. His action is so swift as if it were from Heaven. Spontaneously, his hand responds and his mind follows. All at once clouds and mists are completed; wind and rain are painted. Yet, when one looks carefully, one cannot find any marks of demarcation in the ink.[20]

Like the Chinese artist, the goals of the clinician vary during the body of the interview depending upon the various clinical landscapes with which the clinician is presented.

If the interviewer intends to see the patient numerous times, then the data needed from the first interview may represent a relatively small body of knowledge, for several sessions are available before a treatment plan will be evolved. Consequently, the clinician's pace can be correspondingly leisurely, the emphasis being upon a less structured approach in many respects similar to the processes seen during a dynamic-oriented psychotherapy.

On the other end of the continuum, the clinician may frequently face a true intake interview, in which both triage decisions and initial treatment plans are expected, at times demanded, by the end of sixty minutes. In this situation, perhaps the most demanding of all interviews, the data base requirements are considerably more extensive, requiring a corresponding shift in the interviewer's style.

In this section, the focus will be upon these full intake assessments. To begin the inquiry, we must first acknowledge that one of the major dilemmas confronting the intake clinician concerns the realization that large volumes of data often need to be gathered in short periods of time. Stated differently, good clinicians do not merely empathically listen, they actively explore. Patients do not necessarily know which information is relevant for their treatment planning. It is the clinician who must provide the gentle structuring and guidance that will establish a valid foundation for action.

The apparent "magic" with which a skilled interviewer accomplishes this task is not really magic. It is a skill. It is a skill based on the knowledge of which questions to ask and when to ask them during the body of the interview. This craft emerges directly from a study of the dynamic interactions creating the informational flow of the interview. These principles determine why one interviewer moves smoothly and efficiently, while another proceeds more awkwardly.

In Chapter 1 we discussed the observation that an interview in which the blending is high seems to take on some of the characteristics of a conversation. A natural flow emerges. The two participants appear to move with one another. Common hallmarks of a flowing conversation appear, such as humor and natural body posturing as the two become "engaged" in conversation.

The engagement process, spontaneously developed during natural conversation, holds within itself some pertinent clues as to methods of enhancing the flow of a clinical interview. Consequently it is of value to look briefly at the processes involved in an everyday conversation as they may pertain to the clinical interview itself.

To begin with, if one observes two close friends chatting over some coffee and cheesecake, one will quickly notice, depending upon whether one possesses a habit of eavesdropping, that their conversation is not simply a potpourri of unrelated statements. Quite to the contrary, such conversation usually possesses a gentle structure, determined, albeit unconsciously, by its participants. In general, one friend brings up a topic, which both friends animatedly expand. Many times the second member of the conversation will ask questions, in an effort to more thoroughly understand the first while also showing an appropriate increase in interest.

Once the topic has been discussed, one of the friends will move the conversation to a new topic. This transition is often prompted by something that has already been discussed. Frequently the new topic is triggered directly by a preceding statement. And so the conversation between the friends moves, swelling and ebbing, as more or less interesting topics arise. The basic structure of the conversation consists of succeeding topics connected by transitions.

A smoothly flowing interview possesses many of these same structural elements. One of the keys to generating a natural flow of speech during the body of the interview consists of learning to move gracefully from topic to topic while taking cues from the interviewee's statements. The interviewer is aware of which topics are most pertinent for a triage interview and can gently guide the conversation to these topics. Once within a desired topic, the interviewer takes advantage of the natural conversational mode in order to fully expand that topic. When done well, the interviewer has structured the interview imperceptibly. The clinician establishes a powerful engagement with the interviewee while efficiently gathering a strategic data base for decision-making.

This ability to structure patients naturally is one of the most, if not the most, difficult set of skills for most clinicians to acquire. The problem is that many trainees have no method to their madness, in the sense that no principles and techniques for structuring are utilized. Without a concrete language with which to understand the process of structuring, the trainee is faced with vague admonitions, such as "Work faster," hardly a useful criticism.

The trick for successful structuring lies in developing and understanding a language of structuring that spells out practical applications. This conceptual framework can be gained from a study of the everyday conversation described above.

Specifically, we will focus upon a series of concepts, including topics on which information is needed during a clinical interview (called "regions"), the method of exploring these topics once they are entered (a process referred to as "expansion"), and the methods of transition used between topics (a structure called a "gate"). This language, which allows us to study the intricate movements and transitions used to structure the interview process, is called "facilics." The term "facilics" is derived from the Latin root *facilis* indicating grace in movement. An understanding of facilic principles provides the sound framework that allows interviewers to structure effectively.

A Region of Dialogue

One of the first problems facing the novice interviewer remains the issue of what information is important in a full intake assessment. In this regard the first facilic concept to investigate is the region.

A region is defined as any section of an interview, lasting at least several sentences, in which there exists a unified topic of discussion or a unified process of interaction. In this general sense, a region may be described as either a content region or a process region.

CONTENT REGIONS

As discussed earlier, as with a conversation, an interview tends to revolve around discrete topics. Ten general content regions of frequent practical use in an assessment interview are as follows: (1) the history of the present illness, (2) the diagnostic explorations, (3) the psychological perspectives of the interviewee, (4) the formal mental status exam, (5) the social history, (6) the family history, (7) the determination of suicidal/homicidal potential, (8) the past psychiatric history, (9) the developmental and psychogenetic history, and (10) the medical history.

In order to explore these regions effectively, one must become familiar with their intricacies. In later sections of this book we will look at these regions in more detail. At present it is only important to emphasize that most topics of discussion occurring during an interview can be categorized within one of these ten regions.

In order to ensure a common, initial understanding of these critical informational regions, they will be briefly summarized here.

1. The History of the Present Illness. This region examines the chronological development of symptoms. It emphasizes the types, characteristics, and severity of the symptoms and their duration. Naturally, the history of the present illness frequently includes one or more of the diagnostic regions as well.

2. The Diagnostic Regions. The diagnostic regions are defined by the DSM-III-R criteria. As a rule of thumb, a diagnostic region has been well-explored if one can state whether or not the diagnostic criteria for a particular entity are fulfilled.

3. The Interviewee's Perspective. The interviewee's perspective was discussed earlier, when dealing with the scouting period. It generally includes an attempt to understand the interviewee's views on his or her problems and how help can be utilized, as well as the fears, pains, and expectations uncovered in the interview. This region remains the cornerstone of crisis intervention.

4. The Formal Mental Status Examination. This section represents observations concerning the following broad topics: appearance and behavior, speech and language, thought process and content, mood and affect, and cognitive functioning (including such processes as orientation, concentration, memory, and intellectual functioning). Naturally, many elements of the mental status are evaluated simultaneously with the exploration of the other regions. The more specialized cognitive mental status, in which a clinician examines orientation, attention span, memory functions, and general intellect, tends to form a more discrete region that is easily identifiable during an interview.

5. The Social History. Broadly speaking, the social history includes both interpersonal and environmental information. With regard to interpersonal history, one is interested in interaction with family, friends, employers, and even strangers in both the past and the present. Concerning environmental history, a clinician is interested in such factors as living conditions, neighborhood, economic status, and availability of food and shelter. This region often includes current and past stressors. A careful examination of possible alcohol and/or drug abuse can also be included here.

6. The Family History. This region includes an exploration of psychiatric and other medical illnesses in the patient's blood-related family. It commonly includes a survey of entities such as schizophrenia, affective disorders, suicide, alcoholism/drug abuse, mental retardation, and seizure disorders, as well as any other major medical illnesses such as diabetes, cancer, and hypertension.

7. The Determination of Suicidal/Homicidal Potential. This lethality region requires a careful and sensitive expansion by the interviewer and should never be omitted.

8. The Past Psychiatric History. This region explores previous mental health problems, as well as previous interventions, such as forms of treatment (e.g., medication, psychotherapy, counseling, hospitalization).

9. The Developmental and Psychogenetic History. This region traces the development of the individual from birth onwards, and it includes topics such as birth trauma, developmental milestones, toilet training, schooling, and early object relationships.

10. The Medical History. This region includes past and present illnesses as well as a medical review of systems. Other areas, including allergies, medications, and current physicians, are also examined.

This brief survey illustrates that despite the immensity of an initial data base, the contents tend to fall into relatively discrete regions. Many of these regions tend to overlap. In general, however, a given section of an interview tends to focus upon a single region, much as a conversation tends to focus upon a single topic at a time. In the following excerpt the general region concerning drug and alcohol abuse is readily apparent.

Clin.: . . . So right now you haven't been using alcohol?
Pt.: No.
Clin.: You talked about using drugs in the past. I'm wondering what kinds of things you used then and now.
Pt.: Right now I'm only using pot. I don't mess around with anything else.
Clin.: Are you using it every day?
Pt.: Almost every day.
Clin.: How many joints might you have in a day?
Pt.: Maybe split two; me and Jack might split two.
Clin.: Uh, huh.
Pt.: Because it really does calm me down. It doesn't make you sick like alcohol can make you sick, or give you a bad head the next day. It just relaxes you.
Clin: Any type of pills you're taking now?
Pt.: No.
Clin.: Nothing but the marijuana . . . What kinds of drugs were you using in the past?
Pt.: Well, I never got into any one drug real heavy.
Clin.: Uh, huh.
Pt.: But I have taken LSD, speed, different goofballs, and stuff . . . but I never injected any drugs like dope.

PROCESS REGIONS

In addition to focusing upon content, thereby gathering factual data, the interviewer may opt to focus on the process of the interview itself. Three such "process regions" include the following:

1. Free Facilitation Regions. This region remains one of the foundations of all interviewing. It is the traditional method of nondirective listening. In it, the interviewer invests effort in creating an atmosphere optimally conducive for the interviewee to feel safe enough to begin sharing his or her problems. The interviewee is free to wander freely to whatever topics chosen, while the interviewer maintains a nondirective attitude. The major interventions of the interviewer are usually facilitating head nods, uh-huh's, and simple facilitory statements.

These facilitation regions can appear anywhere in an interview, and are often a very useful method of enhancing engagement. As noted earlier, during the opening phase of the interview the clinician frequently utilizes a free facilitation region. In actuality, the scouting phase is a combination of content regions intermixed with facilitory activities. Furthermore, a psychotherapeutic interview may consist almost entirely of free facilitation regions strung together. Naturally, most content regions have many attributes in common with free facilitation regions; but a facilitation region differs in the goal of its use, which remains the uncovering of information that the patient reveals spontaneously without direction from the interviewer.

A brief example may help to clarify when a section of an interview can be labeled as a free facilitation region.

> **Pt.:** I don't know what's coming over me . . . I just feel sort of crazy.
>
> **Clin.:** How do you mean?
>
> **Pt.:** All my thoughts seem to be mixing like a wet rainbow; distinctions are blurred, people distorted . . . (pause) I feel this way when I'm with my mother. She . . . (pause).
>
> **Clin.:** Go on.
>
> **Pt.:** She seems so oppressive, so large, like a giant machine always pushing, always pulling. Honestly, I don't know where to go with her.
>
> **Clin.:** In what sense?
>
> **Pt.:** She wants me to be a success, lord knows what *that* means. I think she wants me to be a college professor or some dean of this or that. But she's not interested in what I need, never was. A baby without a bottle, that's what I am . . .

A free facilitation region often helps to lower the defenses of the interviewee so that his or her major concerns will surface. It can also be utilized to foster the uncovering of psychotic process, as will be described later.

2. Resistance Regions. In a resistance region the interviewer actively attempts to decrease a specific resistance to the engagement process. Such resistances may arise from any number of factors, including the interviewee's fears, expectations, or other ramifications of the self system. Without a resolution of these resistances, the validity of subsequent data and the power of the therapeutic alliance may be greatly reduced. In any case, the defining characteristic remains that in a resistance region, the interviewer consciously attempts to resolve a resistance shown by the patient.

In the following selection we see an interviewer in the midst of a resistance region:

> **Pt.:** My boss was really into my work and thinks I may be a little . . . you know . . . I don't really think I ought to go on. Do you have a supervisor around?
>
> **Clin.:** You seem concerned about something . . .
>
> **Pt.:** Well, I'd just feel a little better if I were talking to someone a little older.
>
> **Clin.:** What do you think an older clinician would be able to do to help you?
>
> **Pt.:** He'd understand what I've gone through better.
>
> **Clin.:** You know, it's true I'm younger than you and, consequently, I haven't experienced the same things, but I can try to gain some understanding of what you're experiencing. You could help me by telling me a little more about how people have been pressuring you about your age.
>
> **Pt.:** It all started with my wife. She left me about three years ago . . .

3. Psychodynamic Regions. In a psychodynamic region the interviewer asks questions in which the clinician is more interested in how and why the patient responds, as opposed to the content of what the patient says. In general, the clinician attempts to answer questions such as the following: How reflective is the patient? Does the patient have much insight? How does the patient respond to interpretive questions? Answers to these questions may help determine the suitability of the patient for psychotherapy, as well as provide insight into the patient's intellectual development, ego strength, defense mechanisms, and self concept. To answer questions in a psychodynamic region the patient must reflect and offer an opinion.

The following excerpt may clarify when a psychodynamic region is occurring:

> **Pt.:** My father always kept a strangle hold on me. He wanted to know my every move. God pity the boy who wanted to take me out. It was like a gestapo interview for the guy.

Clin.: What kind of impact do you think your father's behavior has had on you?

Pt.: He's made me scared. I'm afraid of him, and who knows, maybe I keep my distance from him because of it . . . Sort of strange though, 'cause when I was a kid I always wanted to be around him. I even would wait for him when he was at work.

Clin.: Go on.

Pt.: Oh, it's sort of silly, but I wondered if he had a toy or something for me . . . I remember a small doll he brought home once, with big black eyes. Just a little doll, but important to me.

Clin.: Go on.

Pt.: Not too much more to say, except that it's sort of sad the way things have turned out between us.

Clin.: What are you feeling as you talk about your father right now?

Here, content is clearly taking a second place to process. The interviewee's responses suggest a willingness and a certain degree of proficiency at self-exploration. This type of region can occur anywhere in an interview, often appearing frequently between content regions.

Thus far, three types of process regions have been illustrated: (1) the free facilitation region, (2) the resistance region, and (3) the psychodynamic region. In actuality, other types of process regions are common, including regions focusing on interviewee ventilation of emotions, interviewee education, or phenomenological regions of questioning as discussed in Chapter 1. These process regions often provide windows through which an understanding of the patient gradually emerges.

Equipped with a facility to move freely among both content regions and process regions, the clinician possesses a powerful flexibility with which to approach any given interviewing task. It is not a matter of only learning to interview in a fairly structured fashion (emphasizing content) or learning to interview in a nondirective style (emphasizing process regions). One needs to master both styles, at times delicately interweaving them. There does not exist a single "correct style" of interweaving these regions. Instead, one finds styles that may be more or less useful for any given clinical situation. Too frequently students learn only one approach, while building an unfounded bias that other styles of interviewing are inferior. No surer method of handicapping one's clinical flexibility can be found.

Having reviewed the type of data base needed in a full intake interview, the focus can be shifted towards a discussion of techniques for exploring these numerous regions in a fruitful fashion.

In the first place, many interviews are made or broken before a word is spoken, for the preinterview planning frequently determines the success of the subsequent interaction. As discussed above, the clinician needs to ascertain what demands on information gathering are needed by the clinical situation. In an intake interview situation, most, if not all, of the content regions discussed earlier may need to be addressed, many of them thoroughly. In contrast, an emergency room evaluation of a patient well known to the system may require a significantly different strategy. In this emergency room situation the clinician may only have twenty to thirty minutes available. Consequently, a conscious decision will need to be made as to which content regions to decrease or eliminate.

One of the most common complaints voiced by supervisees can be summarized as, "I didn't have enough time to gather the information I wanted!" This complaint is often paralleled by harried clinic directors mumbling phrases such as, "My god, how much longer is he going to take with that patient!" Both exclamations represent the end product of a poorly structured interview.

To counteract this problem an understanding of facilics provides the clinician with an awareness of "where he or she is at" with regard to the thoroughness of the data base during the interview itself. From this heightened awareness, the clinician develops an ability to control the pace and flow of the interview.

When discussing the scouting period we examined the problem of the wandering interview in which a patient with a loquacious manner encounters an interviewer incapable of focusing the flow of the dialogue. The result can be a disappointing experience for both participants. But many times a patient with a normal verbal output, who could be easily directed, meets an interviewer with poor focusing abilities. Even in this case, the interview may become quite unproductive, for the patient does not know which information is most needed. The resulting hodgepodge of dialogue can best be called an unguided interview.

One may wonder why unguided interviews are so common. The answer is relatively simple and hinges upon the concept called "tracking." Tracking refers to a clinician's ability to sensitively follow up the statements of a patient with questions pertinent to the area discussed. At a more sophisticated level, good tracking also requires the ability to follow up with questions pertinent to the patient's immediate emotional state. This ability to track well is one of the main attributes of a good listener. Indeed, the ability to track well is a prerequisite if one is to become a good interviewer.

And here lies the catch, for good tracking must be accompanied by an equally good ability to focus the patient sensitively. Many mental health trainees have developed good techniques for tracking through the process of attentively listening to family and friends. But few have learned equally effective methods of focusing. Fortunately, this crucial ability to focus sensitively can be learned.

Generally speaking, once within a content region, it is frequently best to expand that region relatively fully, for the patient will generally find such expansions natural, the topics of discussion being essentially related. If one leaves a specific content region prematurely, one will have to return to that region, sometimes many times. Obviously, if the interviewer makes a habit of approaching most content regions in this haphazard manner, it becomes very difficult to monitor what information has been adequately gathered. Consequently, mistakes of omission occur more frequently. This haphazard approach also tends to decrease the sense of conversational flow.

Considering these pitfalls, one can begin to delineate a general approach to the body of the interview that will decrease the frequency of both wandering and unguided interviews. During the scouting period the clinician should formulate a tentative plan for the interview, utilizing the data gained from PACE. From this analysis, an initial content or process region will be chosen as an entrance into the main body of the interview. Frequently, the patient's own spontaneous discussion will have naturally led into a specific content region, such as the history of the present illness, or a diagnostic area, such as the depression region. If so, the clinician can expand this region fully and then proceed to the next pertinent region as desired. Wandering patients are gently refocused if they prematurely leave regions.

To the degree that the clinician determines which content regions are pertinent for a particular patient in a particular clinical situation, subsequent regions are successfully entered and expanded as the main body of the interview unfolds. Naturally, as deemed necessary, the clinician may pepper the content expansions with process areas such as psychodynamic regions or facilitation regions. Slowly the patient's story emerges and with it an increasing sense of understanding.

Problems tend to arise when clinicians lose awareness of the pacing of the data collection. One of the most frequent problems occurs during the second fifteen minutes of the interview. In this critical region, "the dead quarter," clinicians often utilize too many free facilitation regions instead of focusing upon appropriate content regions.

When this approach is used, the clinician often finds that in thirty minutes very little of the needed information for a sound triage decision has been gathered. This early mistake in the structuring of the interview begets a second error. In reaction to the first misjudgement the clinician will proceed to force a rigid structure into the remaining part of the interview in an effort to catch up. Phrases such as "Let me ask just a few other questions here" or "Oh, I forgot to ask this" frequently appear en masse, as the scramble for needed information takes over. The result may be a patient who begins to perceive that the clinician is more interested in data gathering than in listening.

This vicious circle of disengagement can be eliminated if the interviewer begins gently structuring as soon as he or she emerges from the scouting period somewhere between five and ten minutes into the interview. As the second fifteen minutes closes, the clinician should be nearing the completion of the four or five content regions that seem most pertinent to a particular patient. When such a gradual approach is utilized, rapid focusing is seldom required, and the pace of the interview seems appropriately unrushed to the patient.

If this has been accomplished, the third fifteen minutes can be utilized for expanding content regions deemed more important than originally expected, as well as for gathering data from the remaining content regions felt to be pertinent for treatment planning and triage. It is in this third fifteen minutes that regions such as family history, medical history, social history, and the more formal mental status are often explored.

During the last fifteen minutes, these regional explorations are continued, and new questions, generated by the unfolding information, may be asked. Psychodynamic regions may be explored more intensively and clarifications of previous points may be pursued. The last five to ten minutes are generally utilized for the closing and terminating phases.

As can be seen, the body of the interview represents a delicate organism, whose growth and development warrant careful attention by the interviewer. Perhaps a review of the basic facilic principle utilized to move gracefully through this area of the interview would be useful.

1. Before beginning the interview, make a tentative determination of which content regions are most appropriate considering time constraints, the needs of the patient, and the goals of the interview.

2. During the interview occasionally monitor the progress of your data gathering and adjust your pace as needed.

3. Avoid the overuse of facilitation regions during the body of the interview.

4. Begin gently but persistently structuring as soon as you leave the scouting period and during the second fifteen minutes.

5. Keep in mind that an inadequately structured second fifteen minutes often forces a more rigid and potentially disengaging structuring later in the interview as a means of catching up.

6. Generally speaking, once within an appropriate content re-

gion, it is often useful to expand it fairly fully, unless the patient gives you good reason to move out of it.

Thus far we have focused upon the general strategy needed to determine and monitor the regions of dialogue encountered in an interview. Next we will examine the actual process of exploring a given region once it has been entered.

The Expansion of Regions

The process of exploring a given content region is referred to as the expansion of the region. Different interviewers may approach this expansion in radically different ways.

Speaking broadly, two methods, forming somewhat opposing extremes, can be defined as "stilted expansions" and "blended expansions." In stilted expansions the expansion lacks a feeling of conversational flow. Instead, the interviewee is asked a series of questions that appear somewhat forced, because the interviewer is rigidly attempting to ask specific questions. This type of expansion may cause interviewees to experience the unpleasant feeling that they are "being interviewed," as opposed to talking *with* someone. I suppose one could call this process a "Meet the Press" type of expansion. Rigidly structured interviews sometimes foster a style of expansion such as illustrated below:

> **Pt.:** The pressures at home have really reached a crisis point. I'm not certain where it will all lead; I only know I'm feeling the heat.
>
> **Clin.:** What's your appetite like?
>
> **Pt.:** I guess it's okay . . .
>
> **Clin.:** What's your sleep like?
>
> **Pt.:** Not too good. I have a hard time falling asleep. My days are such a blur. I never feel balanced, even when I try to fall asleep. I can't concentrate enough to even read.
>
> **Clin.:** What about your sexual drive?
>
> **Pt.:** What do you mean?
>
> **Clin.:** Have you noticed any changes in how interested you are in sex?
>
> **Pt.:** Maybe a little.
>
> **Clin.:** In what direction?
>
> **Pt.:** I guess I'm not as interested in sex as I used to be.
>
> **Clin.:** And what about your energy level? How has it been?
>
> **Pt.:** Fairly uneven. It's hard to explain; but sometimes I don't feel like doing anything.

This particular interviewer seems decidedly intent on expanding the depression region, specifically the neurovegetative symptoms of depression. This style of expansion exhibits a mechanical quality, as if the interviewer has a list of questions to reel off. Such rigidity characterizes stilted expansions.

As a study in contrasts, in a blended expansion the interviewer once again focuses on a specific region. However, in this expansion the interviewer attempts to blend the questions into the natural flow of the conversation. Rather than feeling like they are "being interviewed," this type of expansion creates in interviewees a sense of gentle flow, which tends to foster the engagement process. Moreover, this type of interviewing, by decreasing the anxiety of the patient, may enhance both the quantity and validity of the data base as well.

In the following excerpt, a blended expansion unfolds, once again exploring the depression region:

Pt.: The pressures at home have really reached a crisis point. I'm not certain where it will all lead; I only know I'm feeling the heat.

Clin.: Sounds like you've been going through a lot. How has it affected the way you feel in general?

Pt.: I always feel drained. I'm simply tired. Life seems like one giant chore.

Clin.: What about your sleep? Has that been affected as well?

Pt.: Absolutely. Perhaps that's the reason I'm drained. I just can't rest. My sleep is horrible.

Clin.: Tell me about it.

Pt.: I can't fall asleep. It takes several hours just to get to sleep. I'm wired. I'm wired even in the day. And I'm so agitated I can't concentrate, even enough to read to put me to sleep.

Clin.: Once you're asleep, do you stay asleep?

Pt.: Never, I bet I wake up four or five times a night. And about 5 A.M. I'm awake, as if someone slapped me.

Clin.: How do you mean?

Pt: It's like an alarm went off, and no matter how hard I try, I can't get back to sleep.

Clin.: What do you do instead?

Pt.: Worry . . . I'm not kidding . . . My mind fills with all sorts of worthless junk.

Clin.: You mentioned earlier that you have problems with concentration. Tell me a little more about that.

Pt.: Just simply can't function like I used to. Dictating letters, reading, writing notes, all those things take much longer than usual. It really disturbs me. My system seems out of whack.

Clin.: Do you think your appetite has been affected as well?

Pt.: No question. My appetite is way down. Food tastes like paste; really very little taste at all. I've even lost weight.

Clin.: About how much and over how long a time?

Pt.: Oh, about five pounds, maybe over a month or two . . .

In the above process the same region as before was expanded, but this time the questioning appeared to flow naturally, generating an increasing flow of information. The interviewer's questions seemed to relate directly to what the interviewee was saying, thus creating a sense that the interviewer was "with" the interviewee.

This example also illustrates an important point. While expanding the content region, one continuously attends to the engagement process. For instance, early in the above selection the interviewer sensitively utilized a complex empathic statement, "Sounds like you've been going through a lot." And later, facilitative open-ended techniques were used, such as the gentle command, "Tell me about it," and the open-ended question, "How do you mean?" Such a consistent and effective use of engagement techniques coalesces to create a feeling in patients that the interviewer is moving with them in a relatively unstructured fashion, while, in actuality, the clinician is gently structuring the interview, harvesting an ever more meaningful field of information.

A further point to consider concerning the expansion of regions is the usefulness of brief excursions out of a region. For instance, while expanding the anxiety disorder region, the patient may mention the use of Valium. At this point, the clinician may choose to expand the medication history briefly, after which the interviewer can return to the anxiety disorder region to complete its expansion. Such short excursions offer yet another flexible option for the clinician. Humor can also be utilized to further the natural feeling of the interview.

The clinician may also opt to utilize split expansions, with a single region expanded at several different locations during the interview. Although useful, these split expansions can lead to serious omissions if the clinician does not keep track of what information has been gathered. But on a limited basis, split expansions further increase the interviewer's adaptability.

The over-riding point remains the clinician's need to develop an active and conscious awareness of the data flow while simultaneously creating the sensation of the natural flow of conversation. Perhaps a few facilic principles warrant review at this point:

1. Generally speaking, an effort should be made to achieve blended expansions as opposed to stilted expansions; such blended expansions move with the patient.

2. As long as one remembers to monitor the completeness of his or her data base, then techniques such as split expansions and brief excursions can be very useful.

3. Always attend to engagement during the expansion of content regions both on a verbal and nonverbal level.

Before ending our discussion of the various methods of expanding regions, one more point warrants attention. Although stilted expansions generally tend to disengage patients, some patients may, ironically, prefer them. This peculiar preference may surface in the case of a patient suffering from hypochondriacal concerns, associated with the belief that, "Nothing is wrong with my head." Some of these patients may actually prefer the check-list flavor of a stilted expansion, for it parallels the feeling generated by a medical review of systems. Hence, the patient feels more at home with an interaction more redolent of a medical exam than of a psychiatric assessment. Once again, the art consists of adapting one's style to the needs of the patient.

At this time, we can move to the third and last major concern of facilics, the transition utilized between regions. The ability to master these transitions will determine the clinician's ultimate ability to create a smoothly flowing dialogue.

Gates: The Pathways of Transition

As a conversation or an interview passes from one topic to another, different types of transitions occur. We will refer to the actual statements joining two regions as "gates." Although there exist numerous types of gates, five major forms are most common: (1) the spontaneous gate, (2) the natural gate, (3) the referred gate, (4) the implied gate, and (5) the phantom gate. An understanding of the use of these gates provides interviewers with a simple but elegant method of gracefully maneuvering an interview.

The Spontaneous Gate. The spontaneous gate, as its name suggests, initially unfolds without any effort by the interviewer. Instead, the gate results from a change in course unilaterally taken by the interviewee. The gates consist of two parts: a cue statement and a transitional question. The cue statement consists of a spontaneous entrance into an entirely new content region by the patient. If the clinician decides to expand this new region, then he or she will only have to cue off the patient's statement with a follow-up question or a simple facilitating statement such as "Go on." These follow-up questions or facilitating statements made by the clinician represent transitional questions or statements. In the following example, a spontaneous gate provides an essentially unnoticeable movement into a new region:

Pt.: The past two months have been so horrible. I think it's the worst time of my life. I just can't get away from the feeling.

Clin.: Which feelings are you referring to?

Pt.: The sadness; the heaviness.

Clin.: Earlier you had mentioned that you've lost your appetite and always feel tired. What else have you noticed when you're feeling sad and heavy?

Pt.: Nothing seems worth doing. It's late November and my yard is covered with leaves. Usually they'd all be gone into neat little piles, like a little farm, but not now . . .

Clin.: Besides not having energy for chores, do you find you can still enjoy your bridge club or other hobbies?

Pt.: Not really. Things seems so bland. I haven't even gone to bridge club for several months. It is all so different from before. In fact, there were times in the past when I could barely keep still, I was so active.

* Clin.: How do you mean?

Pt.: Oh, I used to be super active, into bridge, tennis, golf, and everything. I was a real dynamo.

Clin.: Did you ever move too fast?

Pt.: In what sense?

Clin.: Oh, sometimes one can get so energized that it gets difficult to get things done.

Pt.: Actually, there were a couple of odd times when people kept telling me to "slow down, slow down."

Clin.: Tell me a little about one of those times.

Pt.: About a year ago I got so wound up I hardly slept for almost a week. I'd stay up most of the night cleaning the house, washing the car, and writing furiously. I didn't seem to need sleep.

Clin.: Did you notice if your thoughts seemed slowed down or speeded up then?

Pt.: Speeded up. I was flying. Everything seemed crystal clear and moved like lightning. It was strange . . .

In this example, two topics are being discussed sequentially. In the first region, the interviewee's feelings of depression are being explored. In the course of this exploration, the interviewee brings up a statement that suggests a different diagnostic region dealing with mania. The cue statement was, "In fact, there were times in the past when I could barely keep still, I was so active."

The interviewer then used this cue to enter the region exploring manic symptoms by simply asking, "How do you mean?" which functioned as the transitional question (indicated by an asterisk). Once within the diagnostic region of mania, a blended expansion was begun. This movement into a new topic was practically imperceptible.

Spontaneous gates create movement that seems unblemished by effort or resistance. In this sense, a clever interviewer will frequently make use of such gates whenever transitions into new regions are desirable. But herein lies a potential pitfall, for it is frequently not desirable to leave a region before it is fully expanded.

In this light spontaneous gates represent critical areas in which the interviewer should consciously decide whether to stay within an expansion or move to a new one. If the clinician can gain conscious awareness of such "pivot points," then the clinician will gain considerable control over the flow of questioning. One does not and should not follow every spontaneous cue with a transition into a new region.

Indeed, the concept of spontaneous gates and pivot points provides us with a new way of conceptualizing both the wandering interview and the unguided interview. These interviews occur when spontaneous gates are followed by the clinician whenever they appear, resulting in a consistent pattern of incomplete expansions. To prevent this wandering process, the clinician must apply the refocusing techniques described earlier.

It should also be noted that at times the clinician may wisely decide to follow a spontaneous gate even in the middle of an incomplete expansion. Such times include situations such as the following: (a) the patient may have unexpectedly related highly emotionally charged material that needs to be ventilated; (b) the patient may have spontaneously mentioned highly sensitive material that may best be approached immediately; and (c) specific memories may warrant immediate follow-up, such as screen memories, dreams, or traumatic events.

Of course, during process regions, such as psychodynamic regions or free facilitation regions, the clinician generally follows most spontaneous gates as they appear, utilizing an occasional restraint. The scouting period is also often filled with spontaneous gates. Along these same lines, during periods of free association, as may appear in therapy itself, spontaneous gates are essentially always followed; indeed, they are nurtured. But no matter what the facilic situation, we return to the all-important realization that clinicians can exercise significant choice as to the pattern any given interview will pursue.

The Natural Gate. The natural gate consists of two parts: the cue statement and the transitional question. The cue statement represents a comment made by the interviewee that contains content material that can be creatively related to a new region by the interviewer. If the interviewer cues off of this statement to enter a new region, the interviewee will feel that the conversation is flowing from his own speech, as, indeed, it is. Such a transition seems both natural and caring to the interviewee.

The transitional question represents the actual question made by the interviewer, which was prompted by the cue statement of the interviewee and leads into a new region. As opposed to the spontaneous gate, the clinician, not the patient, is entering a new region.

In the following excerpt we will see a transition made from the region covering depressive symptoms into the drug and alcohol region. This smooth transformation will be made via a natural gate.

> **Clin.:** Have you been able to enjoy your poker games or your shop work?
>
> **Pt.:** No, I just don't feel like doing anything since I've been feeling depressed. It's a really ugly feeling.
>
> **Clin.:** Tell me more about what it feels like.
>
> **Pt.:** Really pretty miserable. Life doesn't seem the same. I'm tired all the time; no sleep.
>
> **Clin.:** How do you mean?
>
> **Pt.:** Over the past several months sleep has almost become a chore. I'm always having trouble getting to sleep, and then I wake up all night. I must wake up five times and it took me two hours to fall asleep in the first place.
>
> *** Clin.:** Have you ever used anything like a nightcap to sort of knock yourself out?
>
> **Pt.:** Yeah, sometimes a good belt really relaxes me.
>
> **Clin.:** How much do you need to drink to make yourself sleepy?
>
> **Pt.:** Oh, not too terribly much. Maybe a couple of beers. Sometimes more than a couple of beers.
>
> **Clin.:** Just, in general, how many drinks do you have in a given day?
>
> **Pt.:** Probably . . . Now, I'm just guessing, but probably a six-pack or two, maybe three. I hold liquor pretty well. I don't get drunk or nothing.
>
> **Clin.:** What other kinds of drugs do you like to take to relax?
>
> **Pt.:** Well, I might smoke a joint here or there.

In this excerpt, the cue statement was, "I must wake up five times and it took me two hours to fall asleep in the first place." The clinician, wanting to change content regions, sensed that this statement could be used as a springboard into a new topic. The succeeding transition question (indicated by an asterisk) imperceptibly achieved this desired transition into the drug and alcohol region with the phrase, "Have you ever used anything like a nightcap to sort of knock yourself out?"

Transitions of this sort are seldom perceived as focusing mechanisms, for the patient generally feels as if he or she brought up the new topic. This type of smooth transition can greatly enhance a conversational feeling in the interview, slowly bringing the patient into a more powerful sense of safety and spontaneity. The interview begins to take on a self-perpetuating momentum, unique to its own nature.

In Figure 2, the immense power of the natural gate is demonstrated. We shall assume that the expansion of the stressor region has been winding down. The patient then provides a cue statement, which can be utilized by the clinician to enter one of any number of new content regions as illustrated. The flexibility of the natural gate is essentially only limited by the awareness and creativity of the clinician. This figure also provides an introduction to an extensive system for schematically illustrating the flow of any interview. This schematic system has been invaluable in teaching interviewing and is currently

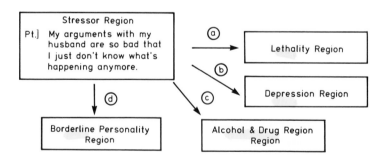

Transition Questions:

a) With all these tensions mounting, have you had any thoughts of wanting to kill yourself?

b) How have all these stresses affected your mood?

c) With all these stresses, have you been drinking at all in an effort to calm yourself?

d). Some people hold all their anger in and others really let it out, maybe even throwing things like glasses or plates. How do you handle your anger?

FIGURE 2. Natural gates utilized as smooth transitions.

being utilized as a research tool. (See appendix for example of supervision performed using facilic diagrams.)

One helpful device, with regard to the use of natural gates, consists of the so-called "manufactured gate." Suppose the clinician has reason to suspect potential homicidal ideation in the patient. In order to get to this delicate topic, the interviewer can set up or manufacture a natural gate as follows:

> **Pt.:** I've really been feeling out of sorts. Frankly, I don't know if I'm coming or going.
>
> **Clin.:** Does it ever help you to relax by drinking?
>
> **Pt.:** . . . Uh, that's hard to say. Sometimes a few calm me down, like after a good Steelers game with Terry Bradshaw (professional football quarterback) throwing passes all over the place. The beer just goes well with it. But at other times it just upsets me more.
>
> **Clin.:** Sometimes when people drink they notice an increased desire to just let off steam, you know, let out the anger, maybe have a good time with a barroom brawl.
>
> **Pt.:** Oh, yeah. I've been in my share of brawls. Won a few, too.
>
> **Clin.:** Has that ever carried over into other areas? Like getting mad at your wife and wanting to hit her?
>
> **Pt.:** Yeah. Just a few weeks ago I wanted to beat the hell out of my wife. She can be such a royal pain in the ass.
>
> **Clin.:** Have you ever really wanted to hurt her, in a more serious way?
>
> **Pt.:** (pause). Once in a while I guess I have. And sometimes I still think she deserves it.
>
> **Clin.:** Deserves what?
>
> **Pt.:** To be killed. It's crossed my mind, I have to admit it.
>
> **Clin.:** What have you thought of doing?
>
> **Pt.:** Cracking her outside the head with a hammer. One real quick snap, like Terry Bradshaw releasing a long pass.

In this excerpt, the clinician was expanding the depression region and wanted to get unobtrusively into the homicidal region. This appears at first glance to be quite a task. It is not exactly easy to ask people if they are murderers. But this clinician makes the difficult seem surprisingly easy. From previous experience, he knew that the homicide region could be frequently entered by a natural gate from the drug and alcohol region, by relating the homicidal thoughts to the poor impulse control commonly associated with drinking. Consequently, the clinician steered the conversation into the drug and alcohol region, thus setting up a natural gate through which he entered the region of homicidal ideation with barely a hint of structuring.

The Referred Gate. A referred gate occurs when the interviewer enters a new region by referring back to an earlier statement made by the interviewee. To the interviewee, a referred gate suggests that the interviewer has been carefully registering what is being said. Also, it allows the interviewer to enter a fresh region smoothly at almost any place in an interview. It remains extremely useful for re-entering a region that was not fully expanded earlier. Structurally, a referred gate lacks an immediate cue statement, for the cue has been taken from a previous area of the interview.

In the following illustration we will enter the interview at the end of a psychodynamic process region in which the patient's feelings concerning his siblings have been explored. As this process region winds down, the interviewer will enter the content region dealing with psychotic phenomena by using a referred gate.

> **Clin.:** What was it like for you when your brother would come home from college?
> **Pt.:** Sort of odd; a little bit like a trespass. You see, when he was gone I had the room all to myself, even the phone was mine alone. As soon as he came back, boom, the room was his again.
> **Clin.:** What other feelings did you have?
> **Pt.:** Some excitement. I really did look up to him, and when he'd come home he'd tell me all about college, frat parties, smoking grass; and it was exciting.
> *** Clin.:** Earlier you had told me that sometimes when you were alone you'd have scary thoughts. Tell me a little more about those moments.
> **Pt.:** O.K. It's sort of like this. I might be sitting late at night listening to some music and things seem sort of weird, almost like something bad is going to happen. And then I have thoughts that keep coming at me and they tell me to do things.
> **Clin.:** Do the thoughts ever get so intense they sound almost like a voice?
> **Pt.:** They *are* voices. They seem very real. In fact, sometimes I try to cover my ears. I just don't know. I don't know . . .

Referred gates, such as the one illustrated above (indicated by asterisk), are deceptively powerful. They can be used for entering new regions essentially at will as well as for re-entering incompletely expanded regions. Moreover, when coupled with a creative sensitivity, the clinician can utilize referred gates to enter potentially disengaging regions gracefully. One of these awkward regions, which frequently poses problems for clinicians, remains the formal mental status exam, or cognitive exam as it is frequently called. While asking questions about orientation and checking digit spans or serial sevens, clinicians frequently worry that patients will feel insulted by the simple nature of the questions. To this end, clinicians may utter phrases such as, "I'm going to ask you some silly questions now, I hope you don't mind," or "Now I have to ask you some routine questions that I have to ask everybody." These phrases are usually accompanied by an apologetic tone of voice or an insecure rustling of the clinician in his or her chair.

The irony of such introductions lies in the fact that rather than dispelling anxiety in the patient, they sometimes create it. The patient can sense that the clinician feels insecure with the subsequent material. All that remains for the patient to wonder is why the clinician needs to apologize. What do these *routine* questions mean and why does a professional ask questions if they are silly? In short, the clinician's sudden obsequiousness serves to signal the patient that something odd is underfoot.

It is here that one of the many uses of the referred gate becomes apparent. By referring to earlier statements of the patient concerning problems of concentration or thinking, the interviewer can enter the cognitive exam smoothly and without a need to apologize. Quite to the contrary, the interviewer's interest indicates a sincere concern to the patient as well as a display of professional knowledge in the sense that these cognitive questions are serving a specific function, a joint undertaking between patient and clinician. Let us take a look at such an approach in action. The patient is suffering from an agitated depression and had complained earlier in the interview of "problems concentrating":

> *Pt.:* Overall, I know it's all my fault. I should never have retired, it's ruined everything. But life goes on. I only hope I feel better some day.
>
> *Clin.:* Earlier, you had mentioned the one thing that was bothering you was your lack of concentration. Tell me a little more about that.
>
> *Pt.:* It's a big problem. I have problems even reading the newspapers, which I used to love to do. Now I read a paragraph and I might as well have my eyes closed. I don't register any of it.
>
> *Clin.:* Has this affected your memory as well?
>
> *Pt.:* Yes, I think so, simple things, just don't remember them well, like names and telephone numbers or even paying my bills.

>   ***Clin.:*** It sounds like you are having some significant problems. I'd like to get a clearer idea of exactly how your thinking has been affected. To do this I'd like to ask you a series of questions that can help us sort out some of the specific problems with concentration and memory you have been having. Some of the questions will be very simple while some of them may get fairly challenging. Why don't we start with some of the simple ones first.
>
>   ***Pt.:*** Sure.
>
>   ***Clin.:*** What day of the week is this?
>
>   ***Pt.:*** I think it's Wednesday.
>
>   ***Clin.:*** That's correct. What city is this?
>
>   ***Pt.:*** Pittsburgh.

This interview dyad moved into the formal mental status exam with a sense of purpose and no hint of uneasiness on the part of the clinician. Even if the patient does not pick-up on the referred gate, an easy transition can be made as follows:

>   ***Clin.:*** Earlier you had mentioned how depressed and out of it you sometimes feel at dusk. I am wondering if during this period of the day you notice any problems with concentration or your memory?
>
>   ***Pt.:*** No, I don't think so. No problems with my concentration.
>
>   ***Clin.:*** That's very fortunate, because frequently when people feel depressed, they have problems with concentration or organizing their thoughts. In fact, I would like to ask some questions designed to pick up even subtle problems with concentration, because if we find some subtle problems, it may give us some idea of how we can best help you. Does that sound okay to you?
>
>   ***Pt.:*** Yes. I don't think I've got any problems here, but I guess it's worth taking a look.
>
>   ***Clin.:*** Good, we'll start with some very simple questions and move towards some harder ones. To start with, what is today's date?

Once again the mental status exam has been entered unobtrusively. Perhaps at this time a few other comments concerning the formal mental status exam are in order. Some authors will state that the formal cognitive exam should not be done unless the clinician strongly suspects a true cognitive deficit, since the questions may be disengaging. I disagree with this point of view for a variety of reasons. First, as we have just seen, when approached with a referred gate the cognitive exam is seldom significantly disengaging. Second, one cannot effectively learn the implication of answers to these questions until one has learned, through experience, the range of answers normally functioning people make. For instance, it is not at all unusual for normal people to make a mistake on serial sevens. In short, to interpret abnormal answers well, one must first become familiar with normal replies. The only way to achieve this familiarity is to perform a brief cognitive exam frequently on patients. Moreover one may also actually uncover early signs of a true cognitive deficit, as seen in the first stages of dementia or in a simmering delirium.

And the third reason, one of the most important justifications, remains the fact that these questions are not asked solely to check cognitive functioning. To the contrary, they represent one of the few areas in the interview in which the clinician receives an opportunity to observe the patient directly solving problems and coping with a potentially anxiety-arousing situation. In short, the clinician gets a first-hand look at the patient dealing with a challenge. This glimpse can be revealing with regard to the patient's psychodynamic defenses.

This psychodynamic window provided by the formal cognitive exam was highlighted to me during an initial interview with an honor student in physiology from a prestigious university. Bruce, as we shall call him, walked into my office with a mildly hesitant step. He was conservatively dressed with an alligator riding his chest. Short-cropped hair framed a reasonably handsome face. Not only was he an honor student; he was also a star athlete. At first, Bruce seemed ill at ease and tended to avoid eye contact. During the preceding months, he had grown increasingly stressed, relating, "I've never been happy, this has been eating at me my whole life." As would be expected, during the main body of the interview he demonstrated no evidence of cognitive dysfunction. He was articulate and reflective. But as the cognitive exam proceeded, an interesting change occurred. More specifically an interpersonal process emerged, a process that apparently plagued him practically on a daily basis. In order to observe this process we will enter the dialogue a short time after the cognitive exam was begun:

> *Clin.:* I am going to ask you to remember four items and I'll ask you to repeat them in about five minutes. Do you understand?
>
> *Pt.:* Yes. (He looked anxious and sat up in his chair.)
>
> *Clin.:* Purple, football, oak tree, and hope. Can you say these words back to me?
>
> *Pt.:* Purple, football, oak tree, and hope. (Said quickly and assertively.)
>
> *Clin.:* Now I'd like to check your concentration by asking you to

	repeat some numbers for me. I will say a line of digits and when I nod you say them back . . . 8–6–1–5.
Pt.:	8–6–1–5 (looking even more intense).
Clin.:	7–9–5–6–3.
Pt.:	7–9–5, uh, uh, 6–3.
Clin.:	2–1–4–5–3–8.
Pt.:	2–1–4–3, uh, 5–8.
Clin.:	Not quite right. Let's try another one.
Pt.:	(Looking very intense) I'm going to beat you at this.
Clin.:	(Pause) Bruce, you seem like you're sort of feeling uptight about this. What are you actually feeling at this time?
Pt.:	You're not going to beat me on this — that's what I'm feeling — I'm going to get this right.
Clin.:	You seem very competitive right now.
Pt.:	I am. I get this way anytime I take a test.
Clin.:	Does that ever interfere with your performance?
Pt.:	Oh yeah, sometimes I get so upset I almost feel like I'm going to run from the room. It's one of the problems I need help with. I'm very competitive.
Clin.:	Just now, it seemed like that feeling was making you feel very uptight with me. What kind of effect does it have on you with other people, if any?
Pt.:	I feel it very frequently. Any time I meet new people, I wonder if the new guy is a threat, somebody who can beat me. It's rough out there. Everybody wants to get ahead of you. And they'll cheat if they have to . . . (pause) but I even feel this with Jennifer, my girlfriend, not much, but it's there, like a sharp stick in my gut.

This interchange generated by the cognitive exam revealed several striking characterological traits in this young college student. His world was one brimming with enemies created in large part by his own mind. Besides uncovering these processes, this exchange provided a reference topic for many of the following psychotherapy sessions. With time, he began to perceive a less threatening environment, one not overrun with hostile figures. In any case, it was the mental status examination that led into this rich vein of psychopathology, while allowing me to watch the patient's reaction to the task at hand.

Perhaps it would be expedient to return to the main topic of referred gates at this time. We have just seen the usefulness of the referred gate in guiding the discussion into a cognitive exam. In a similar way, referred gates can frequently decrease the awkwardness of entering sensitive regions of discussion such as the drug or sexual history. This effectiveness probably results from the fact that relating the sensitive material to previous statements by the patient decreases the perceived social inappropriateness of the question. This principle may seem a bit abstract at present, but the following illustration will clarify the concept.

In this interview, the patient was an attractive woman of about thirty. She had her blonde hair pulled back in a bun, giving an impression of a young professional. Her hands punctuated her words like a well struck typewriter key. She described her various plights in a dramatic and telling manner. After thirty minutes, numerous soap opera vignettes had been laid out on the table, including many years of heavy drug abuse in the past, a striking lack of any stable relationships, five abortions, over two-hundred sexual encounters, and a current investigation by the FBI of her old friends.

She stressed her sexual freedom early during the interview stating, "I'm not hung up on having to like the person I have sex with. Sex is something I can easily divorce from my feelings." Later in the interview, as the facts of her life became clearer, I began to wonder if I was talking with someone who one might call a "slick sociopath." To this end I wanted to expand the antisocial personality region in more detail.

I wondered if she might be involved in prostitution. Needless to say, asking a person during the initial interview if she may be a prostitute can be a delicate matter. In this case a referred gate provided a smooth entry into this sensitive topic.

> **Pt.:** All of my men have ended up leaving me. None of them want to be fathers. We always fight. I'm bored by it all now.
>
> **Clin.:** Earlier you had mentioned that you have been able to successfully separate your sexual feelings from your emotional ones as you've matured. I'm wondering if, because of this ability, you've been able to use your own body in a more practical sense, for instance, by selling sexual favors.
>
> **Pt.:** Yeah, I've done that too. Back in New York I used to be a prostitute for about four or five months, not much longer though.
>
> **Clin.:** What was that like for you?
>
> **Pt.:** Not really that tough. It's a dirty business though and I'm glad I'm out of it. But it helped when I needed it and believe me I needed the money.
>
> **Clin.:** Did you ever sell drugs back then to help pay the rent and other needs?
>
> **Pt.:** No. I never really sold drugs, I would use them like crazy,

> my life has been a wild one. In fact, someone ought to write a novel about me. I've seen it all, but I never got into pushing drugs.

This referred gate, voiced matter of factly, seemed to flow quite naturally. She did not appear particularly flustered, and the blending remained high. Once again, to the interviewee, referred gates suggest that the clinician has been listening carefully in an effort to piece together the patient's story. One can imagine how differently the above situation may have unfolded if the clinician had abruptly asked without a referred gate, "By the way, are you a prostitute?" This method of transition certainly needs a little more polish. Such abrupt gates are the next topic of discussion.

The Phantom Gate. A phantom gate appears to come from nowhere. It lacks a cue statement and also lacks previous referential points, as seen in referred or natural gates. In short, it jolts the spontaneous flow, as the following example will show:

> **Pt.:** I haven't felt the same for months. I'm always down and I'm sick of it.
> **Clin.:** What does it feel like to be down?
> **Pt.:** Very unsettling. I'm like a slab. I don't want to do anything. I miss doing things with my best friend, silly as that may sound. I really haven't been the same since she died.
> *** Clin.:** Was your father an alcoholic?
> **Pt.:** No . . . (pause) I don't think he was. He drank every once in a while.
> **Clin.:** What about your brothers, sisters, or blood relatives? Have any of them had drinking problems?
> **Pt.:** Not that I know of.
> **Clin.:** What about depression? Have any of your relatives been depressed?

This interviewer's sudden leap into the family history region certainly appeared abrupt and ill-timed. Obviously, if such phantom gates (indicated by an asterisk) occur frequently throughout the interview, engagement can be seriously hampered. Even in milder forms, they can quickly produce the "Meet the Press" feeling discussed earlier. They often pop up toward the end of interviews, when interviewers suddenly realize several things they forgot to ask. If important regions have been incompletely expanded, then referred gates, as opposed to phantom gates, can often return the interviewee to these unanswered questions without substantially interrupting the flow of the interview.

In the meantime, a phantom gate placed here and there will probably not cause much of a problem especially if the blending appears high and the content of the question is not sensitive in nature. In general though, one should avoid them, since it seems senseless to risk damaging the flow of the interview by their use.

With regard to the utility of phantom gates two instances come to mind. First, when dealing with a wandering interview, phantom gates may be useful in focusing the patient, especially if milder forms of focusing have been unsuccessful. A second use of phantom gates arises during the exploration of certain psychodynamic regions. Specifically, if one wants to catch a patient off guard in order to observe the patient's spontaneously occurring defenses, then an unexpected phantom gate may be very effective. Phantom gates may also help one break through the resistance caused by a patient bent on manipulating the interviewer or during a rehearsed interview.

In a less antagonistic sense, phantom gates may also be utilized when attempting to help patients reflect upon themselves through the use of interpretive questions. Interpretive questions may assume more bite if asked at an unexpected moment. These latter uses of phantom gates find minimal applicability during initial interviews, but they are more commonplace during psychotherapy interviews, once the therapeutic alliance has been solidified.

The Implied Gate. To round out our summary of transitions used during the body of the interview we can turn our attention to implied gates. These gates are frequently used during chit-chat between friends and may have been the predominant gate overheard as we listened in upon the cafe conversation mentioned earlier.

In an implied gate, the movement into a new region is characterized by asking a question that seems to be generally related to the region already under expansion. Thus, it is somewhat "implied" that the interviewer is simply expanding a topic already germane to the interviewee. Similar to the referred gate, an implied gate lacks a true immediate cue statement. In the following example, movement is made from the region dealing with immediate stressors into past social history. The transition (indicated by an asterisk) seems smooth, an effect that's probably secondary to the similarity in content between these two regions.

> **Pt.:** We're living in a fairly nice house now. It has three bedrooms and a couple of acres. Believe me, we need the space with our four kids.
>
> **Clin.:** How are the kids getting along?
>
> **Pt.:** The two oldest, Sharon and Jim, get along pretty well, on different tracks. They stay out of each other's way.

	But the two little ones — oh my! They live to torture each other . . . Pulling each other's hair, yelling, screaming. It's a zoo.
Clin.:	I'm wondering if, with all those mouths to feed, money is a problem?
Pt.:	In some respects, yes; but my husband is a lawyer, and is doing well. In fact, if anything, our income has increased recently.
* *Clin.:*	Tell me a little bit about what it was like for you when you grew up back in Arkansas.
Pt.:	First of all, I came from a large family of eight children. So we sometimes, many times, had to do without. I remember all the hand-me-down's and, believe me, I appreciated them. My mother was a loving woman, but beaten down by life. She was tough, but her pain showed through.
Clin.:	Do you remember a specific time when her pain showed through?
Pt.:	Oh, yes. I was about five, I think, and . . .

It may be of value to spend a few moments comparing implied gates to the gates previously discussed. As mentioned earlier, unlike a natural gate, an implied gate does not cue directly off the preceding statement. Furthermore, unlike a referred gate, the interviewer does not directly refer back to earlier statements. And, in contrast to the phantom gate, the implied gate seems to fit in very naturally with the current flow of the dialogue. Indeed, when the newly entered region appears very similar to the preceding one, an implied gate is practically imperceptible and rivals a natural gate for smoothness of transition (as in this example).

As the regions connected increase in disparity, the implied gate becomes increasingly more abrupt. Thus, with regard to smoothness, implied gates range on a continuum between natural gates and phantom gates. When the two regions are closely related, implied gates approach the gracefulness of natural gates. On the other hand, if the topics are poorly related, an implied gate may approach the awkwardness of a phantom gate.

Implied gates can be frequently used to enter new regions smoothly. In fact, not infrequently, the clinician may simultaneously expand two regions whose contents are similar in nature. For instance, one can easily expand the anxiety disorder region and the affective disorder region in a parallel fashion, since the symptoms in these disorders frequently overlap.

At this junction, we are nearing the end of our discussion of the various methods by which one can structure the body of the interview. Some of these principles are summarized below:

a. When the patient brings up a spontaneous gate into a new region, the clinician always has the choice of whether to follow it or not. These decision moments are called pivot points.

b. If a premium is put upon efficient data gathering, then it is often best not to follow these gates into new regions. Instead, the clinician can gently continue the expansion of the region currently being explored.

c. If a premium is put upon a dynamic understanding of the patient, then these spontaneous gates are frequently followed by the interviewer, as the patient's wanderings can provide valuable information. These gates are also followed if it appears that the patient has begun spontaneously discussing sensitive areas or seems to need to ventilate disturbing emotions.

d. Natural gates, in which the clinician enters a new region by cueing directly off the patient's preceding statement, offer another method of smooth transition and should be employed frequently.

e. These natural gates offer a means of effectively structuring an interview while conveying an unstructured feeling to the interviewee.

f. Referred gates, in which the clinician literally refers back to earlier statements by the patient, offer effective methods of re-entering poorly expanded regions or bringing up new regions.

g. Referred gates are particularly useful for tying in sensitive or awkward regions such as the mental status exam, for once again the patient feels that this "new topic" appears to relate naturally to the spontaneous dialogue.

h. Implied gates allow one to join similar regions and can also provide parallel expansions of related regions.

i. Phantom gates should be generally avoided unless used for a specific purpose such as focusing a persistent wanderer.

Once a clinician understands these principles of facilics, then the body of the interview can be developed and altered almost at the whim of the interviewer. These tricks of the trade can greatly increase the engagement with the patient, the effectiveness of the data gathering, and ultimately the validity of the data base itself.

In short, initiated by the conscious decisions of the interviewer, the clinical dialogue unfolds. With each unfolding, the initial resistance of the interviewee gradually recedes, for the interviewer, instead of opposing this resistance, moves with it. The natural gates and blended expansions discussed in this section generate interviews that move with the gentle dynamics of a conversation. The patient feels more relaxed, defenses drop, and the interviewer finds a rich field of pertinent information opening before him.

This section on the body of the interview began with a quotation concerning a master artist of China, Wang Hsia, who painted in the eighth century A.D. He worked in a different time and in a different medium than we have discussed. Yet, he, too, was a student of movement. Like ours, his work was based on a few simple principles, practiced until discipline had transformed them into art. Our "painting" is the clinical dialogue we leave behind us. We, too, strive for sensitivity and subtlety. Perhaps, with work, fellow students of interviewing will study one of our future transcripts and find, to their admiration, that "when one looks carefully, one cannot find any marks of demarcation in the ink."

THE CLOSING OF THE INTERVIEW: PHASE FOUR

As the interview steadily moves towards its closure, certain tensions may arise in the interviewee. These tensions arise from the patient's concern as to whether or not help is at hand. From the patient's perspective, the question becomes one of "What have we accomplished here?" or "Was this worth my time?" A variety of questions may be formulating in the patient's mind, either consciously or unconsciously. Not every patient will have all of these concerns, but many patients will be seeking answers to a significant number of them, such as:

1. What is wrong with me?
2. Am I crazy?
3. Did I tell the interviewer what he or she needed to know?
4. Does this interviewer understand my problems?
5. Did this interviewer like me as a person?
6. Do I have a diagnosis?
7. Will I get better?
8. Can I be helped?
9. What are my treatment options?
10. What will happen to me next, and will I see this clinician again?

All of these questions are appropriate and natural. Indeed, the patient, in a sense, has a right to a discussion of these issues with the clinician. The clinician will possess only tentative answers to many of these questions, and the patient should be made aware of this fact, but even tentative answers may provide a powerfully reassuring experience for the patient. If answered sensitively, the clinician can help decrease the patient's fear of the unknown, including the plaguing question of "What's happening to me?"

Addressing this point, Sullivan has stated that a patient should gain something from the assessment process itself.[21] He emphasizes that patients frequently gain a considerable sense of relief merely by exploring their problems in an orderly fashion with a concerned listener. An orderly inquiry frequently begets a more orderly and calming perspective. Over and above this benefit patients may literally come away with tentative answers to some of the disturbing questions raised above.

It should be kept in mind that one of the major goals, perhaps the major goal, of the clinician during the closing phase of the interview consists of solidifying the patient's desire to return for a second appointment or to follow the clinician's referral. Indeed, if the patient decides not to comply with the clinician's recommendations, then the interview has in many respects failed. The clinician may have an extremely accurate diagnosis, but if no patient returns, the utility of the diagnosis is certainly of dubious value.

Towards achieving a better understanding of compliance it is valuable to look at some of the reasons that would motivate a patient to return. Although many reasons exist, the following seem to be most telling:

a. The patient feels that something was gained from the interview.
b. The patient feels comfortable with the interviewer.
c. The patient feels that the interviewer also feels comfortable with the interaction.
d. The patient trusts the clinician.
e. The patient feels that the clinician may be able to help in the future.
f. The patient feels that the clinician appears to be down to earth and accessible.
g. The patient feels that the clinician appears balanced and calm.

To a significant extent, the presence of such favorable "compliance feelings" will at least partially be determined by the manner in which the clinician has handled the introduction, the opening, and the body of the interview. But it remains the closing phase in which many of these compliance feelings can be significantly enhanced. One of the major methods of enhancing these favorable feelings consists of taking the time to carefully address the questions mentioned earlier.

The very fact that the clinician addresses these issues may convey to the patient that the clinician can be trusted and seems to understand the patient's needs. Indeed the clinician's actions represent a direct acknowledgment of the patient's needs at the moment.

One could discuss the issues concerning the closing phase in great detail, but I think it may be of more value to look at a closing phase as it unfolds. This dialogue will represent only one approach to the closing, but it illustrates many of the principles discussed earlier.

In the following illustration, the clinician has been interviewing a middle-aged woman at a local mental health center. The clinician is functioning as an assessment clinician and has decided that the patient is most likely suffering from a major depression. We will pick up the dialogue near the end of the body of the interview. In order to highlight the various aspects of this interview phase, the entire closing phase is included.

> *Pt.:* I don't think any other members of my family . . . let me see . . . no, I don't think anyone else besides my sister and my uncle have been depressed like this. My mother certainly never went through anything like this, perhaps that's why she doesn't seem to understand.
>
> *Clin.:* Well, it doesn't seem like too many people in your family have been depressed, but at least two people have. We've covered a lot of ground so far. At this point, we are coming to the close of our interview today. I'd like to spend some time summarizing what we've talked about and discussing some ways of possibly helping you to help yourself. But first, you mentioned that your mother doesn't seem to understand. I'm wondering how you put together what is happening to you?
>
> *Pt.:* Hmmm . . . it all seems so complicated. I think I may have reached a time of life when my bad qualities are catching up with me. Certainly I'm becoming a burden for my husband and I'm not really doing my share.
>
> *Clin.:* Why do you think it's happening now?
>
> *Pt.:* Maybe because I deserve it, I don't know. Or maybe because the kids are starting to leave the nest as they say.
>
> *Clin.:* Do you think there is anything you might want to add as we close that we haven't covered, that might help us to understand what is going on?
>
> *Pt.:* No, not really, we've covered an awful lot . . . well, one thing though, I didn't mention this because it was so long ago, but in college I had one semester in which I did very poorly in school. Now that I think about it, maybe I was suffering from the same type of thing.
>
> *Clin.:* What were you feeling back then, that makes you feel these experiences were similar?
>
> *Pt.:* Many of the same things. I couldn't sleep well and I was

constantly worried, I was so worried about flunking out I almost did.

Clin.: Did you seek help back then?

Pt.: Are you kidding! My parents didn't think anything was wrong except I was lazy. It never even crossed my mind to get help.

Clin.: But you've come for help today and I'm wondering what kinds of ways you thought we might be able to help you?

Pt.: I'm not really certain. Maybe I thought you might have some magic pill that would take all this away (patient smiles and begins a subdued chuckle). I'll tell you one thing though, it was hard to come here.

Clin.: I'll bet it was . . . tell me a little about what it was like actually coming here today.

Pt.: Oh, I felt very self-conscious walking in off the street. In fact, I looked around first to see if anybody I knew was around. When the coast was clear, I shot in like a dive bomber . . . while I was waiting to see you, I felt very awkward. I didn't know what I was getting into. I almost left.

Clin.: What made you stay?

Pt.: I think I realized I needed help of some sort. I really am at a loss. What do you actually think is happening?

Clin.: First, let me reassure you, most everyone who comes for a first appointment feels much as you have. That's totally normal. It's difficult to share with a stranger. You've done an excellent job of helping me to get a good picture of what you've been experiencing. From what you said I have some ideas of what might be going on. I agree with you that you seem to be dealing with a lot of stresses within your home, including a changing relationship with your children as they leave, and a fair amount of tension with your husband.

Pt.: Yes, I really didn't emphasize the problems with Jack but they are there and have been for years. It's not just the kids.

Clin.: These problems are certainly worth trying to understand so that you can cope with them more effectively. And sometimes some of the pains we feel from the past, like your leaving home at an early age, may also be contributing to the present. Because of this, I think it would benefit you to talk with one of our clinicians perhaps on a weekly basis for a while, to try to sort things out. But, I think there is more to the picture as well. You described a variety of symptoms such as an inability to sleep, a loss of energy, decreased enthusiasm, and a loss of sexual drive. All these symptoms suggest that you may be suffering from a major depression.

Pt.: How do you mean?

Clin.: Over the past ten or so years, we have made tremendous advances in understanding various forms of depression. It used to be thought that depression was only caused by psychological problems, but now we have discovered that some forms of depression are caused, or at least partially caused, by chemical imbalances in the brain. No one thinks about how incredibly complicated the brain is, it is no wonder that sometimes minor chemical imbalances arise. In any case, the symptoms you have are commonly seen in these forms of depression. Another item pointing that way is the fact that two members of your family seem to have also suffered from a very similar depression, and we have found that the biological forms of depression are frequently seen among family members.

Pt.: What does all this mean?

Clin.: Well, some of these depressive symptoms, perhaps caused by your biology, make it difficult for people to effectively work on the psychological problems and even to cope with daily chores. Fortunately, we have found a variety of medications that frequently help to get rid of these depressive symptoms. There are no magic pills though, nor are there promises for success, but these antidepressant medications can be very effective with some people. Because your symptoms do suggest that you may also have a biological depression, I'm going to make a referral to our mood disorders clinic. If you are interested in going there, you'll find the therapists are very skilled in both talking therapy and medications. After they get to know you better, they will let you know exactly which therapy may help you the most. (pause) I've given you a lot of information, I'm wondering if this is making any sense?

Pt.: Yes, yeah, I think so at least.

Clin.: Try to tell me in your own words what I've been explaining to make sure that I'm being clear.

Pt.: Let me see, you think that there may be something wrong with the chemistry in my brain and that's making me feel depressed. And you think some medications may help.

Clin.: That's right. Now this doesn't mean you don't want to look at the psychological stresses as well. This means that there may be more than one way to help you feel better. Do you think you'd be interested in seeing our therapist, I think it could really help.

Pt.: Yes, I think I would like to give it a try, at least. I'd read about depression being caused by chemical problems, I just really never recognized myself as being depressed.

Clin.: Sometimes depression is hard to recognize. Perhaps back in college your parents didn't recognize it in you just as you didn't recognize it yourself today.

Pt.: I never thought of it that way, but I guess it's actually possible.

Clin.: In any case, as we wrap up here, I'm wondering what this interview has been like for you, was it what you were expecting?

Pt.: For the most part, yes. I really didn't know exactly what to expect. I really felt we covered a lot of important ground. It seemed very thorough.

Clin.: Is there anything I could have done differently that might have made you feel more comfortable?

Pt.: No, no . . . I felt, I feel very comfortable with you. I do think you could use more magazines out in the lobby though. It really gets uncomfortable sitting out there.

Clin.: Hmmm . . . that might be a good idea.

Pt.: Will I be working with you again?

Clin.: No, I only work over here in the Assessment Clinic, but I think you'll find the therapists in the Mood Disorders Clinic very knowledgeable and also very nice. Like myself, they will try to gain a broad knowledge of how things have been going for you over the years, in an effort to understand you better.

Pt.: Good, do I call them or what?

Clin.: I'll give you a card here (hands card to patient). This has their number on it, and you can call later today for an appointment. This card also has our number on it, if there are any other unexpected problems before your appointment. I think you made a very good decision coming here today. I think they'll be able to help you to help yourself.

Pt.: Well, thank you. I actually feel a little better.

Clin.: Good, I hope things go well. Give us a call if there's a problem.

Pt.: Thank you very much (patient exits).

This was a nice example of a straightforward closing phase. The first thing to note is that the closing phase takes time. To have this time available, the clinician must leave appropriate time for the closing to occur. One of the most frequent problems I see in supervision remains the over-extension of the main body of the interview, thus forcing the clinician to rush through the closing phase.

This rushed closing can leave the patient feeling disjointed and uncertain as to what just happened. To the contrary, during this phase, where engagement looms so critical for compliance purposes, the clinician should appear unhurried, concerned, and calm. There is a give-and-take element to the closing phase. The clinician is truly interested in the patient's opinions, and this respect helps the patient to feel a sense of trust and control.

If one looks through this dialogue, most of the questions listed earlier as being pertinent to the closing phase were addressed. The clinician added a nice touch by asking for comments about his own performance. I frequently ask this type of question for several reasons. Sometimes patients literally provide very good constructive criticism. Secondly, the metacommunication of the clinician to the patient is reassuring, for the clinician is stating, "I care about how I come across to you and am aware that I make mistakes and can improve as well." This type of metacommunication can help the patient feel that they will be listened to and not just ordered about.

Naturally, each closing phase will be different, but the basic principles outlined above offer at least one practical approach. The reader may discover many others. The important thing remains the realization that the closing phase is different from other sections of the interview, its character being formed by the changing needs of the two co-participants.

Before ending our discussion of the dynamic structure of the interview, one short phase of the interview warrants some attention.

THE TERMINATION OF THE INTERVIEW: PHASE FIVE

The termination phase consists of the actual closing words and gestures of the interviewer and interviewee. As with the introduction, the clinician frequently shakes hands and smiles appropriately. It is not uncommon, if the clinician is functioning as a triage agent and will not be seeing the patient again, to wish the patient good luck with a simple phrase such as, "I hope things go well for you."

The only problems that tend to arise here occur when the clinician feels, for some odd reason, the need to be overly formal and cool. Once again, such pseudo-professionalism only runs the risk of creating alienation in the patient. Instead, a quiet warmth seems more appropriate, a warmth generated by two people who have worked together in an attempt to increase understanding.

I would only like to add that if the clinician will be seeing the patient again, perhaps as the patient's therapist, then increased attention to the actions of the patient at termination may be valuable. Indeed, termination functions as a mini-loss to the patient. In responding to such a loss phenomenon, the patient may betray behaviors suggesting dependent feelings and difficulties with separation. These behaviors may offer early clues to more far-reaching psychodynamic processes.

For instance, some patients may dawdle at the door, looking anxiously back at the clinician for one more sign of approval or acceptance. Other patients may suddenly become cooler, as if they resent the ending of their hour. Such a display may be an early sign of narcissistic entitlement or borderline rage. In any case, a sensitive clinician can gain some insight from even a small piece of patient behavior, ranging from a peculiarly soft knock on the door to an unusually rapid series of departing footsteps.

CONCLUSION

In this chapter we have studied the subtle transformations that evolve as the clinical interview proceeds. The interview was described as a dynamic process, an event born from the immediate needs of the clinician and the person seeking help. At times the agenda of these two people appear vastly different and the art becomes one of moving through this world of opposites in such a manner that the agenda seem less antagonistic or even become unified.

In this chapter we have seen two quotations from Eastern disciplines, ink brush painting and the graceful martial art of T'ai Chi-Chun. These references were not chosen simply to produce a more literary work, for the similarity between interviewing and these other highly skilled activities stands as a striking one. An understanding of this similarity lies at the center of mastering the art of interviewing.

One will find that in order to master these Eastern disciplines, the dedicated student may spend months or years practicing the basic brush strokes and body movements from which these arts were born. Through rigorous emphasis upon learning basic principles, mastery gradually occurs. At first these movements may appear artificial and somewhat limiting, but through intensive practice the pupil eventually develops a creative intuition not possible without first learning the basic maneuvers. One need only watch a T'ai Chi master sparring in order to comprehend the immense creativity cultivated through years of discipline.

In a similar fashion, this chapter has presented a highly analytical approach to interviewing, as if studying the process through a microscope. The use of these techniques may seem awkward at first, but with practice they become a natural and integral part of the clinician's style. A new and more penetrating intuition emerges from the balance, poise, and confidence that characterize an interviewer who understands not only patients but the interview process itself. Moreover, patients sense this internal balance and are powerfully attracted to it. As we pointed out in Chapter 1, talented interviewers are neither solely intuitive nor solely analytic. They are both.

With interviewing one is reminded of a fictional art form described by the writer Herman Hesse in his novel *The Glass Bead Game*. This so-called game was, in reality, the most highly evolved of all art forms. In it, an artist attempts to synthesize two totally opposing views into a unified statement. The more graceful the metamorphosis, the more brilliant the artist. One cannot help but see the parallel between this fictional art form and the craft of clinical interviewing. In this context the reward is not artistic adulation but increased understanding of the patient and a more powerful sense of caring.

I mention Hesse's game because the following excerpt, depicting the qualities sought for in a glass bead player, illustrates the very essence of a talented and flexible interviewer.

Remember this: One can be a strict logician or grammarian, and at the same time full of imagination and music. One can be a musician or Glass Bead Player and at the same time wholly devoted to rule and order. The kind of person we aim to produce, would at any time be able to exchange his discipline or art for any other. He would infuse the *Glass Bead Game* with crystalline logic, and grammar with creative imagination. That is how we ought to be. We should be so constituted that we can at any time be placed in a different position without offering resistance or losing our heads.[22]

And so it is with interviewing: flexibility and creativity are born from understanding and discipline.

References

1. Storr, A.: *The Art of Psychotherapy.* New York, Methuen Inc., 1980, p. 9.
2. Lazare, A.: *Outpatient Psychiatry Diagnosis and Treatment.* Baltimore, The Williams & Wilkins Co., 1979.
3. Campbell, A. A.: "Two problems in the use of the open question." *Journal of Abnormal and Social Psychology* 40:340–3, 1945.
4. Converse, J. M.: "Strong arguments and weak evidence: The open/closed questioning controversy of the 1940s. *Public Opinion Quarterly* 48:267–282, 1984.
5. Dohrenwend, B. S.: Some effects of open and closed questions on respondents' answers. *Human Organization* 24:175–184, 1965.
6. Elliot, R., Hill, C. E., Stiles, W. B., et al.: Primary therapist response modes: Comparison of six rating systems. *Journal of Consulting and Clinical Psychology* 55:212–223, 1987.

7. Friedlander, M. L.: Counseling discourse as a speech event: Revision and extension of the Hill counselor verbal response category system. *Journal of Counseling Psychology* 29:425–429, 1982.

8. Hill, C. E.: Development of a counselor verbal response category system. *Journal of Counseling Psychology* 25:461–468, 1978.

9. Lazarsfeld, P. F.: The controversy over detailed interviews — An offer for negotiation. *Public Opinion Quarterly* 8:38–60, 1944.

10. Marquis, K. H., Marshall, J., and Oskamp, S.: Testimony validity as a function of question form, atmosphere, and item difficulty. *Journal of Applied Social Psychology*, 2:167–186, 1972.

11. Metzner, H., and Mann, F.: A limited comparison of two methods of data collection: The fixed alternative questionnaire and the open-ended interview. *American Sociological Review* 17:486–491, 1952.

12. Naik, R. D. Responses to open and closed questions: An analysis. *The Indian Journal of Social Work*, 44, 1984.

13. Rockers, O. S. F. Dolore: The effects of open and closed inquiry modes used by counselors and physicians in an initial interview on interviewee perceptions and self-disclosure. Ph.D. dissertation, 1976.

14. Rugg, D., and Cantril, H.: The wording of questions. *Journal of Abnormal and Social Psychology* 37:469–495, 1942.

15. Schuman, H.: The random probe: A technique for evaluating the validity of closed questions. *American Sociological Review* 21:218–222, 1966.

16. Schuman, H., and Presser, S.: The open and closed question. *American Sociological Review* 44:692–712, 1979.

17. Singelman, C. K.: Evaluating alternative techniques of questioning mentally retarded persons. *American Journal of Mental Deficiency* 86:511–518, 1982.

18. Singleman, C. K., Schoenrock, C. J., Spanhel, C. L., Hromas, S. G., Winer, J. L., Budd, E. C., and Martin, P. W.: Surveying mentally retarded persons: Responsiveness and response validity in three samples. *American Journal of Mental Deficiency* 84:479–486, 1980.

19. Benjamin, A.: The Helping Interview. 2nd edition. Boston, Houghton Mifflin Company, 1974.

20. Chung-yuang, C.: *Creativity and Taoism, A Study of Chinese Philosophy, Art, and Poetry.* New York, Harper Torchbooks, 219, 1963.

21. Sullivan, H. S.: *The Psychiatric Interview.* New York, W. W. Norton and Company, 1970.

22. Hesse, H.: *The Glass Bead Game.* New York, Holt, Rinehart and Winston, Inc., 1970, p. 68.

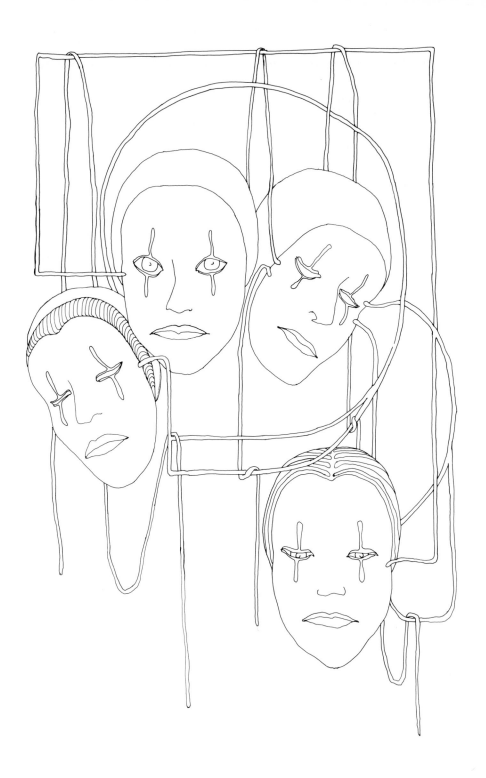

3

Nonverbal Behavior: The Interview as Mime

And now a dark cloud of seriousness spread over her face. It was indeed like a magic mirror to me. Of a sudden her face bespoke seriousness and tragedy and it looked as fathomless as the hollow eyes of a mask.

Herman Hesse, Steppenwolf

In this chapter we will explore the intricate processes known as nonverbal behavior. Few studies are more intriguing or more pertinent for the clinician. Our study will include not only body movements but also those elements of verbal communication that are concerned not with the content of spoken word but with how the words are spoken. Indeed, the noted social scientist Edward T. Hall has commented that communication is roughly 10 percent words and 90 percent a "hidden cultural grammar." He continues, "In that ninety percent is an amalgam of feelings, feedback, local wisdom, cultural rhythms, ways to avoid confrontation and unconscious views of how the world works. When we try to communicate only in words, the results range from the humorous to the destructive." [1]

The practical relevance of Hall's words can be readily seen in the following clinical vignette. During an afternoon of supervision, I had the opportunity to watch two interviewers interact with the same patient in back-to-back interviews. The patient, a male in his early twenties, sat with a slumped posture, his head seemingly pulled to his chest by an invisible chain. His legs were open, and his hands lay resting quietly on his lap. The interviewer was a young woman, who spoke in a quiet but persistent voice. The blending between the two was weak at best, provoking an occasional upward nod from the patient, rewarding the starved interviewer with a momentary scrap of interest.

When the second interviewer entered the room, an intriguing process unfolded. Within five minutes the patient sat more alertly in his chair. Eye contact improved significantly and was accompanied by actual animation, albeit mild, in his voice. By the end of the interview, the conversation was proceeding naturally, and a reasonably good therapeutic alliance had been formed. Both interviewers were relatively young women, both of whom conveyed a caring attitude. One wonders what factors resulted in the clearly more powerful blending of the second interview.

Some of the answers may lie in the communication channels each of these interviewers used in an effort to engage the patient. The first interviewer spoke in a quiet tone of voice intermixed with numerous nods of her head. Such head nodding frequently appears to facilitate interaction. Unfortunately, visual cues lose their impact if the patient refuses to look at the clinician. In short, her facilitory efforts were on the wrong sensory channel. To the contrary, the second interviewer spoke in a more lively tone of voice, which appeared to perk the patient's attention. More importantly, her words were frequently punctuated with auditory facilitators such as, "uh huh" and "go on." In contrast, the first interviewer verbalized few such auditory facilitators. The patient had been stranded in the room, responding with detachment to the clinician's monotone voice. Like the first clinician, the second interviewer also utilized head nodding, but her nods became progressively more effective as the patient met her eyes more frequently.

This example demonstrates the usefulness of flexibly employing different communication channels depending upon the receptiveness of the patient. If the patient's head is down, one can increase the number of facilitory vocalizations. With a deaf patient, one can increase head nodding. Perhaps more importantly this example emphasizes the overall influence of the interviewer's nonverbal communication on the patient. It suggests that we may be able to consciously alter our nonverbal style in an effort to create a specific impact on the patient.

This fact brings us to one of the most important challenges of this chapter. In order to flexibly alter their styles, interviewers must become familiar with the baseline characteristics defining their own styles. From such a self-understanding, flexibility emerges.

Thus a study of nonverbal behavior provides two distinct avenues of exploration. First, as the opening quotation from *Steppenwolf* suggests, one can learn an immense amount about the patient by studying nonverbal cues. This aspect of nonverbal behavior is the most commonly acknowledged. Hesse's protagonist quickly perceives his companion's change of affect as "a dark cloud of seriousness spread over her face." Second, as our clinical vignette illustrates, one can discover the impact of one's own nonverbal behavior on the patient and subsequently alter it as deemed appropriate.

Before proceeding it may be expedient to examine the definition of nonverbal behavior, for this term can have different meanings. In their excellent book, *Nonverbal Communication: The State of the Art*, Harper, Wiens, and Matarazzo explore some of the ramifications of defining this term.[2] In the first place, it is of value to make a distinction between the terms nonverbal communication and nonverbal sign. Nonverbal communication consists of an actual attempt to communicate a message using an accepted code between an encoder and a decoder.[3] A nonverbal sign does not involve an attempt at communication but represents a nonverbal behavior to which the observer infers a meaning.

Although developed as a refinement of research theory, this distinction between nonverbal communications and nonverbal signs can be adapted to provide a sound background through which to discuss clinical work. Specifically, in this book nonverbal behavior is viewed as the general category of all behaviors displayed by an individual other than the actual content of speech. In this context, tone of voice and the pacing of speech are also considered as examples of nonverbal behavior.

This broad category of nonverbal behavior can then be split into two subcategories, nonverbal communications and nonverbal activities. In the first category, nonverbal communications, the patient is using a commonly accepted symbol associated with a specific meaning. An irate football fan "throwing the finger" to the quarterback of the visiting team is displaying a piece of rather vivid nonverbal communication. In the second category, nonverbal activities, the overt behavior does not have a single commonly agreed upon meaning, and the sender may not be consciously trying to convey a message. The act of chain smoking cigarettes would represent a nonverbal activity. This activity may indeed be usefully interpreted by the observer as having a meaning, perhaps indicating anxiety. But this interpretation is inferred and may be wrong. In short, nonverbal activities may have numerous meanings.

As clinicians we are interested in attempting to understand the significance of both nonverbal communications and nonverbal activities. It is important to keep in mind that nonverbal activities are generally multiply determined. It seems unwise to begin assuming that one "knows" exactly what any given activity means. In this regard Wiener and associates criticized some psychoanalytically oriented researchers as immediately positing unwarranted unconscious meanings to nonverbal activities.

Considering this context one is reminded of the old psychoanalytic saw in which the astute clinician observes that the patient is experiencing severe marital discord because the patient is playing with her wedding band. Such interpretations of nonverbal activities are invaluable if kept in perspective. The clinician needs to think about other possible causes of the stated activity. For instance, this patient may be playing with her wedding band because she feels intimidated by the interviewer. She releases her anxiety by playing with objects in her hands. Normally she rolls a pencil back and forth, but since no pencil is available, she twists her ring. Other interpretations may be equally correct. To ignore these other possibilities while assuming the marriage is troubled is to ignore sound clinical judgment. On the other hand, having considered the various possibilities, the experienced clinician may gently probe to sort out which is correct and may indeed uncover marital discord.

From this discussion, the following general principle emerges. Nonverbal communications are relatively easily deciphered, whereas nonverbal activities should be cautiously interpreted, for more than one process may be responsible for the behavior. This point deserves emphasis because both clinical literature and popular literature sometimes read as if the authors felt they knew the exact meanings of nonverbal activities. They imply that one can read a person like a book. In a similar vein, the concept of "body language" suggests that nonverbal activities are more codified than behavior actually is.

A similar element of caution emerges as one surveys the research concerning nonverbal behavior. The body of research appears both vast and promising, but there exist many limitations. Nonverbal interactions are so complex that it remains difficult to successfully isolate variables to study. For instance, suppose research was designed to prove that it was the paralanguage (how the words were said) of the second interviewer in our clinical vignette that directly increased blending. Attempting to isolate this single variable would prove difficult, for a variety of other variables could have had an impact, such as the interviewer's physical attractiveness, the distance between seats, and even the fact that there were two interviews.

Even when one successfully isolates the relevant variables, the very act of isolation poses serious problems. Nonverbal elements seldom function as isolated units.[4] Instead, the various nonverbal elements exert their influences jointly, making the findings of research based on single channels such as paralanguage or eye gaze somewhat artificial. A different approach, the functional approach, attempts to study the various nonverbal elements as they function in unison.

These research issues are worth mentioning because it is important for the clinician to realize that little knowledge exists on nonverbal activity that can be called "factual." It is safe to say that this body of exciting research is in its childhood. In this regard the material of this chapter is best viewed as opinion concerning an evolving craft or art. The subsequent material is culled from a variety of sources, including clinical work, supervision, research literature, personal communications, and even popular literature[5] if it seems to shed light on clinical issues.

The following chapter is divided into two sections. In the first section three of the main categories of nonverbal behavior are briefly surveyed. As with the previous chapter, we shall develop a practical language through which to study the phenomena in question. Specifically, the following three areas are addressed: (1) proxemics (the study of the use of space), (2) kinesics (the study of body movement), and (3) paralanguage (the study of how things are said).

In the second section we shall adopt a functional perspective, carefully investigating the interplay of these three areas as applied to clinical practice. The broad clinical tasks studied include assessing the nonverbal behaviors of patients, actively engaging patients, persuading and focusing patients, and calming hostile patients.

THE BASIC PRINCIPLES OF NONVERBAL BEHAVIOR

Proxemics

Edward T. Hall was quoted at the beginning of the chapter. Few people would be more suitable for introducing topics such as nonverbal behavior, for Hall literally coined the term "proxemics." It was in his book *The Hidden Dimension* that he defined proxemics as "the interrelated observations and theories of man's use of space as a specialized elaboration of culture."[6]

Proxemics deals with the manner in which people are affected by the distances set between themselves and objects in the environment, including other people. As Hall notes, humans, like other animals, tend to protect their interpersonal territories. As humans move progressively closer to one another, new feelings are generated and new behaviors are anticipated. Hall postulates that people learn specific "situational personalities" that interact with the core traits of the individual, depending upon the proximity of other individuals. This set of expected behaviors and feelings can be used by the clinician to improve blending. By observing the patient's use of space, the clinician may even uncover certain diagnostic clues.

Hall delineated four interpersonal distances: (1) intimate distance, (2) personal distance, (3) social distance, and (4) public distance. With each of these distances different sensory channels assume various levels of importance.

At the intimate distance (zero to eighteen inches), the primary sensory channels tend to be tactile and olfactory. People feel at home with the specific scents they associate with lovers and children. At these close distances, thermal sensations also play a role, especially when making love or cuddling. Visual cues are of diminished importance. In fact, at the intimate distance, most objects become blurred unless specific small areas are focused upon. Voice is used sparingly. Even whispered words can sometimes create the sensation of more distance.

As one moves to the personal distance (one-and-a-half feet to four feet), kinesthetic cues continue to be used but olfactory and thermal sensations diminish in importance. With their decline the sense of sight begins to assume more importance, especially at the further ranges of this interpersonal space.

Upon arriving at the social distance (four to twelve feet), we have reached the region where most face-to-face social interchange occurs. Touch is less important, and olfactory sensations are markedly less common. This region is the playland of the voice and the eyes. Most conversations and interviews unfold within the range of four to seven feet.

At the public distance (twelve feet or more), vision and audition remain the main channels of communication. Most importantly, as people move further and further away, they tend to lose their individuality and are perceived more as part of their surroundings.

A respect for these spaces is of immediate value to the initial interviewer. In general, people seem to feel awkward or resentful when strangers, such as initial interviewers, encroach upon their intimate or personal space. With this idea in mind it is probably generally best to begin interviews roughly four to six feet away from the patient. If an interviewer is by nature extroverted, by habit the interviewer may sit inappropriately close to the patient, intruding upon the patient's personal space. Obviously such a practice can interfere with blending and should be monitored.

It should be kept in mind that patients do not determine a sense of interpersonal space by slapping yardsticks down between themselves and clinicians. As observed by Hall, it is the intensity of input from various sensory channels that creates the sensation of distance. An interviewer with a loud speaking voice may be invading a patient's personal space even when seated at six feet. Once again clinicians must examine their own tendencies in order to determine how they come across to patients.

To emphasize the point that it is sensory input, not geographical distance, that determines interpersonal space, one need only consider the impact of a patient who seldom bathes. Such patients frequently create a sense of resentment, for, in essence, olfactory sensations are supposed to occur only at intimate and personal distances. These patients invade the intimate space of those around them even when seated at a distance. The same principle can explain why even pleasant odors such as perfume can also be resented if they are too strong.

If a clinician intrudes into a patient's personal space, the clinician can set into motion the same awkward feelings and defenses commonly encountered in elevators. The artificial intimacy created by invading the patient's space results in a shutdown of interactive channels, so as not to further the intimate contact. Like a person in an elevator the patient will avoid eye contact and move as little as possible. The patient's uneasiness may even predispose the patient to decreased conversation. In effect, the clinician might just as well be conducting the interview on an elevator, hardly the image of an ideal office. This "elevator effect" can also occur if the clinician ignores cultural differences.

Hall's distances were determined primarily for white Americans. These distances may vary from culture to culture. One piece of research found that Arab students spoke louder, stood closer, touched more frequently, and met the eyes of fellow conversants more frequently.[7] Sue and Sue relate that Latin Americans, Africans, and Indonesians like to converse at closer distances than most Anglos.[8] They go on to describe that when interviewing a Latin American, an interviewer may push away, for the situation may feel crowded. Unfortunately this need for distance by the clinician could be perceived as an element of coolness or indifference by the client. In a similar light, the clinician may make the mistake of immediately feeling that the client is socially invasive, when in reality the client is merely interacting at the appropriate distance for Latin American culture.

Race may also play a role during the interview. Research suggests that blacks may prefer greater distances than whites.[9] Moreover, Wiens discusses the finding that the sexes of the participants can affect the preference for interpersonal distance.[10] One study demonstrated that male-female pairs sat the closest, followed by female-female pairs. Male-male pairs sat the furthest apart.

Kinesics

Kinesics is the study of the body in movement. It includes "gestures, movements of the body, limbs, hands, head, feet, and legs, facial expressions (smiles), eye behavior (blinking, direction and length of gaze, and pupil dilation) and posture." [11] In short, kinesics is the study of how people move their body parts through space with an added attempt to understand why such movements are made. As a field, it is a natural companion to proxemics. And like proxemics it had its own avatar of sorts, Ray T. Birdwhistell, who first elaborated his work in 1952 with the book *Introduction to Kinesics: An Annotation System for Analysis of Body Motion and Gesture.*[12]

Birdwhistell is an anthropologist and emphasized understanding body movements in the context of their occurrence. He also pioneered the study of videotapes in an effort to decipher the subtle nuances of movement. Through his microanalysis he attempted to define the basic identifiable units of movement. For instance, he coined the word "kine" to represent the basic kinesic unit with a discernible meaning.[13]

Albert Scheflen, a student of Birdwhistell's, expanded these notions to the study of broad patterns of kinesic exchange between people. In this context Scheflen postulated that kinesic behavior frequently functions as a method of controlling the actions of others.[14] By way of example, hand gestures and eye contact may be used to determine who should be speaking at any given moment in a conversation.

Kinesics plays a role in all interviews. Specific activities may shut down or facilitate the verbal output of any given patient. Besides yielding information that may help the clinician to foster engagement, the study of kinesics can provide valuable insights into the feelings and thoughts of patients. Freud phrased it nicely when he stated, "He that has eyes to see and ears to hear may convince himself that no mortal can keep a secret. If his lips are silent, he chatters with his finger-tips; betrayal oozes out of him at every pore."[15]

Paralanguage

The study of paralanguage focuses upon how messages are delivered. It may include elements such as tone of voice, loudness of voice, pitch of voice, and fluency of speech.[16] The power of paralanguage is immense and popularly acknowledged. Phrases such as, "It's not what you said, but the way you said it that I don't like," are considered legitimate complaints in our society. One can easily picture John Wayne snarling out such a phrase to some unruly bandit. Moreover, actors and comedians are well aware of the power of timing and tone of voice as it impacts upon the meaning of a statement.

By way of illustration, the phrase "that was a real nice job in there" appears complimentary at first glance. But one cannot determine its meaning unless one hears the tone of voice used in its conveyance. It could be far from pleasant if it was said with a sarcastic sneer by a displeased supervisor following an interview observed via a one-way mirror.

Besides the tone of the voice, speech is characterized by a number of other vocalizations. Although not words per se, vocalizations can play an important role in communication. One set of vocalizations consists of "speech disturbances." [17] Under the heading of flustered or confused speech, these disturbances include entities such as stutters, slips of the tongue, repetitions, word omissions, and sentence incompletions, as well as familiar vocalizations such as "ah" or "uhm." Such disturbances occur roughly one time for every sixteen spoken words. As would be expected, under stressful conditions these disturbances increase significantly. Thus they can serve to warn the clinician of patient anxiety as the interview proceeds.

There is more to vocalizations than just their appearance or lack of it. Some vocalizations serve to enhance blending, as seen with the frequently used facilitory statements "uh-huh" and "go on." But once again the way in which these vocalizations are used can significantly alter their effectiveness, as shown in the following vignette.

The interviewer in question possessed a pleasant and upbeat personality. He was a caring clinician, but found patients shutting down at times during his interviews. Videotape analysis revealed an interesting phenomenon. As he listened to patients he frequently interspersed his silences with the vocalization "uh-huh." His "uh-huhs" were said quickly with a mild sharpness to his voice as if chopping off sausages. He also used vocalizations such as "yep" and "yea," also stated with a curt tone of voice.

The net result was the creation of the feeling that he was in a hurry, wanting just the facts. And that is exactly what his patients gave him. This habit, coupled with a tendency to overutilize note-taking, fostered a businesslike persona, despite his natural warmness in daily conversation. It was a habit well worth breaking and once again highlights the power of paralanguage.

Cross cultural differences also affect paralanguage. Sue and Sue describe the variations in paralanguage that can interfere with the blending or assessment process when working with people outside the clinician's culture. For instance, silences are frequently interpreted as moments when the patient, for conscious or unconscious reasons, is holding back. Silence may also signal that the patient is ready for a new question. At other moments silence can create a feeling of uneasiness in both interviewer and interviewee.

But as Sue and Sue clearly state, the obvious may be too obvious.

Although silence may be viewed negatively by Americans, other cultures interpret and use silence much differently. English and Arabs use silence for privacy, whereas the Russians, French, and Spanish read it as agreement among parties. In Asian culture silence is traditionally a sign of respect for elders. Furthermore, silence by many Chinese and Japanese is not a floor-yielding signal inviting others to pick up the conversation. Rather, it may indicate a desire to continue speaking after making a particular point. Oftentimes, silence is a sign of politeness and respect rather than lack of desire to continue speaking. A counselor uncomfortable with silence may fill in and prevent the client from elaborating further. An even greater danger is to impute false motives to the client's apparent reticence.[18]

Many other cultural subleties exist, but they are beyond the scope of this text. Clinicians frequently working with other cultures should make it a point to understand the cultural characteristics of their clients.

CLINICAL APPLICATION OF NONVERBAL BEHAVIOR

Assessment of the Patient

Sir Denis Hill made the following observations during the Forty-seventh Maudsley Lecture in 1972:

Many experienced psychiatrists of an earlier generation believed that they could predict the likely mental state of the majority of the patients they met by observations within the first few minutes of contact before verbal interchange had begun. They did this from observation of nonverbal behavior — the appearance, bodily posture, facial expression, spontaneous movements and the initial bodily responses to forthcoming verbal interaction.[19]

Sir Denis Hill was concerned that the ability to observe nonverbal behavior astutely represented a skill that had fallen by the wayside. Let us hope this demise is not the case, for experienced clinicians today as much as yesterday need to utilize nonverbal clues throughout their clinical work. The knowledge available today concerning nonverbal behaviors is significantly more advanced than forty or fifty years ago. It is to this knowledge that we now turn our attention.

To begin our discussion we will look at another statement by Sir Denis Hill: "An important difference between the disturbed mental states which we term 'neurotic' and those we term 'psychotic' is that in the latter, but not in the former, those aspects of nonverbal behavior which maintain social interactional processes tend to be lost." [20]

An awareness of these potential deficits in the psychotic patient can alert the clinician to carefully probe for more explicit psychotic material in a patient whose psychotic process is subtle.

Perhaps an example will be useful at this time. I was observing an initial assessment between a talented trainee and a woman in her mid-twenties. The patient had been urged to the assessment by her sister and a close friend. Apparently the patient's mother was currently hospitalized with a major depression.

By the end of the interview, the clinician seemed aware that the patient was probably also suffering from a major depression or some form of an affective illness. But the severity of the patient's condition did not seem to have registered. Instead the clinician was about to recommend outpatient follow-up. The patient's nonverbal behavior was telling the clinician to take another look. In the second interview, which I performed, the patient disclosed a recent weekend brimming with psychotic terror. She had felt that her long-dead father had returned to the house to murder her. She was so convinced of this delusion that she had shared her secret with several young siblings, not a good idea if one is trying to get baby brother and sister to sleep. Eventually she ran from her house to escape her father's wrath. Even in the interview she could not clearly state that her father's return was an impossibility, although she hesitatingly said she thought it was.

Let us return to the interview in order to uncover the nonverbal cues that suggested the possibility of an underlying psychotic process. The patient, whom we shall call Mary, answered honestly and appeared cooperative. She displayed no loosening of associations or other overt evidence of thought process disorganization, but she demonstrated some oddities in her communicational style. With regard to paralanguage, she demonstrated long pauses (about four to eight seconds) before beginning many of her responses. This gave her a somewhat distracted appearance as if muddled by her thinking. This effect was heightened by a mild slowing of her speech and a flattening of the tone of her speech as well.

As we have seen, silences, especially of this length, are generally avoided in daily conversation. Everyday social protocol would ordinarily pressure Mary to answer more quickly. This breakdown in normal communicational interaction was one suggestion that all was not well and represents a disruption of the empathy cycle. Her body also spoke to her internal turmoil.

Although for the most part she had reasonably good eye contact, there existed protracted periods of time when she looked slightly away from the interviewer in a distracted fashion, whether she was talking or listening. This lack of "visual touching" during conversation is unusual.[21,22]

Frequently, before beginning to speak, the intended speaker glances away briefly. As he or she looks back, speech will begin. While talking the speaker will frequently look away. But as the end of the speaker's statement is reached, the speaker will look towards the listener. This glance signals the listener that the speaker's message is over. The speaker and the listener glance at each other's eye regions in varying lengths, usually between one and seven seconds, the listener giving longer contact. This complex eye duet was frequently missing with Mary. In depression the eyes are frequently cast downwards, but it is the peculiar manner in which Mary tended to stare past the clinician that hinted at the possible presence of psychotic process. As Sir Denis Hill had suggested, Mary had lost some of the nonverbal cues that maintain social interaction.

Other kinesic indicators of speech pattern have been called "markers of speech." [23] For instance, hand gestures are generally made as one initiates words or phrases. As the speaker finishes commenting, the hands may tend to assume a position of rest. To keep one's hands upwards, in front of oneself, can indicate that one is not done speaking or will soon interrupt.

In Mary these markers of speech were generally diminished. She sat stiffly with her feet flat on the floor. Her head seemed to weigh her body down as she sat slightly hunched over with her fingers interlocked. She displayed little hand gesturing, leaving the interviewer with the odd sensation that it was not clear when Mary was going to start or stop speaking. Most likely, Mary's lack of movement was an associated aspect of her major depression, but it may also have been a ramification of her psychotic process.

A more striking nonverbal clue to the degree of Mary's psychopathology lay in her method of dealing with unwanted environmental input, in this instance the questions of the interviewer. Apparently Mary had been concerned for some time that she might be "just like her mother," who was currently in the hospital. In addition, her sister had undergone a psychotic depression roughly six months earlier. Mary had been attempting to hide from herself the evidence of her own psychotic process, while the fear of an impending breakdown nagged at her daily. During the interview, as questions directed her back into her paranoid fears, she began to realize the extent of her problems. At this moment she did something out of the ordinary.

Mary leaned forward slowly, her elbows perched upon the tops of her knees with her head cupped between her hands. In this position her hands literally covered her ears, as if keeping out unwanted questions or thoughts. All eye contact was disrupted. Mary remained in this position for a good five minutes, answering questions slowly but cooperatively. She appeared detached from the world around her. This type of behavior has been studied under the rubric of "cut-offs." [24] Cut-offs represent nonverbal behaviors made to dampen out environmental stress. When exaggerated to the degree of appearing socially inappropriate, as was the case with Mary, they may be indicators of psychotic process. Indeed, catatonic withdrawal represents a prolonged and drastic cut-off.

One must also attempt to compare nonverbal activities to the patient's baseline behavior. Mary was normally a high-functioning secretary and most likely possessed better than average social skills. In this light, her preoccupied conversational attitude, and in particular her prolonged cut-off, represents very deviant behavior for her. A subsequent interview with Mary's friend revealed that Mary had been observed at work sitting and staring at the phone for hours.

For a moment I would like to elaborate on the issue of cut-offs. We have been discussing dramatic forms of cut-off behavior, which may indicate underlying psychotic activity, but mild forms of cut-off behavior occur routinely in our work with nonpsychotic individuals. These more subtle forms of cut-off are not without meaning and warrant some discussion. Morris[25] described four such visual cut-offs, to which he attaches some descriptively poetic names.

With the "Evasive Eye," the patient shuns eye contact by looking distractedly towards the ground, as if studying some invisible object. It can create the feeling that the patient is purposely not attending to the conversation and may frequently accompany the speech of disinterested adolescents. In the so-called "Shifty Eye," the patient repeatedly glances away and back again. With the "Stuttering Eye," the patient now faces the interviewer directly, but the eyelids rapidly waver up and down as if swatting away the clinician's glance. Finally, in the "Stammering Eye" the patient once again faces the clinician but shuts the eyes with an exaggerated blink.

These four eye maneuvers represent nonverbal activities whose meaning may be multiple. They may indicate that the patient at some level no longer wants to communicate. Perhaps a specific topic has been raised that is disturbing to the patient, resulting in a nonverbal resistance. At such moments a simple question such as, "I am wondering what is passing through your mind right now," may uncover pertinent material. Such cut-offs may also represent objective signs of decreased blending and movement into a shut-down interview. Exaggerated examples of these cut-offs can also be part of a histrionic presentation and in this sense could also be seen in both wandering and rehearsed interviews.

Investigators have also looked at the promising possibility that nonverbal activities could provide even more specific diagnostic clues, but at this point the research results remain tentative.[26,27] Moreover, the results appear to be in accordance with what common clinical sense would predict.

Concerning the diagnoses found on Axis I, schizophrenia appears to be accompanied by some distinctive nonverbal behaviors. Studies show that schizophrenic presentations are marked by a tendency for gaze aversion. A flattening of affect with decreased movement of the eyebrows was noted (which could alternatively be secondary to antipsychotic medication). Patients' postures were slumped, and they had a tendency to lean away from the interviewer. Naturally the type of schizophrenia and the stage of the process could significantly affect the type of nonverbal behavior present, emphasizing a cautionary note to these generalizations.

Depression has also been investigated. Researchers have noted that nonverbal behaviors vary depending on whether one is observing an agitated depression or a retarded depression. In the agitated depression, patients demonstrated "a puzzled expression, grimacing and frowning, gaze aversion, agitated movements, a crouched posture, and body leaning towards the interviewer. Subgroup 2 (retarded depressives) showed some increase in gaze, slowed movements, self touching, an emotionally blank expression, and a backward lean away from the interviewer." [28] In many respects, these findings have limited usefulness, for they simply seem to confirm the obvious.

But at a different level, especially with depressive patients, these findings emphasize the importance of nonverbal behaviors as clinical indicators of improvement.[29] The return of routine hand gesturing may herald an oncoming remission even before the patient admits to much subjective improvement. As the clinician becomes more aware of such behaviors as spontaneity of facial expression, smiling behavior, and eye contact, the informal monitoring of such cues to improvement can become a routine element of clinical follow-up.

With regard to Axis II, less research is available. Consequently, we will emphasize principles derived from clinical observations. Observations made during the first five minutes of the scouting period may provide important diagnostic clues. In this sense, these cues can help determine which diagnostic regions to emphasize in the body of the interview, for in the limited time available, it is generally not feasible to explore all areas of Axis II pathology. The following three clinical vignettes illustrate the usefulness of nonverbal activities in suggesting the presence of possible character pathology.

In the first example, I was observing an interview performed by a psychiatric resident during morning rounds on an inpatient unit. The patient was an adolescent girl with a head of curly light-reddish hair. The interviewer was sitting on a couch in a group activity room. The patient pertly entered the room and promptly plunked down beside the clinician. At first she leaned towards him with her right arm straddling the back of the couch behind his shoulder, but she quickly withdrew the arm. Her final perch was with her right knee up on the couch resting a few inches from the clinician's body.

In a proxemic sense, she had positioned herself well within the personal distance zone and actually very close to being within the clinician's intimate zone. Her speech was bright and snappy, percolating from a face rich with expressions and playful eyes. All this activity occurred in a matter of a few seconds. The clinician immediately responded by leaning away from the patient and crossing his legs by placing his left ankle over his right knee. This brief territorial excursion by this patient is not a typical initial interaction, even with adolescents who frequently feel more comfortable with "chummier" interpersonal distances. Instead, this type of interpersonal game may be seen in people with underlying histrionic personality traits or borderline personality traits.

The second patient was a woman in late middle age, with graying hair pulled back in a bun. Before the interview, she had had to wait longer than usual before entering the room. Initially, the clinician gently apologized for the inconvenience with a warm smile on his face. She made cool eye contact. Her lips did not so much as consider returning his smile. She fluctuated between a baseline of mildly cooperative answers, with a reasonably lengthy DOU, and brusque shutdown remarks.

A peculiar piece of body movement gradually evolved as she continued with her acerbic tone of voice. She tended to lean back in her chair, and gradually proceeded to stretch her legs out in front of her towards the interviewer. The movement was ingeniously slow but as steady as a barge pulling into a dock. As usually happens, the dock was gently bumped by her feet, at which point she did not pull away. Instead, the dock recoiled, with the interviewer quickly tucking his feet beneath his chair.

Her nonverbal activities may be multiply determined, but one possibility well worth exploring would be underlying passive-aggressive traits. Later historical information from the interview tended to further substantiate this diagnostic hunch.

The third and final patient carefully orchestrated a relatively unappealing opening gambit. She was a tall woman in her mid-twenties with long black hair hanging limply about her body. She was dressed in jeans and a black pullover sweater. Her first noticeably unusual action consisted of reaching over to pull up a chair, which she promptly used as a footstool. She stretched her body out, making herself conspicuously at home. This settling in did not signify the beginning of an easy engagement, for she proceeded to visually cut the female interviewer off throughout most of the interview. She would look down at her hands, frequently using the Evasive Eye movement described earlier.

All of this display was topped with a convincingly dour facial expression. Concerning paralanguage, she managed to push through her disinterested facial mask an equally disinterested and mumbling voice. Her attitude visibly disturbed the interviewer. She also demonstrated one other nonverbal communication with a set meaning. Specifically, she held her coat on her lap throughout the interview, perhaps communicating an eagerness to leave.

Her collection of behaviors, all present during the first few minutes of the interview, suggested a variety of personality traits worth exploring later. Her unconcern for making the interviewer feel more at ease could suggest a possible hint of antisocial leanings. Along similar lines her obvious attempt to display disinterest could be part of the manipulative trappings of a borderline personality or perhaps of a narcissistic personality. And as we saw with our previous example, some passive-aggressive tendencies may be present. Her behaviors in no way prove that she has any of these disorders, but they do provide suggestions of which disorders warrant additional consideration, further highlighting the importance of noting nonverbal behavior.

Let us now move from away from diagnostic issues, and look at some of the nonverbal clues that may suggest that patients are feeling uncomfortable or anxious.

One of the most well-known indicators of increased anxiety remains the activation of the sympathetic nervous system, the system geared to prepare the organism for fight or flight. During the activation of this system a variety of physiological adaptations occur that can serve as hallmarks of anxiety. The heart will beat faster and blood will be shunted away from the skin and gut to be preferentially directed towards the muscle tissue that is being prepared for action. This shunting accounts for the paleness so frequently seen in acutely anxious people, who look like they have seen a ghost. Saliva production decreases, and the bowels and bladder are slower to eliminate. Breathing rate increases, as does the production of sweat.

This last sign, increased sweating, reminds me of one of the more striking and humorous examples of autonomic discharge I have encountered. A medical student was doing one of his first physical exams on a real patient, which can truly be an upsetting experience, as the student frequently feels painfully inept. In this case, the patient was a child about nine years old, who could be generally classified under the label "brat." As the exam labored onward, with the worried mother looking increasingly fretful, the student began to sweat profusely. As the student leaned over to listen to the child's heart, a bead of sweat fell from his forehead directly onto the child's chest. Being a subtle kid, he immediately looked the student in the eye and in a loud voice said, "What's a matter with you, you're sweatin' all over me!"

If the poor student was not already uptight, that little proclamation did it. He sheepishly turned to the increasingly upset mother and produced a quick-witted white lie, "Don't worry, I've got a thyroid condition." I know this story all too well because I was the poor panic-stricken medical student. It clearly shows the truth that the autonomic system does not lie. With our patients, subtle signs of anxiety such as sweating, damp palms, and increased breathing rate can help us detect anxiety. If the anxiety represents evidence of poor blending, we may be able to purposely attend to the patient's fears. If it represents the presence of unsettling thoughts, we may be inclined to probe deeper.

If the sympathetic system is not presented with a chance to actually get the organism into action soon enough, the parasympathetic system may try to counterbalance with a discharge of its own. In these cases, one may find a sudden urge to urinate or defecate, as people frequently feel before public performances or job interviews. If a patient begins a session by immediately requesting the need for a restroom, this may represent a clue to a higher anxiety level than the patient may verbally admit.

Other good indicators of anxiety are described by Morris under the rubric of "displacement activities." [30] These activities are those bodily movements that release underlying tension. I recently watched a businessman waiting for a meeting. As he sat in the lobby, he nervously tugged at his tie and picked at his clothes. He then hoisted his briefcase onto his lap and meticulously unloaded it piece by piece, after which he gingerly repacked the case, carefully feeling each object as he delicately reassembled his "peripheral brain."

These behaviors were accomplishing very little in the way of needed physical functions, but they offered a calming effect of some sort for the businessman. Other typical displacement activities include smoking, twirling one's hair, picking at one's fingers, nailbiting, playing with rings, twitching one's feet, tugging at the ear lobe, self-grooming activities, tearing at paper cups, and twirling and biting pens. The list could certainly be extended. For instance, Morris points out that serving drinks and holding them in one's hands at cocktail parties probably serve to decrease people's anxiety, as they "have something to do." [31]

Clinically speaking, displacement activities are worth noting during both the initial interview and subsequent psychotherapy. Each patient seems to display a unique set of displacement activities. Once decoded by the clinician, these activities can be unusually reliable indicators of patient anxiety. When suddenly increased, they may represent a more reliable indicator than the patient's facial expression or verbal response that an interpretation was on the mark.

It is also of interest that anxiety will sometimes display itself not through the appearance of displacement activities but in their conspicuous absence. When engaged in an active conversation, most people will display a normal amount of periodic displacement activities. If these suddenly stop or are not present from the beginning, then the person may be experiencing anxiety. In a sense they may be trying to avoid mistakes by doing nothing.

This "still-life response" frequently appears when people are videotaped or interviewed in public. It seems to afflict interviewers even more than patients. Supervisors need to be aware that this response may be more of an artifact than a stylistic marker.

Another area of interest revolves around facial clues that the patient is visibly shaken or on the verge of tears. I am sure the reader is well aware of the faint quiverings of the chin and glazed quality of the eyes that frequently indicate that a patient is close to tears. But a fact not as well publicized is the tendency for people to demonstrate extremely fine muscle twitches across their faces when stressed. These frequently occur beside the nostrils and on the cheek. In people who demonstrate this tendency, these fine twitches can be extremely accurate indicators of tension.

By way of example, I was working with a young businesswoman during an initial interview. She had been referred to me for psychotherapy. She was attractively dressed with a bright disposition and her speech was accompanied by a collection of animated gestures. When asked to talk about her history, she launched into a detailed review of her life since age sixteen. Of note was her striking avoidance of any events prior to age sixteen.

When asked why she had done this, she responded that she did not know and had not noticed it. I asked her if any aspects of her life seemed different before the age of sixteen. She commented, "Not really, although I spent more time with my father back then." At that point a few muscle twitches appeared by her left nostril. I commented that I had a feeling she was feeling upset, and she burst into tears. Subsequent therapy revealed a complex and ambivalent relationship with her father and other male figures. Throughout therapy, those faint twitches were a sure sign of tension.

This issue of tension leads directly to another important aspect of nonverbal behavior, the detection of deception. In one piece of research a group of nursing students were asked to participate in a study in which they would be asked to deceive a person.[32] They were told that gentle deceptions were sometimes needed in clinical work, as when comforting frightened patients. Thus the nurses felt a need to perform well in the testing situation.

In the research itself the nurses were exposed to two different types of films. Some films were pleasant in nature, such as an ocean scene, and other films depicted unpleasant scenes such as a burn victim and a limb amputation. After seeing the pleasant film segments, the nurses were asked to describe their feeings to the listener. This task was obviously not problematic. But after viewing the unsettling film, in one experimental design, the nurse had to convince the listener that the gory film was pleasant and enjoyable to watch. This task was not so easy. Indeed, it so reproduced the sensation of lying that some nurses dropped out of the study.

All of these interactions were videotaped. Segments of these videotapes were then shown to subjects, who were supposed to determine from the visual images who was indeed lying. It was an ingenious experiment and represents the foundation work upon which further research on deception proceeded.

The original researchers, Ekman and Friesen, predicted that subjects would state that while lying they would focus upon making their faces "look natural." This prediction proved to be true. The deceivers did attend to their faces more, which suggested that nonverbal activities from the neck down may provide a better lead concerning deception. Interestingly, trained observers could pick up clues of deception from videotaped facial expressions. These microexpressions represent accurate clues but are too difficult to pick up routinely.

On the other hand, the body of the deceiver had a tendency to betray its own head, so to speak, and further research has substantiated many of these initial findings as described in Ekman's fascinating book *Telling Lies*.[33] Apparently, changes in below-the-neck movements may be of the most practical significance for accurately detecting deception. Direct communications or emblems, as Ekman refers to them, can sometimes be useful indicators of deceit. Emblems represent nonverbal behaviors that carry a distinct meaning, such as a yes or no head nod or pointing to an object. Just as slips of the tongue may betray hidden feelings, slips of the body can occur. With the nursing students in the above study, many felt a helpless sensation that they were not hiding their feelings well. This feeling of helplessness was sometimes inadvertently conveyed by a shrugging movement.

When representing indicators of nonverbal leakage, emblems usually appear in part. Thus only one shoulder may partially rise or one palm turn up during a shrug. Another good indicator that an emblem represents a deceitful mannerism is the display of the emblem in an unusual placement. An angry fist will not be raised towards an antagonist but will quietly appear by the side of the patient.

Hand gestures, which people make while speaking, have been called illustrators by Ekman, and they tend to decrease when deceit is under way. This decrease is particularly true if the patient has not had time to rehearse the lie and must carefully attend to what is being said. The clinician can monitor behaviors such as those described above while exploring regions in which resistance and deceit may be high. For example, when eliciting a drug and alcohol history from a typically active interviewee, a sudden decrease in associated hand movements may suggest that deception is occurring. Several other studies have also found supportive evidence for the idea that below-the-neck clues are best for detecting deceit on a practical level.[34,35]

Besides kinesic indicators of deception, the clinician can look for paralanguage clues that deceit is occurring.[36] For instance, a higher pitch to the voice has been associated with deception as well as emotions such as fear. In a complementary sense, lower pitches have been associated with judgments by observers that the subject is more relaxed and sociable. Another possible clue to deception involves the RTL. Deceptive subjects were found to demonstrate a longer RTL and to give longer answers when in the act of deceiving.

It should be kept in mind that most of the kinesic and paralanguage clues to deception mentioned so far represent nonverbal activities, not nonverbal communications. Thus these behaviors may be multiply determined and do not in any way ensure that the patient is being deceitful. In many cases, they may simply indicate that the patient is feeling more anxious. Each activity must be interpreted in the interpersonal matrix in which it was born. By way of example, one researcher found that an increased latency of response could be interpreted in different fashions. If it was followed by a self-promoting comment, then it was often interpreted as being an indication of deception. On the other hand, if the pause was followed by a self-depreciating comment, it was often registered in the opposite direction as evidence of a truthful remark.[37]

It is probably best to conclude the discussion of cues of deception at this point. Clearly the research is somewhat tentative, but it suggests that some changes in the baseline behavior of the patient may provide useful hints that deception may be at hand. Two practical points warrant mentioning. First, as the interview proceeds, it is generally a good idea to ascertain the baseline body movements that are typical of the patient. Second, during sensitive inquiries, it is best to avoid note-taking. Note-taking can completely eliminate the ability of the interviewer to observe the subtle nonverbal clues that may be the only warnings of deception.

In the same sense that nonverbal activities may indicate that the patient may be deceiving the clinician, a variety of important mixed nonverbal messages may be sent to an interviewer. These mixed messages are not necessarily deceptions. Instead, they may represent hallmarks of patient ambivalence and confusion.

In order to explore this fascinating area, the work of John Grinder and Richard Bandler[38] offers a wellspring of practical and sound clinical observation. Although controversy has arisen over their later work, their first two books provide some pioneering insights into engagement techniques.

Their work follows naturally from the principles we have been discussing thus far. Put simplistically, they state that as a person communicates a message, the message is transferred through a variety of communcational channels simultaneously. The patient's message may be conveyed through the content of the spoken words, the tone of voice, the rate of speech, the amount and type of hand gesturing, the posture, and the facial expression. These messages are termed paramessages. When all paramessages have the same meaning, the paramessages are said to be congruent. But if some of the channels convey discordant information, then the paramessages are said to be incongruent.

The underlying theory is simple; perhaps that is why it proves to be so powerful therapeutically. People who consistently communicate with an incongruent style can frequently create a confusing impression. Their incongruence may make the people around them feel ill at ease and uncomfortable. If the clinician can detect this self-defeating interpersonal style, he or she may be able to help the patient modify it. In a more immediate sense, incongruent paramessages may indicate underlying mixed feelings of which the patient is unaware. Once again, the therapist may be able to cue off this incongruence, leading the patient into an exploration of the uncovered mixed feelings.

More germane to the topic of the initial diagnostic interview, episodes of incongruent communication may alert the clinician to areas worthy of more immediate investigation or perhaps regions pertinent to explore in later sessions.

I am reminded of a woman in her early thirties who I was evaluating for possible psychotherapy and/or medication. Ms. Davis, as we shall call her, was coping with a variety of stresses, not the least of which was the loss of her mother several months earlier. For years she had been her mother's caretaker and verbal whipping post. Ms. Davis was mildly overweight with stocky legs, offset by a face embraced by a full head of black hair. As she spoke, her conversation turned to her bitter relationship with her boyfriend, who apparently enjoyed her sexually but found marital ceremonies not to his liking. She commented, "I hate him, I'll never go back to him. He's not worth it."

Harsh words, but one should be wary of taking them too seriously, for Ms. Davis' body spoke differently. The words were spoken with a tone of pained resignation, not biting anger. They had the quality of the child-like pout, "Daddy's not bringing home a present from his vacation." Not only did her voice lack self-indignation, but her hands played a martyr's role. Rather than the more typical pointing and jerking movements of an angry accusation, they were held low towards her lap with the palms upwards. This type of hand positioning is frequently associated with a tone of supplication and need.

Put more precisely, Ms. Davis was communicating with an incongruent set of paramessages. As Grinder and Bandler point out, all of these messages may have elements of truth to them. In Ms. Davis' case, she certainly did have angry feelings towards her boyfriend, as suggested by the content of her words. But she also had extremely powerful needs to be accepted by him; indeed, these needs bordered on a masochistic willingness to be verbally beaten by him. Her tone of voice and hand gestures suggested her strong need for acceptance. Even her breathing rate did not increase or become more spurt-like, as is frequently seen as someone becomes increasingly angered. This set of incongruent messages was one of the first clues to her deeply rooted problems concerning hostile dependence, which became central working issues in the remaining therapy. Indeed, her relationship with her mother was in reality no different from her relationship with her boyfriend.

In any given initial interview, periods of incongruent communication may occur. If noted, they can serve as road signs that significantly guide the interviewer towards a deeper understanding of the patient.

In a similar fashion the work of Albert Scheflen, who I mentioned earlier, deserves more detailed examination, for it too focuses on the nonverbal interactions that serve as communication scripts for people.[39] Scheflen discusses the idea that humans, like other animals, engage in certain shared behaviors that tend to escalate into specific actions. Such actions include fighting behavior, mating behavior, and parenting behavior. Frequently, these mutually arousing actions serve to eliminate the actual need to engage in the final activity. In such a manner animals will frequently avoid actual combat by undergoing a territorial display of sorts. Scheflen calls such escalating patterns of behavior "kinesic reciprocals."

Kinesic reciprocals can frequently be seen in clinical interactions. If the patient begins the reciprocal, the clinician may inadvertently continue the process. I have certainly seen this process occur within the realm of the courting or mating reciprocal. I remember watching a videotape of a session of psychotherapy. The patient was a young woman interacting with her therapist, who was a relatively young male with about seven years of clinical experience. The patient sat pertly forward, cigarette hanging esthetically from her fingers. The therapist, who was dressed casually in a sport shirt, sat rakishly back, also with a cigarette in hand. Their voices possessed a spritely coyness.

It was unclear whether I was watching the beginning moments of a therapy session or the opening sequences of a grade B movie. In any case, the therapist and his patient were engaging in the courting reciprocal, otherwise known as flirting. Inadvertent participation in such reciprocals can create a variety of problems. Obviously it can stimulate an erotic transference. Moreover, if initiated unconsciously by the therapist and then reciprocated by the patient, it can lead the therapist towards the inappropriate perception that the patient is histrionic.

I am reminded of one clinician who tended to be pleasantly flirtatious and bouyant with staff. She was surprised when male patients, following initial evaluations, would ask her out. On videotape the answer was obvious in that some of her flirtatious qualities appeared in her clinical work, albeit in a much toned down fashion.

Scheflen provides a good description of kinesic behaviors utilized by both sexes in the courting reciprocal:

> The full-blown picture of the female courting posture is well known to us, for models and actresses simulate it continually in being seductive or attractive. The head is held high and cocked. The "mark" is looked at from the corners of the eyes. The chest is brought out so that the breasts protrude. And the legs appear "sexy" as the foot is extended and the calf musculature is tightened. . . . An actively courting woman may present her palm, a highly affiliative act, in many ways; e.g., when she pushes back her hair, when she smokes, or when she covers her mouth while coughing.
> . . . The man's state of high tonus is evident most clearly in the thoracic-abdominal behavior. He moves from a slump, with abdominal protrusion to thoracic display by sucking in his belly and squaring his shoulders. A man may use some of the same behavior in courting that he uses in dominance. He may draw up to full height, protrude his jaw, stand in close, and display what is generally regarded as a masculine stance.[40]

Other reciprocal behaviors besides the courting reciprocal can occur in an initial interview. A striking example was provided by a videotape made of an initial interview for use in supervision.

The interviewer was a young woman. Across from her the patient sat with eyes occasionally cast downwards. As the interview unfolded, the patient produced a folded piece of paper, and she asked the clinician to read the paper before proceeding. Her voice seemed to step meekly away from her lips. In the meantime the patient began fumbling with the microphone. She had correctly wrapped it around her neck but had problems attaching it to her blouse. Noticing her problems the clinician looked over and asked if she needed help. The patient did not look up for a moment as she continued to fumble. Then with her head cocked downwards, she innocently glanced upwards shaking her head "yes." She gazed with the helpless eyes of a little girl and said not a word. The clinician promptly leaned over and fixed the microphone.

The parenting reciprocal had emerged as naturally as if enacted between a true mother and her child. In this brief vignette, the power of the first few minutes of the scouting period to provide clues for further diagnostic probing is once again amply demonstrated. This patient's manipulative style and dependent behavior suggested the possibility of some form of character pathology. Indeed, further interviewing revealed a mixed personality disorder with histrionic, passive-aggressive, and dependent characteristics. Apparently this patient had perfected the art of eliciting parental responses as a method of garnering attention.

This patient also displayed another type of nonverbal activity, auto-contact behavior. Auto-contact behavior consists of movements involving self-touching.[41] Such behaviors may consist of grooming behaviors, defensive-covering behaviors, and self-intimacies.

Self-intimacies are defined as, "movements that provide comfort because they are unconsciously mimed acts of being touched by someone else."[42] These self-intimacies appear frequently during interviews. Patients may hold their own hands or sit with their knees pulled up to their faces, arms literally hugging their own legs. In regressed patients, one can see even more extreme forms of self-hugging as patients lay in tightly curled fetal positions.

With regard to frequency, the most common self-intimacies in order of most to least frequent are as follows: (1) the jaw support, (2) the chin support, (3) the hair clasp, (4) the cheek support, (5) the mouth touch, and (6) the temple support. With hair touching there is a three-to-one bias in favor of women. Temple touching demonstrates the opposite bias with a preference in men of two-to-one. Sometimes these kinesthetic comforters can be tied into other sensory modalities as well. I remember one patient who would pull her hair across her cheek. She would simultaneously gently sniff at her hair, which she related as being very comforting. Such activity was a sure sign of her underlying anxiety, much like a displacement activity.

In this manner these behaviors may serve to alert the interviewer that the patient is feeling pained or anxious. It can cue the interviewer that the patient may need some verbal comforting, perhaps prompting an empathic statement. It can also alert the clinician that powerful affective material is being approached, possibly suggesting the need for further exploration.

In summary, in the above material the focus has been upon the power of the patient's body to convey information to the perceptive clinician. It is now time to explore the reverse situation, those moments when the clinician uses his or her body to affect the patient.

Utilization of Nonverbal Behavior to Engage the Patient

SEATING ARRANGEMENT AND PROXEMICS

One of the exercises undertaken in our interviewing class concerns the use of seating arrangement. Two of the trainees sit in the middle of the room on easily rolled chairs. They are given a simple task, to situate themselves so that they feel the most comfortable with regard to conversing with one another. In about 90 percent of the cases, the participants choose a similar position.

They sit roughly four to five feet apart. They are turned towards each other, but do not quite directly face one another. Instead, they are turned about a five to ten-degree angle off the line directly between them, both in the same direction, as shown in Figure 3A. Only about 10 percent choose to face each other directly.

If the participants are asked to turn directly towards each other, they complain of feeling significantly less comfortable. Some will even push their chairs back a bit. The discomfort is related as feeling "too close." More specifically, many of the trainees complain that the head-on position forces eye contact, making it difficult to break eye contact without undertaking a significant head movement. This head-on position fosters a sensation of confrontation.

On the other hand, the preferred position readily allows for good eye contact but also makes it easy to break contact in an unawkward fashion. In my own practice, I have certainly found this position to be the most comfortable and the most flexible interviewing position for me. This last statement is important, for it emphasizes that the most comfortable position may be different for each interviewer and indeed for each interviewing dyad. Each clinician needs to discover a comfort-

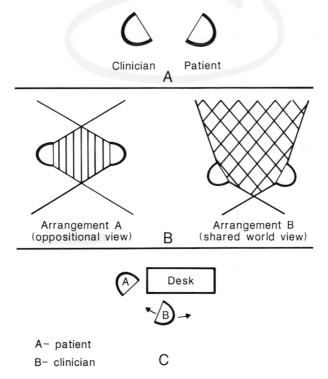

FIGURE 3. A, Preferred seating angle. B, Comparison of shared visual fields. C, Utilization of desk.

able position, keeping in mind that the clinician must also be willing to alter this position depending upon the needs of the patient.

In addition to the nonconfrontational feeling provided by the position described above, another phenomenon may be enhancing its comfortableness. As discussed before, one of the key processes that enhances blending is the ability of the clinician to convey a sense of seeing the world through a shared perspective.

If one looks at the actual fields of vision available to each participant in the interview, an important relationship readily becomes apparent. When two people are directly facing each other, the fields of vision exhibit little overlap. What overlap exists lies directly between the two participants. This situation tends to foster the sensation that "You are over there, and I am here." It seems to work against the sensation of "We are here together." On the other hand, when the two participants are turned slightly away from each other, so that they are subtly facing the same direction, then the feeling that "We are here, and the rest of the world is out there" naturally emerges.

Thus, in a phenomenological sense, the feeling of confrontation is decreased, while the sense of blending is given a gentle boost, as illustrated in Figure 3*B*. It should be noted that the directly oppositional position may be preferred by some people. Indeed, some clinicians recommend it,[43] but I myself do not, for the reasons provided above.

The concept of seating raises the more general issue of furniture arrangement. Some clinicians prefer setting, away from their desk, two large comfortable chairs. Another alternative is to utilize the desk creatively. In general, I believe a desk should not sit between the clinician and the patient, for this creates an authoritarian distance appropriate for chief executive officers, not therapists.

On the other hand, the desk can be placed as shown in Figure 3*C* with only a corner protruding between the clinician and the patient. If the clinician's chair rides on wheels, the clinician can move the chair and alter the resulting interpersonal distance either by increasing or decresing the amount of desk between the participants. A paranoid patient may require more distance from the clinician, which can easily be accomplished by moving only a short way, for the desk quickly provides a protective barrier. On the other hand, the clinician can easily move to a point where essentially no desk intervenes.

The overall concept of the clinical setting warrants attention. When designing a private office, an effort should be made to provide a comfortable and professional atmosphere. The office represents an extension of the clinician's persona, and the patient's first impression in the scouting period may be significantly affected by the decor of the clinician's waiting area or office. Calming prints or photographs, accompanied by several diplomas and shelves of books, provide a reassuring and pleasant environment.

Trainees are faced with limited financial resources. But three or four unframed art posters and a few plants can be bought very reasonably, producing a sometimes startling change in the atmosphere of the room. There is no need for a trainee's room to look like a prison cell. On the contrary, part of the training experience is learning to consider the principles behind creating an appropriate private office.

Outside the office, situations can be a bit more difficult, since the clinician faces crowded hospital rooms and disorganized emergency rooms. It remains important in these situations to consider the comfort of both the patient and the clinician. While performing a consultation in a crowded hospital room, there is nothing wrong with saying, "Before we start, would you mind if I slide your bed over, so both of us can have more room to talk."

This discussion of seating arrangements leads to the issue of determining an optimum distance between the clinician and the patient, which will vary for each interviewing dyad. There does seem to exist a small region in which the clinician's presence respects the patient's sense of personal space while still allowing the movements of the clinician to have an immediate impact on the patient. This zone of effective interpersonal space may be referred to as the "responsive zone" (RZ). If the clinician moves out of the RZ towards the patient, then the interviewer risks frightening the patient or creating a sense of discomfort. On the other hand, if the interviewer leaves the RZ by moving too far away from the patient, then the movements of the clinician may have little impact on the patient. For instance, the act of gently leaning forward towards a patient, which can enhance communication during particularly sensitive moments of an interview, may have no effect if done outside the RZ.

Two examples may help clarify the importance of establishing an RZ that seems most comfortable for each patient. First, if one intuits that a patient may be feeling paranoid, it is useful to remember that such patients may require a larger space around them in order to feel more comfortable. In these cases the RZ is larger and it may be wise to begin such interviews sitting further from the patient than one normally would sit or perhaps using a desk or table to help provide a safety barrier as mentioned earlier. As the interchange proceeds the clinician may find that the distance can be gradually decreased; hence the RZ frequently may change as the blending waxes or wanes.

In the second example, one looks at the problem of accurately eliciting a formal cognitive exam in elderly patients who are seriously depressed and withdrawn. To attract and maintain their attention, the interviewer might need to sit considerably closer than normal. This more intimate RZ may help decrease the likelihood of obtaining poor cognitive results secondary to the patient's lack of attention or interest. If a patient is not interested in answering, then the risk of getting artificially low scores becomes very real indeed. In such cases the tendency to suspect a real dementia when only a pseudo-dementia is present can become a true dilemma.

Another way of obtaining the withdrawn patient's attention during the cognitive exam is to speak more loudly, effectively moving closer but not moving one's chair. At times it is also important to ensure attention by literally asking the patient to look at the clinician as the questions are asked. For instance, the interviewer can gently but firmly make statements such as, "It may help you to do well on these questions if you watch me as I actually say the digits to you." In the last analysis, if a withdrawn patient is looking down at the floor as the clinician performs the cognitive mental status, the validity of the results are certainly questionable.

The concept of increasing the validity of the cognitive exam also raises the issue of touching patients. Some clinicians seem to have a block against the idea of touching a patient. And although it is not frequent for me to touch a patient during an initial interview (except for handshakes), I sometimes find touching useful and poignant. With regard to the cognitive exam, some depressed and withdrawn patients may ignore the clinician's attempts to make eye contact and attend to the task at hand. In such instances, one can touch the arm of the patient, offering comments such as, "I know it is difficult for you to concentrate right now, but it really is important." At such points, the patient may glance up at the interviewer and more effective contact will have begun.

Of course, touching, a method of entering the patient's intimate space, as described by Hall, may also be used at points at which the patient may benefit from some simple comforting. I am reminded of a sad, middle-aged man who I interviewed as he was entering the hospital. For all of his life he had been a kind and hard-working mill worker. Unbeknownst to himself he was being exposed to an extremely toxic industrial poison. Over the years he experienced gradual changes in his behavior, including irritability and occasional violent outbursts, which frightened him and produced extreme guilt. Simultaneously he underwent marked changes in his intellectual functioning, to the point that he had problems dealing with everyday activities. Only recently had he learned that his problems were secondary to brain damage.

As we neared the end of the interview, he told me that he was afraid of the hospitalization because "people say mean things to me, they think I'm stupid. Please let me come in, I promise I won't hurt anybody, I promise, and I'm not that stupid." At which point he began to weep. It seemed only natural to reach over and grasp his arm while reassuring him that I believed what he said and that we would help him make the transition to the hospital.

Outside of the types of situations described above, touching patients is not common during initial interviews, for touch is a powerful communication, that may carry numerous connotations, not all of which are appropriate. Patients may misinterpret touch as an erotic gesture or at a minimum as a sign of implied intimacy. Although the clinician may intend the gesture as a sign of caring, a psychotic patient or a histrionic personality may distort the message considerably. Indeed, if a clinician finds a routine need to touch patients during initial interviews, it would be wise for the clinician to determine why such a need is arising. Usually it is not from clinical considerations. Such clinicians frequently have a desire to be perceived as "comforting angels." Ironically, this drive to be perceived as "comforting" may get in the way of effective care giving. Such self-exploration may also reveal flirtatious traits or histrionic qualities in the therapist.

At this point we can turn our attention to another aspect of nonverbal behavior, which frequently emerges if the clinician has effectively determined the appropriate RZ for the patient. At such times the appearance of certain nonverbal behaviors can suggest that the blending process is proceeding well. As mentioned in Chapter 1, several verbal signs, such as an increased DOU, may indicate the presence of improved engagement. In a similar fashion nonverbal activities may also be used routinely to monitor the blending process.

For instance, as blending increases, the patient may begin to make progressively better eye contact, while spontaneous arm gestures and "talking with one's hands" may increase. Along similar lines, if a patient in a shut-down interview begins to talk more with his or her hands, this may be a hint to pursue the present topic more fully in order to further strengthen the engagement process. The clinician can also frequently see the patient turn more towards them as blending increases. Relaxation is also shown by an asymmetry in posture, while tense posture is frequently seen with people who feel threatened.[44]

We have been discussing the nonverbal activities that may suggest powerful levels of blending. It is important to return to a topic approached earlier, namely, the differences seen cross-culturally. With regard to the black culture, eye contact is not considered as important in conveying attention to a listener.[45] Just being in the room or close to the speaker may be considered enough to convey that attention is being given.

Direct eye contact may be considered disrespectful in certain cultures, such as with Mexican-Americans and with the Japanese. In this context, a clinician could be making a serious error in judgment by interpreting poor eye contact with members of these ethnic groups as an indication of rudeness, boredom, lack of assertiveness, or poor blending.

Another process that may emerge more frequently when one has successfully found the RZ is the surprising phenomenon of postural echoing.[46] In postural echoing one finds that two people who are communicating effectively tend to adopt similar postures and hand gestures. At a cafe, two lovers may sit across from each other, both heads perched in their hands, as they animatedly stare into each other's eyes.

A frequent phenomena seen in interviewing occurs when one member suddenly shifts positions and relaxes. Simultaneously the other person will also shift and relax. Moreover microanalysis of videotapes has suggested that as blending increases the minute movements of the interviewer and the interviewee tend to parallel each other as if a miniature minuet were being performed. During moments of discordant interchange this reciprocity decreased.

At one level these findings suggest that the appearance of postural echoing may serve as a clue to the clinician that the blending process is on the right track. In a slightly different vein, the clinician can subtly match some of the patient's postures in an effort to actively increase blending. For example, if a male clinician is interviewing a steel worker who is crossing his legs with his ankle over one knee, the therapist may cross his leg in the same manner, as opposed to crossing his leg at the knees. The latter method could be misconstrued by the interviewee as "feminine." By adopting a style similar to that of the patient, the metacommunication is passed that "we do certain things similarly and we may not be as different as one might first suppose." This discussion of the use of postural echoing, in an effort to actively engage the patient, leads to a consideration of other methods of nonverbally increasing the blending process.

BASIC FACILITATIVE TECHNIQUES

One collection of nonverbal behaviors potentially useful in the art of engagement consists of the so-called affiliative behaviors. Such behaviors include eye contact, smiles, and gesticulations. It has been shown that counselors who demonstrate these behaviors are viewed as significantly more persuasive than counselors who do not.[47] Another commonly encountered affiliative behavior consists of a body lean of about twenty degrees towards the patient.[48]

One of the most well-recognized affiliative gestures is the simple head nod. Morris makes the interesting observation that the vertical head nod indicates a "yes" or "positive" response in all cultures and groups in which it has been observed, including whites, blacks, Balinese, Japanese, and Eskimos. It has been observed in deaf and blind individuals as well as in microcephalic people incapable of speech. He relates that the head nod may convey different types of "yes" messages, such as the following:

The Acknowledgment Nod: "Yes, I am still listening."
The Encouraging Nod: "Yes, how fascinating."
The Understanding Nod: "Yes, I see what you mean."
The Agreement Nod: "Yes, I will."
The Factual Nod: "Yes, that is correct." [49]

Interviewers should make an attempt to learn the frequency with which they typically head nod. This frequency can vary significantly among interviews. From my own observations it appears that interviewers who are particularly adept at engaging patients tend to head nod numerous times during any several minutes of an interview. As obvious as the utility of the head nod may appear, I have found that roughly 20 percent of professionals I supervise tend to underuse it. A few barely head nod at all.

The power of the head nod became apparent to me in an unexpected fashion during a session of psychotherapy. I had been working with a middle-aged male patient for several months. I decided to try a brief exercise in which I would purposely stop my typical head nodding for several minutes, in order to see what this practice would feel like to me. To my surprise I found it difficult to do, for it had become habitual in nature. But more to my surprise, the patient broke off his spontaneous conversation after about two minutes and asked, "What's wrong? Somehow I feel that you don't like what I'm saying." This vignette emphasizes the power of nonverbal cues during clinical interaction.

ENGAGING GUARDED OR PARANOID PATIENTS

In Chapter 1 we discovered that with guarded or paranoid patients, certain changes in approach could enhance engagement. In particular, certain verbal approaches that were effective with most patients could be potentially disengaging with guarded patients. For instance, guarded patients frequently respond better to simple empathic statements rather than to complex empathic statements. In a similar fashion, with certain patients, the clinician's nonverbal behavior may be too empathic or intimate.

As mentioned earlier when discussing proxemics, guarded and paranoid patients may appreciate being provided with more space than most other patients. Along these lines, some of the affiliative gestures, when done too frequently, may prove disruptive to the guarded patient. I have heard paranoid patients comment that they have disliked frequent eye contact, perhaps twisting the attentive gaze of the "good listener" into the stark gaze of a potential persecutor. In this context, one may purposely break eye contact more frequently with paranoid patients, providing them with visual space.

Even head nodding and arm gestures can be unsettling when done too frequently with guarded or paranoid patients. I vividly remember one patient whom I interviewed in an emergency room. He was an intoxicated male about thirty years old, who wore a frequent sneer. He challenged me frequently with not-so-subtle sniper's remarks such as, "I bet you think you're a good listener Doc." And at one point he suddenly began mocking my head nodding by aping it, with his jaw jutting outwards while grunting out loud "Uh-huhs." Not one of my more rewarding interviews. He was the patient who later, while waiting for his disposition, spontaneously attacked one of our safety guards.

This patient also illustrates the point that if the clinician finds a patient giving negative responses to typically engaging nonverbal behavior, then the interviewer should consider the idea that the patient may be guarded, hostile, or potentially violent.

The Clinician's Self-Awareness of Paralanguage

Each clinician has a unique personality. In particular, clinicians will vary on such parameters as tone of voice, rate of speech, and loudness of voice. It is important for clinicians to discover their own typical way of coming across. This knowledge is of value, for certain patients may respond better to different approaches. Understanding one's own natural style offers the clinician the chance to modify it, if necessary, to enhance the blending process.

With this idea in mind, it is of value for clinicians to practice exercises such as speaking more gently and slowing down their rate of speech. If an interviewer tends to speak loudly and quickly, a toning down of these parameters may prove more effective with a frightened or guarded patient. By way of example, my own personality is somewhat upbeat, with a mild pressure to my speech and a slightly louder voice than many people. When beginning interviews, I purposely adjust to a calmer middle ground until I understand the specific needs of the patient. Adjustments can then be made as deemed necessary. In instances when I have not made this adjustment, I have certainly come on too strongly for certain patients.

There exists another area in whch tone of voice can frequently disengage a patient. Specifically, when talking with geriatric patients, clinicians often unconsciously adopt a rather distinctive tone of voice. They talk as if they were speaking to a helpless child. This tone of voice, which is often mildly slowed, can easily be perceived as condescending. It is an extremely frequent phenomenon, and clinicians must guard against it carefully. It is sometimes even done with psychotic patients and adolescents. In both cases the clinician is flirting with trouble.

THE NONVERBAL CUES OF THE CLINICIAN

We are generally well trained to observe the behavior of others, but the value of self-observation is frequently underplayed. As we have seen, the interview represents a dyadic process in which an understanding of one component depends upon an understanding of the impact of the other component. The clinician's nonverbal activity always has the potential to significantly alter the behavior of the patient, as we have seen in our discussion of reciprocal behaviors.

With regard to gestures, as with paralanguage, clinicians need to develop a sound sense of their natural nonverbal style. One exercise that helps clinicians in developing self-awareness consists of repeatedly picturing a mirror descending during the interview itself. This mirror is to drop into place between the clinician and the patient. Such a visualization exercise rather rudely awakens clinicians to the fact that their every move is potentially an object of scrutiny to an inquisitive patient. As a complement to this visualization exercise, videotaping provides invaluable objective self-observation.

In any case the clinician wants to foster an awareness of those nonverbal activities that may inadvertently decrease blending. I am reminded of an interview, which I supervised, of an adolescent boy. The patient sat in a pool of brooding preoccupation. He wore a worrisome expression more suited to a sixty-year-old man coping with an agitated depression than to a boy poking at adolescence. Curiously he had referred himself to the evaluation center, not wanting his mother to be contacted.

During the interview he moved about anxiously in his chair and had considerable difficulty looking at the interviewer. He had a rounded face framed by a bowl of sandy hair neatly clipped around his ears. It was about one of these ears that his discussion soon focused. Apparently he had the misfortune of watching a television documentary on cancer several days earlier. Since that time he had become fixated on a small bump on his right ear, to which he gingerly pointed. He was convinced that he had developed a malignant tumor. This gnawing obsession, which may very well have reached delusional proportions, was nestled amidst a variety of depressive symptoms and difficult life circumstances.

As the interview proceeded the boy became progressively more ill at ease. At several points he stopped talking, asking the interviewer, "You don't understand, do you?" To which the interviewer responded in a reassuring fashion that he was trying to understand and wanted to hear more. This type of response generally might have decreased the tension, but in this case it seemed of no avail.

What the interviewer did not realize was the message conveyed by his own face. Each time the boy discussed his "tumor" the clinician furrowed his brow in a not-so-subtle fashion, forming two small vertical lines between his eyebrows. Apparently the patient interpreted this facial gesture as a look of disbelief or condemnation. The clinician had no conscious awareness of this particular expression, which frequently cropped up as a habit during his interviews. It is just this type of habit that can lead to recurring problems with poor blending.

These habits are difficult to recognize unless the clinician is directly supervised or videotaped. They are also sometimes hard to accept. The clinician above seemed unimpressed with my explanation for the poor engagement until several weeks later. He then approached me sheepishly and said, "You'll never believe what a patient just did. In the middle of the interview he cut me off and asked me why I was frowning. My God, I must actually do it!"

One of my own habits illustrates another category of clinician movement that can become problematic. As I become anxious, I begin to twist my hair behind my ears. This nonverbal activity represents what we have discussed earlier as a displacement activity. These displacement activities can be used to monitor patient anxiety, but on the flip side, they can be a useful self-monitor, indicating anxiety in the clinician.

The clinician may not even have been aware of the presence of stress, but the appearance of numerous displacement activities warns that anxiety is present. At such points of self-awareness in the interview the clinician can explore the origins of the tension. Sometimes the interviewer is concerned about personal matters not related to the interview, including countertransference tensions. At other times the clinician may be intuitively registering patient hostility or even well-hidden psychotic process. In any case the recognition of clinician displacement activities can provide yet another avenue for understanding.

Another good reason for studying displacement activities concerns the eradication of potentially disengaging gestures. For the most part, displacement activities are natural and help to create a feeling of spontaneous communication. As such there is no need to eliminate them; indeed, they may actually foster good blending. But there exist certain displacement gestures that are porbably best eliminated. We can return to my own habit of twisting my hair. This displacement activity has the potential to be disengaging. To some patients it may appear effeminate, for as mentioned earlier women touch their hair three times more frequently than men. To others it may simply be distracting. In either case it serves no purpose and is probably best discarded.

In a similar vein, certain categories of patients may not respond well to demonstrations of increased anxiety in the clinician. The immediate category that comes to mind includes patients escalating towards violence. These patients are frequently frightened that they are about to lose control. If they see the clinician becoming progressively more tense as well, they may become even more agitated. The same holds true for paranoid patients, who may appear almost ludicrously hyperattentive to their environments. I remember an older man with marked paranoid process who once asked me why I had just scratched my head. When I said I had an itch, he did not seem particularly reassured.

Two other clinician displacement activities warrant discussion. The first activity is smoking. I personally do not believe that clinicians should smoke cigarettes or even the proverbial "Freudian pipe" while interviewing patients. My bias evolves from the feeling that smoking, at the very least, represents a possible distraction to the patient. More likely, it may sometimes actually function as an irritant. Even if one asks permission from the patient, many patients who do not like smoking may find it difficult to convey such concerns. Pipe smoking is so stereotypic of "a shrink" that it may bias transference or simply turn some patients off.

The second displacement activity is much more of a mixed blessing, for it clearly serves some useful purposes. I had never even viewed it as a displacement activity until I had asked one student what his most common displacement activities were, and he replied, "That's easy, I'm constantly scribbling notes."

There exist many good reasons for taking detailed notes, such as making process notes to be shared with a psychotherapy supervisor. On the other hand, in initial interviews I have become more and more convinced that much of note-taking represents a displacement activity that frequently distracts both the clinician and the patient. No matter how one views it, a clinician looking down at his or her clipboard while actively composing sentences cannot possibly be attending to the fine nuances of patient behavior available to the clinician with undivided attention.

Once again I am sharing a bias that some clinicians would disagree with, but I feel that note-taking should be minimized in the initial interview. It should be utilized to jot down hard-to-remember details such as dates, medication dosages, and family trees. Instead of meticulously making a transcription of the patient's words, the clinician can carefully attend to the patient directly. In particular, during the early scouting period, I believe it is far better to do little, if any, note-taking. At this early stage the emphasis should be upon actively engaging the patient. To this end, I find that patients are more responsive to clinicians who seem more interested in them than in the clinician's clipboard.

I frequently do not even pick up a clipboard until well into the interview. When I do begin to write, as a sign of respect, I often say to the patient, "I'm going to jot down a few notes to make sure I'm remembering everything correctly. Is that all right with you?" Patients seem to respond very nicely to this simple sign of courtesy. This statement of purpose also tends to decrease the paranoia that patients sometimes project onto note-taking, as they wonder if the clinician is madly analyzing their every thought and action. Along these lines, note-taking should be avoided with actively paranoid patients.

THE NONVERBAL ASPECTS OF CALMING POTENTIALLY VIOLENT PATIENTS

Interacting with a patient who is escalating towards violence presents the clinician with one of the most difficult of clinical situations. Although it would be nice to think that violent interactions are rare, the facts speak otherwise. Tardiff reports that approximately 17 percent of patients reporting to an emergency room are violent. He further reports that roughly 40 percent of psychiatrists have reported being assaulted at least once in their careers.[50]

Obviously, it is to the clinician's benefit to review the various approaches that may de-escalate an angry patient. In particular, the nonverbal characteristics of potentially violent dyads are of considerable importance, for issues concerning proxemics, kinesics, and paralanguage can all be of value in handling these situations. The interaction with the potentially violent patient provides an excellent topic with which to close this chapter, for the craft of utilizing nonverbal behavior is seldom put to a more critical test.

I would also like to emphasize that violence is frequently a dyadic process. The clinician and the patient represent a two-person system, and it is this system that becomes violent. Clinicians may inadvertently, with their nonverbal behavior, further escalate an already agitated patient. Fortunately this cycle, representing a violence reciprocal, can frequently be broken.

To begin with I am reminded of a curious story related by an anthropology professor during my undergraduate education. He described an interspecies encounter in which violence was averted by the quick thinking of a field anthropologist. This anthropologist had been extensively studying the behaviors of a baboon troop. One day he accidentally startled a mother baboon and her baby. Within seconds the squawkings of the alarmed mother attracted a swarming bevy of guard males. One can assume their intent was not of a social variety. Indeed, baboons are both intelligent and ferocious when provoked. The appearance of an ugly white ape with a mustache and safari hat was more than ample stimulus to prompt a display of their virility. Indeed, the baboons could have quickly disposed of the anthropologist.

Having observed baboons demonstrating submissive behavior

within the troop, he purposely replicated their submissive gestures, which apparently involved lowering oneself and making certain jaw movements. To his relief, the baboons grunted and snarled but waved off their attack.

Besides representing a delightful tale for college professors to relate to wide-eyed undergraduates, the above story has a valuable message. A group of animals were about to interact violently. The violence was prevented by the use of specific nonverbal behaviors, which functioned as actual nonverbal communications. Similar to these baboons the human animal possesses a repertoire of nonverbal activities and communications that signal the intent to attack and the intent to submit.

For the clinician, the signals of impending attack, when recognized in a patient, can quickly alert the clinician that something needs to be altered in the interpersonal dyad before a violence reciprocal ensues. Through a knowledge of the signals of submission, the clinician may alter behavior in a fashion that appears less threatening to the paranoid or intoxicated patient. In many instances these alterations can break the dyadic cycle of violence, as effectively as the anthropologist supplicating the baboon warriors. It should be kept in mind that in some instances no matter what preventive actions are undertaken, violence will erupt. The goal is not to eliminate violence but to decrease its likelihood.

Towards this endeavor the clinician should consider whether the clinical environment suggests that violence may be a possibility. In the first place, diagnosis can alert the clinician to an increased likelihood of aggression. Most psychotic patients are not violent, but psychotic process as manifested in schizophrenia, bipolar disorder, paranoid disorder, and other atypical psychoses may predispose the patient towards aggression, especially when paranoid delusions are simmering beneath the patient's social facade. If frightened, these paranoid patients may go to great extremes to protect themselves, as we would if we shared their vision of the world. It is always important to remember that such patients may believe that they are literally fighting for their lives.

Other types of psychosis or poor impulse control may present problems. For instance, patients suffering from organic brain disease, as seen in the frontal lobe syndrome, deliriums, and various dementias, may be predisposed towards aggression. A particular red flag should arise in the clinician's mind when interacting with people under the influence of various drugs, including speed, quaaludes, and PCP. Alcohol intoxication remains a major area in which violence erupts, especially in settings such as emergency rooms. Because we frequently deal with alcohol intoxication in social settings in our culture, it is easy to be lulled into underestimating the potential for violence when dealing with an intoxicated patient. Such patients can quickly move from jovial jesting into a fit of rage.

Diagnoses do not tell the clinician that any specific patient is about to be violent. Most people suffering from schizophrenia are not violent, but the diagnosis does alert the clinician to the possibility of aggression. This consideration may represent the first step in preventing violence. In addition, the clinician may note that a patient has a history of assaultive behavior. In such instances, the clinician is well advised to take appropriate precautions, such as having safety officers unobtrusively nearby and aware of the situation.

Besides diagnostic and historical factors, the clinician may be part of a situation in which violence is more likely. If the clinician has been asked to participate in the evaluation of a patient who is being committed involuntarily, then caution is always advised. There are probably few life situations more frightening than to have one's freedom taken away. In this situation patients should always be considered as potentially violent.

I remember one instance in our emergency room late at night. The patient, an agitated woman of about thirty, was being committed. Safety officers had been called down and were appropriately nearby. The patient appeared to have calmed and was quietly sitting with family members by her side. Everything seemed in control. The clinician began to move away from the patient and turned her back as she headed for the staff room. In a matter of seconds the patient was ferociously choking the clinician, for no apparent reason. I mention this vignette because it highlights the need to think cautiously while evaluating committed patients. It also reminds one of the old adage that one should never turn one's back on a patient, an adage as true today as when it was first coined.

One other clinical situation to keep in mind arises when patients are agitated and accompanied by family members. In such situations the clinician should attempt to determine quickly whether the family member is calming or upsetting the patient. In emergency rooms a common mistake is to not separate feuding family members until it is too late. It is often best to separate the antagonistic family members quickly, while allowing different staff members to attempt to calm and understand the perspectives of both parties.

I have strayed from the topic of nonverbal behavior. But in a practical sense, the first step in utilizing nonverbal behavior with violent patients consists of recognizing the violent situation in its infancy, not its adolescence. If the clinician is aware of the potential for violence, then the following nonverbal techniques can be brought into play.

We will first look at various nonverbal activities that may alert the clinician that violence may be incubating. Subsequently we will look at ways in which to change our own behaviors in an effort to avoid confrontation.

The signs of impending aggression can be loosely grouped into two categories, early warning signs and late warning signs. Although it is extremely difficult to predict whether a patient will engage in violence in the future, it is not particularly difficult to tell when a patient may be headed towards immediate violence.

The early warning signs consist of behaviors that suggest emerging agitation. In the simplest examples, one may notice the patient beginning to speak more quickly with a subtly angry tone of voice. These paralanguage clues may be augmented by a display of sarcastic statements or challenges, such as, "You think you're a big shot, don't you!"

These types of early warning signs may appear obvious, which is the exact reason they warrant mentioning. As clinicians we may inadvertently ignore these signs, in the process unintentionally escalating the patient. This seems to occur during periods of intense time pressure or when the clinical situation has become increasingly hectic, as in a busy emergency room. Such obstinancy can unfortunately return as an unwanted gremlin. When these early warning signs are present, it is very important to crystallize in one's mind what the patient's needs may be. If the clinician can move with the patient's needs, hostility will frequently decrease.

Kinesic early-warning signs consist of actual evidence of agitation, such as pacing and refusing to sit down. If patients refuse to sit, it is frequently useful to gently request them to return to their seat. One can use phrases such as, "It might help you to relax some if you sit over here," or "Let's sit down and see if we can sort some things out." If comments such as these fail to elicit compliance, one can more firmly state, "I'd like you to sit over here so we can talk." Some clinicians might quietly add, "It's difficult to have to keep staring up. I think we'll both be more comfortable if we sit." If these maneuvers fail, then it is probably best to let the patient walk around freely, while recognizing that this patient may be seriously impaired with regard to impulse control. In short, the patient may be on the way towards violence, and appropriate steps should be taken. If no one is aware that the clinician is alone with such a patient, it is generally best to let someone know what is going on. It is relatively easy for a clinician to make an excuse for leaving the room at such points. It may not be so easy ten minutes later.

Other kinesic early warning clues include rapid and jerky gesturing. Of particular note is the action of vigorously pointing one's finger at the clinician to "make a point." Such a gesture may be a harbinger of impending hostility. Increased and intense staring may also suggest anger. Finally, the appearance of suspiciousness or other increases in psychotic process, such as an increasing disorganization, should alert the clinician to the possibility of violence.

As a person comes closer to overt violence, specific behaviors may serve as reliable indicators that aggression is imminent. Just like the charging guard baboons with their bared teeth, humans have evolved symbolic signs of threat.

Morris has described behaviors known as intention movements.[50] These intention movements consist of those small gestures that suggest impending movement. For instance, as persons intend to rise from a chair, they frequently lean forward grasping the arms of the chair. This is a clear signal that they want to rise, signaling that the conversation is about to end. The intention movements suggesting possible violence include activities such as clenching of the fists, whitening of the knuckles as one tightly grasps an inanimate object, and even a snarling as the lips are pulled back from the teeth. People may not be as different from baboons as we would like to think.

Perhaps the most common intention movement of attack is the raising of a closed fist over the head. Overhand blows delivered from this position are the most frequent blows seen in street brawls and riots despite the unlikelihood of hurting one's opponent in this manner. This behavior may be instinctual in nature, as it is frequently seen in children who are fighting.

Morris also describes vacuum gestures, which represent completed actions but are not actually carried out on the enemy. Frequent vacuum gestures include shaking the fist, assuming a boxing stance, gesturing as if strangling the opponent, and the pounding of the fist into the opposite palm. All of these intention movements and vacuum gestures serve as late warning signals that violence is near at hand.

It should also be noted that verbal threats or statements that one is about to strike out often accompany the nonverbal behaviors described above. When the above late warning signs are present, violence is a distinct possibility. At this point an application of nonverbal skills may help prevent aggression.

Earlier, reciprocal behaviors were discussed, such as the mating reciprocal, in which two organisms engage in an orderly sequence of events leading to a final outcome. Scheflen describes dominance and submission reciprocals.[52] In our story of the baboons, the anthropologist refused to participate in the dominance reciprocal. If he had, he might very well have been killed. Instead he chose to begin the submission reciprocal, which his would-be attackers fortunately agreed to follow. In a similar fashion, humans can engage in either of these reciprocals.

When faced with a hostile patient, the trick is to avoid engaging in the dominance reciprocal while utilizing some submissive behavior. One avoids the dominance reciprocal by not demonstrating any of the early or late warning signs of aggression. Although this appears to make an obvious point, it is striking to watch the maladaptive behavior of clinicians when faced with an agitated patient. The fear generated by the patient's hostility frequently results in unconscious behaviors that may threaten the patient. The clinician's voice may be raised. At times, the actual movements of the clinician speed up as the waiting area is hurriedly cleared of furniture and other patients. Even frankly antagonistic remarks may emerge. In this respect, it is not an exaggeration to say that clinicians can actually precipitate violence.

There exist no absolute rules for interacting with a patient on the verge of violence, but some principles seem relevant. In the first place, the clinician wants to appear calm. The speaking voice should appear normal and unharried. It is particularly important to avoid speaking loudly or in an authoritarian manner. With regard to kinesics, the clinician wants to avoid an excessive display of displacement activities, which may be misinterpreted as aggressive displays. Moreover, exaggerated displacement activities may create an increasing atmosphere of fear, stoking the patient's own fears of an impending loss of control.

Eye contact should probably be decreased. And the hands should not be raised in any gesture that may signify an intent to attack or defend oneself. Curiously, some clinicians will place their hands behind their backs, a situation that may raise fears in the patient that a weapon is being hidden. With regard to posture, one can purposely stoop one's shoulders a bit in an effort to appear smaller, for humans, when about to attack, frequently raise their shoulders and chests, a bit of gorilla-like display. It is probably also wise to remain in front of the patient, for an approach from behind or from the side may startle the agitated patient.

One of the most important points concerns an issue mentioned earlier when discussing proxemics. At least one study has suggested that potentially violent patients may have significantly altered buffer zones.[53] Specifically, they will feel that their intimate body space is being invaded at distances much further away than for most people. These patients may feel that the interviewer is "in my face" while standing a full six feet away. In general, the agitated patient needs more room and interpersonal space. This can be a tough principle to remember, for some good-hearted clinicians feel a desire to calm the angry patient by touching them. This desire usually goes away after a few unfortunate encounters with feet or fists.

If these principles are followed, accompanied by an intelligent use of safety officers and medication as needed, many violent encounters can be avoided. With regard to avoiding dangerous situations, another point warrants mentioning. When sitting in a room with a patient one does not know, it is probably wise to arrange the chairs so that the clinician is closer to the doorway, while not obstructing the patient's pathway to the doorway. With this arrangement one can always get away if the patient becomes threatening or produces a weapon. It is naive to think that these situations do not arise, especially in emergency rooms. To pretend that they do not probably represents a defensive denial that prevents the clinician from fully thinking about these situations in a manner that could help prevent them in the first place.

In conclusion, nonverbal processes are core elements of human communication during violent interactions. A sound knowledge of these processes can help the clinician to calm the angry or frightened patient. Helping patients to regain a sense of internal control remains one of the fine points of the art of interviewing. It also increases the chances that the clinician will be around to practice his or her art.

Conclusion

In this chapter we have reviewed the basic principles of proxemics, kinesics, and paralanguage. It can readily be seen that these processes are at the very root of communication. As such integral parts of human interaction, they remain pivotal in bringing the initial interview to a successful conclusion.

In these first three chapters, we have reviewed many of the basic principles of both verbal and nonverbal behaviors as they apply to the initial interview. Before proceeding much further, the important topic of treatment planning warrants a thorough discussion. Such a discussion will quickly move us into some of the most complex and fascinating aspects of assessment interviewing.

References

1. Hall, E. T.: Excerpts from an interview conducted by Carol Travis, *GEO* 25(3):12, 1983.
2. Harper, R. G., Wiens, A. N., and Matarazzo, J. D.: *Nonverbal Communication: The State of the Art.* New York, John Wiley and Sons, 1978.
3. Wiener, M., Devoe, S., Rubinow, S., and Geller, J.: Nonverbal behavior and nonverbal communication. *Psychological Review* 79:185–214, 1972.
4. Edinger, J. A., and Patterson, M. L.: Nonverbal involvement and social control. *Psychology Bulletin* 93(1):30–56, 1983.
5. Morris, D.: *Manwatching, A Field Guide to Human Behavior.* New York, Harry N. Abrahms, Inc., 1977.
6. Hall, E. T.: *The Hidden Dimension.* New York, Doubleday and Company, 1966.
7. Watson, O. M., and Graves, T. D.: Quantitative research in proxemic behavior. *American Anthropologist* 68:971–985, 1966.
8. Sue, D. W., and Sue, D.: Barrier to effective cross-cultural counseling. *Journal of Counseling Psychology* 24(5):420–429, 1977.
9. Baxter, J. C.: Interpersonal spacing in natural settings. *Sociometry* 33:444–456, 1970.
10. Wiens, A. N.: The assessment interview. In *Clinical Methods in Psychology,* edited by Irving Weiner. New York, John Wiley and Sons, 1976.
11. Knapp, M. L.: *Nonverbal Communication in Human Interaction.* New York, Holt, Rinehart, and Winston, 1972.
12. Birdwhistell, M. L.: *Introduction to Kinesis: An Annotation System for Analysis of Body Motion and Gesture.* Louisville, Kentucky, University of Louisville Press, 1952.

13. Harper, R. G., 1978, p. 123.
14. Scheflen, A. E.: *Body Language and Social Order.* Englewood Cliffs, N. J., Prentice-Hall, Inc., 1972.
15. Freud, S.: Fragment of an analysis of a case of hysteria. In *Collected Papers* (Vol. 3). New York, Barri Books, 1959 (originally published in 1925).
16. Carmier, W. H., and Carmier, L. A.: *Interviewing Strategies for Helpers, A Guide to Assessment, Treatment and Evaluation.* California, Brooks/Cole Publishing Company, 1979.
17. Wiens, A. N., 1976, p. 27.
18. Sue, D. W., 1977, p. 427.
19. Hill, Sir Denis: Non-Verbal Behavior in Mental Illness. *British Journal of Psychiatry.* 24:221–230, 1974.
20. Hill, Sir Denis, 1974, p. 227.
21. Wiens, A. N., 1976, p. 33.
22. Morris, D., 1977, p. 75.
23. Scheflen, A. E., 1972, p. 46.
24. Morris, D., 1977, p. 164.
25. Morris, D., 1977, p. 165.
26. Pansa-Hendersen, M., De L'Horne, D. J., and Jones, I. H.: Nonverbal behavior as a supplement to psychiatric diagnosis in schizophrenia, depression, and anxiety neurosis. *Journal of Psychiatric Treatment and Evaluation 43:489–496, 1982.*
27. Jones, I. H., and Pansa, M.: Some nonverbal aspects of depression and schizophrenia during the interview. *The Journal of Nervous and Mental Disease* 167(7):402–409, 1979.
28. Pansa-Henderson, 1982, p. 495.
29. Jones, I. H., 1979, pp. 402–409.
30. Morris, D., 1977, p. 181.
31. Morris, D., 1977, p. 109.
32. Ekman, P., and Friesen, W. V.: Detecting deception from the body or face. *Journal of Personality and Social Psychology,* 29(3):288–298, 1974.
33. Ekman, P.: *Telling Lies. Clues to Deceit in the Marketplace, Politics, and Marriage.* New York, W. W. Norton and Company, 1985.
34. Littlepage, G. E., and Pineault, M. A.: Detection of deceptive factual statements from the body and face. *Personality and Social Psychology Bulletin* 53(5):325–328, 1979.
35. McClintock, C. C., and Hung, R. G.: Nonverbal indicators of affect and deception in an interview setting. *Journal of Applied Social Psychology* 5:54–67, 1975.
36. Edinger, J. A., 1983, pp. 42–43.
37. Kraut, R. E.: Verbal and nonverbal cues in the perception of lying. *Journal of Personality and Social Psychology* 36:380–391, 1978.
38. Grinder, J., and Bandler, R.: *The Structure of Magic II.* California, Science and Behavior Books, Inc., 1976.
39. Scheflen, A. E.: *Body Language and Social Order.* Englewood Cliffs, N. J., Prentice-Hall, Inc., 1972.
40. Scheflen, A. E., 1972, p. 16.
41. Morris, D., 1977, p. 102.
42. Morris, D., 1977, p. 102.
43. Egan, G.: *The Skilled Helper: A Model for Systematic Helping and Interpersonal Relating.* California, Brocks/Cole Publishing Company.
44. Wiens, A. N., 1976, p. 35.
45. Sue, D. W., 1977, pp. 420–429.
46. Morris, D., 1977, p. 83.
47. La Crosse, M. B.: Nonverbal behavior and perceived counselor attractiveness and persuasiveness. *Journal of Counseling Psychology* 19:417–424, 1972.
48. Haase, R. F., and Tepper, D.: Nonverbal component of empathetic communication. *Journal of Counseling Psychology* 19:417–424, 1972.
49. Morris, D., 1977, p. 68.
50. Tardiff, K.: The violent patient. In *Manual of Psychiatric Consultation and Emergency Care,* edited by F. Guggenheim and M. Weiner. New York, Jason Aronson Inc., 1984.
51. Morris, D., 1977, p. 173.
52. Scheflen, A. E., 1977, p. 173.
53. Wiens, A. N., 1976, p. 28.

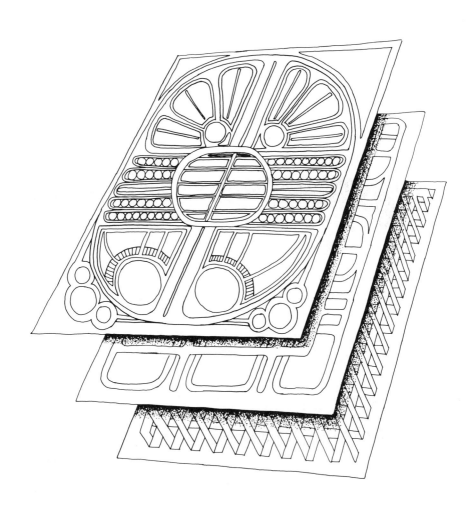

4

The Treatment Plan:
Listening to the Data Base

We shall not cease from exploration
And the end of all our exploring
Will be to arrive where we started
And know the place for the first time.
T. S. Eliot, Little Gidding

In the first three chapters we examined a variety of principles fundamental to the development of the verbal tapestry we call an assessment interview. We focused upon both verbal and nonverbal skills, exploring proxemics, kinesics, facilics, and blending techniques. The interviewer is now faced with the challenging task of resourcefully utilizing the carefully procured information.

One of the most pressing problems for the assessment interviewer remains the need to organize data so that it can be transformed into an effective initial treatment plan or triage decision. To develop a viable plan, the clinician must first recognize which treatment modalities are potentially available for the unique needs of the patient at hand.

Frequently I have seen clinicians falter, not because they lack adequate knowledge about the use of specific treatment modalities, but because the use of certain modalities never comes to mind. They become lost in the data base, emphasizing certain information while ignoring, or not even obtaining, other pertinent data. We are dealing with an information processing problem, a not unexpected dilemma considering the vastness of the information involved in understanding another person's problems.

By way of example, one such instance that comes to mind concerns a clinician who might select an antipsychotic medication for a person suffering from an acute psychotic breakdown. Suppose for a moment that the clinician has not involved the patient's family in the reasoning behind the use of such a medication. Suppose further that the family has a deep-rooted bias that drugs are not good for people. When this patient returns home, there exists a significant chance that the patient's family will support or even instigate noncompliance with the medication. In this instance the family system was ignored during the development of the treatment plan. The result is both disappointing and predictable. More importantly, it is potentially preventable.

In this chapter we will study a common-sense approach to creating a realistic list of viable treatment options. No attempt is made to suggest the pros and cons of any specific treatment; rather the focus is upon making the transition from the interview itself to the initial stage of treatment planning. This is a chapter devoted to a discussion of the process of clinical thinking, based upon the idea that one cannot truly understand how to interview if one does not understand the reason for the interview.

This chapter also demonstrates that the treatment opportunities that come to mind for the clinician appear to be directly related to both the data collected and the method of organizing this data. For example, a clinician who does not learn to ask questions concerning symptoms suggestive of a drug-responsive depression will most likely not think to utilize such a medication. Likewise, a clinician is less likely to think of intervening via social work channels if current stressors are ignored.

To avoid such tunnel vision, clinicians can organize their data into schemata that emphasize conceptualization from multiple viewpoints. In this chapter we will look at three such systems. Through them the power of a well-organized data base to lead to effective treatment planning will become apparent. In an ironic sense, the art of treatment planning returns us to our original starting point, the data gleaned from the initial interview itself. As T. S. Eliot suggested in our opening quotation, significant insight can be gained by learning to listen more openly to what is already familiar.

We shall look at the following three assessment perspectives: (1) the diagnostic perspective provided by the third edition of the Diagnostic and Statistical Manual of Mental Disorders (DSM-III), and its revision, DSM-III-R,[2] (2) the systems analysis perspective, and (3) the perspective provided by understanding the "core pains" of the patient. Although overlapping at their interfaces, each of these perspectives generates unique clues for treatment planning. Consequently it is expedient to create an initial treatment plan utilizing all three perspectives. I have found single-perspective treatment planning unsatisfactory, akin to beginning a watercolor with only half the needed paints.

Each of the three assessment perspectives provides the following approaches for usefully organizing clinical information:

1. An easy and rapid method of checking, during the interview itself, whether pertinent data regions have been explored.

2. A reliable method of reminding the clinician to borrow from different data perspectives when formulating a treatment plan.

3. A flexible approach to actually delineating a list of potential treatment modalities.

4. A method that the therapist can use during the ongoing treatment of the patient in order to review treatment planning, as well as generating new ideas when treatment has reached a setback or an impasse.

The chapter will begin by reviewing a data base gleaned from an actual initial interview. Following this presentation the information from each of the three perspectives mentioned above will be examined, observing the utility provided by each viewpoint.

CASE PRESENTATION

When I first saw Miss Baker she was sitting in the waiting room. Her eyes were hiding behind a pair of large, pink-framed sun glasses. These frames were rimmed by her shortly bobbed brown hair. She had a round face and a rather short frame. She was wearing a T-shirt and a pair of freshly washed jeans. Around her left wrist a wide leather band was wrapped with the name Paul tooled into it.

When I asked if she was Miss Baker she pertly looked up, smiled and replied, "Yes, I'm Miss Baker but not for long." I asked what she meant, and she replied, "Oh, I'm getting married in a month to another woman."

Once in my office she related a story of a longstanding problem with fluctuating moods. She spoke in a quiet voice, frequently casting her eyes to the floor, as if to avoid seeing the impact of her words upon my face. She displayed no evidence of loose associations, thought blocking, pressured speech, or flight of ideas. She gave no evidence of responding to hallucinations and denied both auditory and visual hallucinations.

With regard to her moodiness, she stated that her moods frequently changed throughout the day. It was not at all unusual for her to feel various moods, including anger and rejection, during the course of a single day. Although she reported intermittent periods of feeling decreased energy, decreased interest in activities, decreased libido, and difficulty falling asleep, she denied any periods of two weeks or more in which these symptoms were persistent. She denied manic or hypomanic symptoms past or present.

She lived in a world of imagined fear, persistently worried that she would be abandoned. At nights she would become angered if her partner fell asleep first, for she would quickly become engulfed by her fear of being alone. These fears fostered an intense dependency, which she readily admitted was a major handicap. She went out of her way to please her partner, allowing all major decisions to be made by her, including the upcoming wedding plans. This dependency also surfaced with the string of therapists lying in her wake. Her most recent therapist had had her forcibly removed from his office by the police, an act marking the end of their contact.

As one might have surmised, impulse control was not a strong point. For instance, several years earlier she had managed to toss a picnic table bench through a friend's picture window while enraged. Moreover, she had a history of popping pills in small suicidal gestures about every two to three months over the past three years.

Her relationship with her parents was very strained, and she felt she had always been marked as the black sheep of the family. She had one sister two years older than she who was employed as an accountant and was reported as happily married. One of her earliest memories was of standing behind the front door weeping as her father walked away down the stone path. As she cried her mother shook her violently, pulling her away from the doorway.

To my surprise, the wristband bearing the name Paul had nothing to do with past or present friends or lovers. Instead it referred to herself, for she often fantasized that she was Paul Newman. This vivid fantasy game was fostered by her partner, who would call her Paul, relating to her in this pseudo-identity. At no time did Miss Baker lose sight that this was merely a fantasy, although she longed to be anyone but herself. When talking of her fantasy identities, she would occasionally cry softly, as if punctuating her story with tears.

THE DIAGNOSTIC PERSPECTIVE OF DSM-III AND DSM-III-R

General Diagnostic Principles

For clinicians diagnosis serves one major purpose: to discover information that may lead to more effective methods of helping the patient. A diagnostic schema provides this avenue by allowing clinicians and researchers the opportunity to share their experiences in a common language. For example, when a clinician discovers a treatment plan that is useful in relieving a resistant major depression, these findings may be applicable to a patient being treated by a fellow clinician, who might benefit from the shared knowledge. Diagnosis should not be an intellectual game or a pastime used to placate insurance companies. It is a practical passport to the knowledge housed in journals, books, and the minds of our fellow clinicians.

Like the common language we have developed for discussing the interviewing process, diagnosis allows one to conceptualize more clearly. In particular, diagnosis can provide valuable information concerning prognosis, possible treatment modalities, and pitfalls to be avoided in dealing with certain syndromes. For these reasons the art of diagnostic formulation remains of pivotal importance to the initial interviewer. Basic triage decisions may be dependent upon the diagnostic assessment.

In particular, diagnoses can be valuable in suggesting possible treatment modalities. For instance, major depressions frequently respond to antidepressants. Bipolar disorder (manic phase) is usually approached with lithium, antipsychotic medications, or sometimes antiseizure medications such as carbamazepine. Phobias are frequently alleviated by using behavioral techniques. Milder forms of major depression can be approached using dynamic and cognitive psychotherapies, behavioral approaches, or numerous counseling techniques. The above list merely represents a terse survey, but it nevertheless highlights the power of a diagnostic system to help in developing a diverse treatment approach.

A clinical vignette will make this abstract discussion more concrete. I was working with a couple whose marriage was riddled with a nasty streak of passive aggression and strained communication. After several sessions the marital therapy seemed to be bogging down. The husband, a rather narcissistic man, kept insisting that nothing was being done for him. In reviewing my notes I discovered that the referring clinician had diagnosed the husband as suffering from a dysthymic disorder. To my surprise I had recently read an article in which certain types of dysthymic disorders responded well to antidepressant medication.[2] My patient fit one of these descriptions and consequently was begun on an appropriate antidepressant. He quickly found significant relief. Moreover, to the chagrin of both the patient and his spouse, their marital friction remained painfully present. Up to this point he had balked at couples therapy, for he felt that it was his depression that was causing all the problems. Now he realized the relationship itself needed attention. He no longer had an excuse for avoiding the work of therapy, thanks to the antidepressant, and suddenly the marital therapy could move ahead more effectively.

This vignette illustrates the power of a common diagnostic language to provide a clinician with knowledge discovered by others. Without the diagnostic label, this learning would have been unavailable.

Before proceeding it seems expedient to review some of the important limitations of diagnostic approaches, such as the DSM-III and its revision DSM-III-R. Only through a knowledge of a system's weaknesses can its strengths be utilized safely.

One of the most obvious limitations remains the fact that diagnoses are labels. As labels they can be abused. One such abuse occurs when clinicians fall into the trap of using diagnoses as stereotypical explanations for human behavior. It should be remembered that a diagnosis provides no particular knowledge about any given patient. It merely suggests possible characteristics that may or may not be generalizable to the patient in question.

Moreover, diagnostic formulations are evolving processes and as such should be periodically re-examined. There is a realistic danger that patients can become stuck with inappropriate diagnoses, a problem that can only be avoided through persistent reappraisal. In a similar fashion the clinician should remain healthily aware of the potential ramifications of certain diagnostic labels with regard to the patient's culture and family. By way of example the label schizophrenia can result in the loss of a job or in the development of a scapegoating process within a given family. Considerations of these problematic aspects of diagnosis should be integral parts of sound clinical care.

The issue of the significance of a specific diagnostic label to the patient himself or herself can be of marked importance. For this reason I frequently ask patients if anyone has given them a diagnosis in the past. If the answer is a "yes," one can follow with questions such as, "What is your understanding of the word schizophrenia?" or "Do you think that diagnosis is right?" The answers to these questions can provide valuable insights into the patient's self-image, intellectual level, and previous care.

One of the most important considerations remains the necessity of reminding oneself that a correct diagnosis does not necessarily give one much information about the patient as a unique individual. Other conceptualizations must be used to provide this critical understanding, as we shall discuss later in this chapter and throughout the remainder of this book.

With these ideas in mind we can now explore the DSM-III-R in more detail. The DSM-III introduced many of the innovations such as multi-axial formulation discussed below in 1980. In 1987 the revised edition, known as the DSM-III-R, was published and will be the focus of our subsequent discussion. We will not attempt to review diagnostic criteria, for these are discussed in subsequent chapters. Instead we will look at the principles that help make diagnostic formulation possible in the first fifty minutes.

Multiaxial Formulation

One of the most useful aspects of the DSM-III-R is the fact that the system pushes the clinician to consider various perspectives while formulating a diagnostic picture. Each perspective is placed upon one of five axes, which in a simplified version appear as follows in the DSM-III-R:

Axis I: All clinical syndromes and V codes except for personality disorders and developmental disorders

Axis II: Personality disorders and developmental disorders

Axis III: Physical disorders and conditions

Axis IV: Severity of psychosocial stressors

Axis V: Global assessment of functioning

Axis I

At first glance Axis I may appear confusing because of the large number of diagnostic entities it contains. But there is little need for concern. The craft lies in approaching the task by first uncovering the general diagnostic probabilities and then delineating the specific diagnoses (see Figure 4).

As the initial interviewer listens during the opening phase and the body of the interview, the symptoms of the patient will suggest diagnostic regions worthy of more elaborate expansion. This primary delineation will lead the clinician to one or more of the following easily remembered regions:

1. Mood disorders
2. Schizophrenia and related disorders
3. Anxiety disorders
4. Organic disorders (including dementia and delirium)
5. Alcohol and drug abuse disorders
6. Somatoform disorders (such as hypochondriasis)
7. Adjustment disorders
8. Other miscellaneous disorders (such as sexual disorders, factitious disorders, and impulse control disorders)
9. No disorder
10. V codes

Looked at in this simplified fashion the first step in utilizing the DSM-III-R appears considerably more manageable than at first glance. In order to succeed, the clinician must be well grounded in psychopathology, as will be discussed in the following chapters. This knowledge base will allow the interviewer to quickly determine which of the ten areas are most pertinent. As the interview proceeds the clinician can reflect upon whether each of these broad areas has at least been considered, thus avoiding errors of omission.

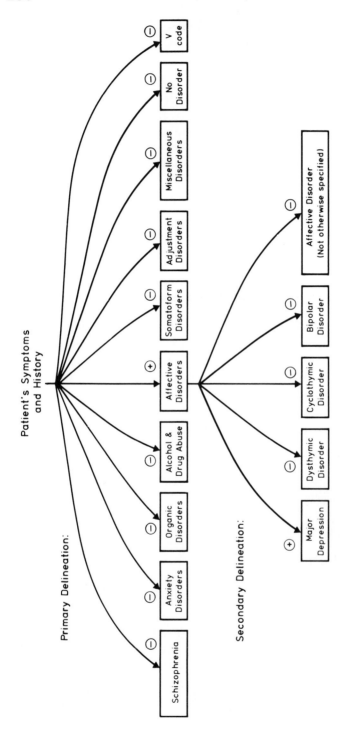

FIGURE 4. *Basic approach to diagnostic utilization (patient with a major depression).*

Once the primary delineation has been made, the interviewer can proceed with the secondary delineation, in which the specific diagnoses subsumed under the broad diagnostic areas are explored and the more exact DSM-III-R differential diagnosis is determined. Thus, if the clinician suspects a mood disorder, the clinician will eventually hunt for criteria substantiating specific affective diagnoses such as major depression, bipolar disorder, dysthymia, cyclothymia, bipolar disorder not otherwise specified, and depressive disorder not otherwise specified. This secondary delineation would be performed in each broad diagnostic area deemed pertinent.

As already described in Chapter 2, these explorations occur during the main body of the interview. Most importantly, they are done in a highly flexible fashion, always patterning the questioning in the fashion most compatible with the needs of the patient and the clinical situation. Consequently the clinician expands these diagnostic regions in a unique fashion with each patient, mixing them with various other content regions and process regions. When done well, the result is an interview that feels unstructured to the patient, yet delineates an accurate diagnosis.

The No Disorder category serves as a timely reminder to the clinician to always look for the strengths and normal coping mechanisms of the patient. Too many clinicians fall into the biasing perspective of only "seeing with the eyes of psychopathology" as opposed to the equally important "eyes of health."

V codes represent conditions not attributable to a mental disorder that have nevertheless become a focus of therapeutic intervention. Examples include academic problems, occupational problems, uncomplicated bereavement, noncompliance with medical treatment, marital problems, parent-child problems, and others. Sometimes these codes are used because no mental disorder is present, and the patient is coping with one of the stresses just listed. They can also be used if the clinician feels that not enough information is available to rule out a psychiatric syndrome, but, in the meantime, an area for specific intervention is being highlighted. Finally, these V codes can be used with a patient who carries a specific psychiatric syndrome but for whom that syndrome is not the immediate problem or the focus of intervention. For example, an individual with chronic schizophrenia in remission may present with marital distress.

Axis II

Axis II emphasizes the realization that all of the Axis I diagnoses exist in the unique psychological milieu we call personality. Indeed, many mental health problems are primarily related to the vicissitudes of personality development. Moreover, the underlying personality of the patient can greatly affect the manner in which we choose to relate to the patient both in the initial interview and in subsequent therapy. Consequently it is expedient to conceptualize which personality characteristics have evolved in any given interviewee.

The basic approach to diagnosis follows the same two-step delineation discussed for Axis I. In the first delineation one asks whether the interviewee's story suggests evidence of long-term interpersonal dysfunction that has remained relatively consistent from adolescence onwards. If so, the patient may very well fulfill the criteria for a personality disorder or disorders.

After determining that a personality disorder may very well be present, the clinician proceeds with the secondary delineation in which specific regions of personality diagnoses are expanded. This secondary delineation will result in the generation of a differential from the following list:

1. Paranoid personality disorder
2. Schizoid personality disorder
3. Schizotypal personality disorder
4. Histrionic personality disorder
5. Narcissistic personality disorder
6. Antisocial personality disorder
7. Borderline personality disorder
8. Avoidant personality disorder
9. Dependent personality disorder
10. Compulsive personality disorder
11. Passive-aggressive personality disorder
12. Personality disorder, not otherwise specified (NOS)

In Chapter 7 we will examine in great detail the many fascinating subtleties involved in exploring personality structure during an initial interview. But at this point I would like to mention an often forgotten point. In many cases the interviewee will not demonstrate psychopathology warranting the diagnosis of a personality disorder. Instead, he or she will possess traits (sometimes adaptive in nature) found in these disorders in smaller degrees. The DSM-III-R is very flexible in such cases, allowing the clinician to simply list the traits that are present. One might simply write on Axis II that "the patient displayed some histrionic and paranoid traits."

Besides personality traits, on Axis II the clinician may also list specific defense mechanisms, which may be pertinent with regard to future treatment. These defense mechanisms range from those commonly seen in neurotic disorders such as rationalization and intellectualization to those seen in more severe disorders such as denial, projection, and splitting. These defense mechanisms are defined in Appendix C of the DSM-III-R.

It should be noted that Axis II was further revised in DSM-III-R to include all forms of developmental delay. Mental retardation is included on this axis as well as specific developmental disorders such as a developmental reading disorder or an articulation disorder. Also included on this axis are the more debilitating pervasive developmental disorders such as infantile autism.

Axis III

On this axis the clinician considers the role of physical disorders and conditions. Stated differently, this axis reminds the clinician to adopt a holistic approach to the patient, one in which both the patient's mind and the patient's body are considered as parts of the same organism.

I do not think this axis can be emphasized too much. In my opinion all patients who exhibit psychological complaints for an extended time period should be evaluated by a physician to rule out any underlying physiologic condition or causative agent. To not perform this examination is to risk a real disservice to the patient, for entities such as endocrine disorders and malignancies can easily present with psychological symptoms.

In this same light a medical review of systems and a past medical history should become a standard part of an initial assessment. Other physical conditions that are not diseases may also provide important information concerning the holistic state of the interviewee. For instance, it is relevant to know if the interviewee is pregnant or a trained athlete, for these conditions may point towards germane psychological issues.

Axis IV

This axis concerns itself with an examination of the current stresses affecting the interviewee. It examines the crucial interaction between the patient and the environment in which he or she lives. All too often interviewers are swept away by diagnostic intrigues and fail to uncover the reality-based problems confronting the patient. These reality-based concerns frequently suggest avenues for therapeutic intervention.

By way of illustration, on this axis the interviewer may discover that secondary to a job lay-off, the home of the patient is about to be foreclosed. Such information may suggest the need to help the patient make contact with a specific social agency or may suggest the utility of a referral to a social worker.

This axis also remains of paramount importance in crisis intervention. Any time a patient presents in crisis, it is generally useful to determine what perceived stressors have brought the patient to the point of seeking professional help. A question such as the following is often useful, "What stresses have you been coping with recently?" or "What thoughts made you decide to actually come here tonight as opposed to coming tomorrow or some other time?" In any case the fourth axis provides another pathway for both understanding and treatment planning.

Axis V

A variety of changes were made in Axis V when the DSM-III was revised into the DSM-III-R. In DSM-III this axis solely differentiated the highest functioning of the patient over a two-month period in the preceding year. This relatively narrow perspective did not provide an abundance of practical information. Consequently, in DSM-III-R this axis was broadened. It now includes not only a rating of the highest functioning in the past year but also a rating of the current functioning, which provides immediate data pertinent to treatment planning and the decision as to whether hospitalization is warranted. These ratings are to be made by combining both symptoms and occupational and interpersonal functioning on a ninety-point scale, the Global Assessment Functioning Scale (GAF Scale).

The first rating, the highest level of functioning in the past year which is sustained for at least a two month period, may help to predict ultimate outcome, for some clinicians feel that higher levels of recent functioning may suggest somewhat better hopes prognostically. Probably of more practical importance to the clinician is the window that this axis opens onto the patient's adaptive skills and coping mechanisms.

Access to this axis can be made with questions such as, "In the past year what two months were best for you?" or "If you were forced to relive two months from the last year, which two months would you choose to go through again?"

The following inquiries, including both open and closed-ended questions, can help the clinician uncover coping skills possessed by the patient:

a. When you are functioning well, what do you do to help yourself relax?

   b. What kinds of things do you like to do in your spare time?
   c. How do you go about making important decisions in your life?
   d. What are some of your hobbies?
   e. How many people have you shared your problems with? (This question may indirectly give the clinician some views on the patient's communication skills and his or her support systems.)
   f. Do you enjoy sports or dancing?
   g. Do you enjoy reading or the arts?
   h. Have you ever kept a journal?
   i. If someone asked you to list two of your best skills or talents, what would you say?

These types of questions may uncover important coping skills of a patient in crisis. For instance one might discover that a patient has frequently kept a journal or diary as a method of sorting out problems. The clinician might use this information to remind the patient of past successes in dealing with problems, thus helping the patient to regain confidence. The clinician may also choose to have the patient solve problems, using his or her journal, before the next session, a therapeutic technique that will utilize the patient's natural skills while rekindling feelings of mastery during a time of crisis.

The second rating, a global assessment of current functioning, pushes the clinician to carefully review evidence of immediate coping skills as affected by symptomatology. It is important to utilize behavioral incidents in this exploration, for patients, if asked for opinions, may give very misleading answers. By way of example, an acutely psychotic patient, who does not want to enter the hospital, may reply with a simple "not often" when asked, "Are the voices bothering you frequently?" Utilizing a behavioral incident approach, the clinician may find that the dialogue develops more along the following lines:

Clin.: Looking at the last two days, how many times have you heard the voices per day, a hundred times, ten times?
Pt.: (Pausing and glancing away for a moment) Probably, well . . . maybe a good 50 times a day.
Clin.: What types of things do they say?
Pt.: (Pause) They tell me I'm ugly.
Clin.: What do you feel when the voices say mean things like that to you?
Pt.: It hurts, but I try to push them out of mind.
Clin.: Do they ever tell you to hurt yourself?
Pt.: You could say that.
Clin.: What exactly do they tell you?

Using the behavioral incident technique, the clinician has found not only that the voices are bothersome but also that they are quite frequent.

Also keep in mind with regard to current functioning that sources outside the patient, such as family and friends, frequently provide more valid information than the patient. Once again, when questioning collaborative sources, behavioral incidents should be elicited to ensure validity.

Case Application of DSM-III-R

To begin using our first assessment perspective, DSM-III-R, we must first organize our data axis by axis. We will then ask ourselves what if any treatment modalities are suggested by the diagnoses we have generated. With regard to the first axis, Miss Baker's presentation suggests several diagnostic entities. The first delineation suggests that her symptoms are those of some type of mood disorder. Regarding the secondary delineation into the specific mood disorders present, she does not appear to currently fit the criteria for a major depression, but she may represent a variant of dysthymia. As mentioned earlier the presence of this disorder might suggest the use of an antidepressant. Dysthymia can also be approached using a variety of psychotherapeutic modalities, including behavioral techniques.

Her history suggests no strong evidence for entities such as schizophrenia or other psychotic processes, although the clinician may want to explore her vivid fantasy productions in more detail to rule out the possibility of delusional material. There is no evidence on Axis I of delirium or dementia. One area not well explored is the area of anxiety disorders, and in a later interview this omission should be corrected.

Along Axis II several possibilities are emerging, which may provide important clues as to how to proceed. Many of her symptoms, such as her deep fears of abandonment and being alone, suggest the possibility of the diagnosis of a borderline personality and perhaps a dependent personality. Both of these diagnoses serve to warn the clinician that Miss Baker may be predisposed to becoming overly dependent upon the clinician. Dependency issues may be important areas for focus in the upcoming therapy. Also of importance is the fact that a large body of literature exists concerning the treatment of the borderline personality, a literature that can be easily tapped by the clinician. As a triage agent, the diagnostic label of a borderline personality may also suggest the wisdom of not assigning this patient to a newly trained or poorly skilled therapist, for such patients are frequently difficult to manage. On this axis one might further explore entities such as a histrionic personality, a schizotypal personality, or an antisocial personality.

An exploration of Axis III brings many important points to mind. In the first place Miss Baker's depressive symptoms suggest the possibility of an organic affective disorder. She needs a medical examination. If the initial clinician is a psychiatrist, then this clinician has omitted a good medical review of systems. This omission, brought to our attention by the use of Axis III, will need to be rectified. Pertinent lab work will be ordered, and a physical exam may be indicated.

But the value of Axis III does not end here. The history of episodic violence may suggest an underlying seizure disorder that has been routinely missed by previous clinicians. Once again the interviewer will want to ask questions pertinent to this diagnosis and may consider ordering an EEG. Her worsening of symptoms near her menstrual periods also adds the possibility of a premenstrual syndrome, which may suggest the use of medications such as motrin to relieve cramping and an antianxiety agent used for a day or two near her periods to decrease her premenstrual tension.

A final consideration on Axis III concerns Miss Baker's obesity. One wonders whether there may be an organic etiology for her obesity as well as whether her weight represents a powerful psychological concern, which she was hesitant to discuss.

Axis IV provides further pertinent information. In particular, one questions what the impact of the upcoming wedding will be. Even for the most stable of people, weddings are far from unstressful. A review of this axis also indicates that the interviewer has not explored stressors very well yet. With regard to triage and the determination of when this patient should be seen next, it would be useful for the interviewer to have a much clearer picture of the current stressors.

As we end our survey of this perspective, we come to the global assessment of adaptive functioning as delineated on Axis V. A clear concept of the best two months of functioning is not readily apparent. In a practical sense this means that the interviewer lacks a well-defined picture of the course of Miss Baker's problems. One does not know whether she is currently getting worse or better or is about the same. A more thorough examination of current functioning would be of value in determining disposition. One also wonders what skills she may possess, which may be utilized in her treatment. For instance, her overactive fantasy life, if toned down, may represent a fertile imagination, which could be an asset in her development as an individual.

The above discussion illustrates the immense power the DSM-III-R represents as a method of organizing data in a fashion that generates treatment options. But this assessment perspective alone yields an incomplete picture. It is now time to move to a different framework with which to understand the problems facing Miss Baker.

SYSTEMS ANALYSIS

Nothing exists in isolation. Whether a cell or a person, every system is influenced by the configuration of the systems of which each is a part, that is, by its environment.

George L. Engel

Basic Paradigm

Systems analysis provides a stimulating method of organizing and utilizing the data gained from the initial interview. In this perspective one conceptualizes the patient not as a static "thing" with permanent characteristics but rather as an intertwining series of processes. Each process or system offers a potential wedge for therapeutic intervention.

George Engel, an internist with many interests in psychosomatic medicine, has been an elegant proponent of utilizing the systems approach.[3] Many of the following ideas parallel his thinking, although the subsequent paradigm is simpler, having been developed specifically for use in conceptualizing data for mental health assessments.

In this approach each person is viewed as representing the conjunction of seven progressively larger systems. These seven systems include (1) the physiological system, (2) the psychological system, (3) the dyadic system, (4) the family system, (5) the group system, (6) the societal system, and (7) the existential system: the patient's framework for meaning. Each smaller system is subsumed by the system above it. Like the axes of the DSM-III-R, each of these systems can be used as a level at which to organize data and subsequently develop a list of potential treatment modalities, each system providing a clarifying lens through which to understand the patient. These seven systems are illustrated in Figure 5.

The Physiological System

On the first level, the interviewer focuses upon the physiological make-up of the patient. This system is identical to the third axis of DSM-III-R. In it the clinician hunts for evidence of medical illness as well as the presence of symptoms suggesting that somatic treatments may be of value. The clinician reviews whether any investigations or interventions can be made at the physiological level. Investigations may include entities such as lab tests, CT scans, EEGs, or a physical exam. Physiologic interventions could include antidepressants, antipsychotics, other medications, relaxation techniques, meditational

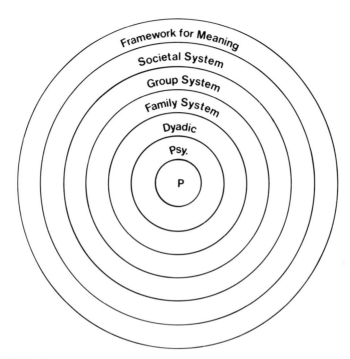

FIGURE 5. Systems analysis. P = physiological system; Psy = psychological system.

techniques, or ECT. The main point centers upon an active inquiry into the workings of the patient's body as well as the patient's mind.

With regard to the physiological system, an analysis of Miss Baker remains essentially unchanged from our discussion with regards to axis III. In this instance there exists a direct overlap between the DSM-III and systems analysis.

The Psychological System

In the second system, the psychological system, one enters an area which only partially overlaps the DSM-III-R as reflected by considerations of personality development on Axis II. Consequently, it is an exploration ripe with implications. At this level the clinician attempts to understand the patient both in a phenomenological sense as a unique human being and in a psychodynamic sense as a product of past development. Each interviewer will have preferences for which psychological theories seem relevant, whether they be Freudian, Jungian, Rogerian, or some combination of the numerous viewpoints available. But the important point remains that the clinician attempts to understand the patient in a human context and not merely as a diagnostic entity. In this system perspective interviewers expand their lists of treatment options by considering the use of individual psychotherapies or counseling techniques.

As the psychological system is reviewed a more personalized view of Miss Baker emerges as she becomes at once more complicated and more human. Several conflictual issues are readily apparent, including (1) fears of abandonment, (2) problems with anger and impulse control, (3) ongoing problems with low self-esteem, (4) suicidal gestures, and (5) problems with identity and a sense of self. By delineating these areas the clinician can begin to generate further options for treatment. For example, her problems with anger and impulse control could be approached using behavioral modification, perhaps training her to self-monitor behaviors suggesting that an angry outburst is imminent, at which point alternate ways of relieving her hostile tension could be implemented. From a different perspective, an analytic viewpoint, one could look at her disturbances in her sense of self as indicating the need for specific psychotherapeutic approaches developed by clinicians such as Kohut, Kernberg, or Masterson.

Furthermore, a survey of the information known at this level reveals that not much psychogenetic data has been garnered yet, a deficit that can be tended to in future sessions. The important point remains that by conceptualizing in the psychological system interviewers prompt themselves to consider areas of intervention utilizing individual psychotherapy, as well as checking to see if this region of highly pertinent information has been adequately tapped.

The Dyadic System

When we move to the third level, the dyadic system, the patient is viewed as one component of the numerous two-person interactions that fill the patient's daily interactions. The patient's interpersonal skills are assessed. For instance, does the patient have adequate verbal skills and social skills? Some patients suffering from schizophrenia may act oddly or may share their delusions with others without realizing the disengaging impact of these activities. Such patients may benefit from social skills training. In a similar vein, retarded patients represent another category of patients with whom social skills training with kits such as TIPPS may yield gratifying results. The interviewer should also bear in mind that the patient's interaction with the interviewer provides direct and immediate information concerning this system. Unfortunately this arena is frequently overlooked by clinicians. Utilizing the systems approach helps to prevent this important omission.

In the case of Miss Baker the dyadic system focuses attention on her style of relating to other individuals. One wonders if her angry outbursts may be reactions to a chronic style of passively deferring to the needs of others. Such a situation may suggest the utility of self-assertiveness training.

This system refocuses attention on the impact of the patient's physical appearance and behavior. Miss Baker's loud sunglasses and old T-shirt, coupled with her obesity, may indeed strike an unappreciative chord upon first contact. Miss Baker may be unaware of the ramifications of her behavior, and social skills training may be useful at some point. In the end all of these interpersonal issues are of relevance to her relationship with her lover, an appropriate invitation to the next level of analysis, the family.

The Family System

As we look at the fourth system, the family, we come upon one of the most powerful systems affecting all humans. To conceptualize patients without considering the dynamics of their family is to see half a picture at best. To plan treatment without considering the needs and opinions of the patient's family may represent an invitation to treatment failure.

Moreover, whether interviewers like to admit it or not, the patient's family is psychologically present in any interview, representing a powerful determining force on the patient's behavior. The interviewer should always consider the utility of a family assessment, or eventual employment of family therapy.

Ideally, a clinician may actually be presented with an opportunity to interact with the family as a unit in a joint interview. For example, in an emergency room situation, the patient is frequently accompanied by family members. On these occasions the clinician can directly observe the process of family interaction.

But even within the confines of an individual assessment, an enormous amount of information can be gained concerning family dynamics by gently probing. Pertinent data will emerge simply by learning some of the background facts and pieces of demographic information. The clinician can begin a familiarization with the family matrix by inquiring into where various family members have chosen to live. It is probably not merely chance that leads to a situation in which all the children have moved thousands of miles away from mom and dad. Nor should one ignore the implications of a family in which most members have chosen to live on the same block.

I remember a young woman seeking help for severe marital discord, who complained that she could not get her mother "to mind her own business." Later in the interview I was surprised to find that the patient had recently moved back into the same apartment complex where her parents lived, ostensibly for convenience. The issue of inappropriate attachment to her parents appeared as a psychodynamic theme throughout the remaining therapy.

Another important area reveals itself when one inquires about which people are living under the same roof with the patient. Such questioning may uncover unexpected findings, such as a domineering grandparent whose ideas of discipline clash with the concepts of the parents.

On a more specific level, further questioning may directly begin to unravel the complexities of the family, such as:

a. What were holidays like at your house?
b. What kinds of things did your brothers or sisters like to do? (often yields clues to sibling rivalry)
c. Describe the physical appearance of your brother. (another nice gate through which to explore sibling rivalry)
d. Whom do you share secrets with in your family?
e. Who makes the decisions in your family?
f. Who do you think you are most like in your family?
g. Tell me a little about what kinds of things your parents used to argue about.
h. Did you go to the same schools as your brother? (and if so, what was that like?)
i. Did you share a room with any siblings? (and if so, what was that like?)

With questions such as the above the initial interviewer can begin to determine whether a family assessment may be indicated.

An analysis of the family system is not emphasized in the DSM-III-R except as an aspect of the stressors on Axis IV, once again highlighting the utility of applying several assessment grids when planning treatment. Some authors have suggested creating a new axis in DSM-IV upon which to conceptualize family pathology. Further discussion of this critical area of assessment would take us out of the topic of the book, but the interested reader may find the writings of Stephen Fleck useful in building a foundation for a more specific approach to family assessment.[3,4]

With regard to Miss Baker, the importance of her relationship with her lover immediately emerges as she boldly announces her upcoming wedding. It is as if she can hardly wait to shed her identity, washing her hands of her own name with a brisk shrugging as she meets the clinician. As the interview progresses the added information that her lover also indulges the patient's fantasy identities is further evidence of a powerful bond between the two, perhaps a bond laced with pathology. This relationship, on the other hand, has endured for several years and may represent a potentially powerful resource in therapy. To increase the light on this relationship the clinician may consider the use of a joint assessment session with the couple.

Turning towards the impact of her nuclear family, Miss Baker's poignant early memory of being tugged away from the door as her father vanishes conveys the sense of a deeply troubled childhood. Clearly, more information in this region will be enlightening, and the clinician is reminded once again of the potential utility of family assessment and/or therapy.

The Group System

In the fifth system, the group system, the interviewer investigates the patient's ability to function within groups outside of the family. In particular one looks at the patient's relationships at work and with networks of friends. A pivotal issue concerns the patient's abilities to handle authority figures such as employers. The clinician keeps an eye open for evidence that the patient is generalizing feelings from family members onto other relationships, such as sibling rivalry reappearing as intense competitiveness at the workplace. It is also valuable to search for subcultures to which the patient may look for values and support. Such cultures could include the drug culture, the bar culture, the jock culture, or ideological entities such as the Ku Klux Klan. An ignorance of a patient's cultural subgroup can lead to major errors in treatment planning. Alcohol detoxification will probably serve little purpose if the patient immediately returns to the bar scene for a rendezvous with drinking buddies. While contemplating this system, the interviewer should consider whether group therapy may be of value. Moreover one is also reminded of utilizing subcultures for therapeutic effect, such as recommending Alcoholics Anonymous.

Little is known about the functioning of Miss Baker at a group level. Indeed, the absence of her mentioning friends perks our attention, perhaps suggesting problematic relationships or none at all. There also seems to be a conspicuous absence of support groups or outside activities. A potentially important subculture worth exploring with Miss Baker remains the impact of the gay culture upon herself and her lover. In reviewing the information gathered at this level concerning Miss Baker, the clinician is reminded of the possible advantages of group therapy. On a behavioral level, as therapy progresses, it may be beneficial to steer her towards rewarding group activities such as volunteer work.

The Societal System

The sixth level represents the societal system. This system can be viewed as consisting of the various social forces shaping the patient's functioning within the community. These forces include economic, political, institutional, and social class factors. As Engel's quotation suggests at the beginning of this section, the patient's environment should always be considered. In particular, an investigation of the patient's financial status, housing, and food availability remains an important area for inquiry. All of these conditions are intimately related to the political climate of the patient's county, state, and federal governments. It is also possible that a patient's society is problematic, disabling the patient through prejudice and/or violence. Once again the interviewer must remember not to focus solely on individual dynamics, for the patient is part of many different systems, any one of which may be malfunctioning. It remains a basic tenet of assessment interviewing that one must understand the patient's culture in order to understand the patient's behavior.

In this light the issue of Miss Baker's sexual preference warrants an understanding of her culture. Further interviewing revealed that she and her lover had been forced to deal with considerable ostracism. At first glance this ostracism seems totally at odds with the further development of Miss Baker, but there may be a curious catch here. In essence this easily identified enemy has served as a common threat around which Miss Baker and her lover have mobilized, thus stabilizing their relationship.

Perhaps a digression is warranted at this point. Thus far we have been using the systems perspective to help organize data into distinct regions, which provide potential approaches to treatment. For the initial interviewer this aspect of systems thinking is very productive. But as therapy progresses, a different characteristic of systems thinking becomes increasingly important, namely, the actual interaction among the seven systems.

A change in any one system may have a potential impact, not always a beneficial one, on all other systems. The clinician needs to weigh the potential impact of intervention at one level upon the overall development of the patient. This ever-changing web of relationships stands at the very heart of therapy. Many a therapist has rued the day he blindly intervened at one level without considering potential ramifications at other levels.

By way of clarification, suppose Miss Baker and her lover lived in a community that was overtly hostile towards homosexuality, as was the case. A clinician might suggest that moving neighborhoods could be beneficial, but such a suggestion could be a serious miscalculation.

One of the most powerful glues for this relationship could be their unified need to protect each other from this community's attacks. If placed in a new and benign community, the relationship itself could begin to collapse, fulfilling Miss Baker's frightening fear of abandonment. In this example it might be better to stabilize the relationship upon more solid grounds before suggesting such a move.

It is well beyond the scope of this book to explore the interactional aspect of systems theory further, but I think it is important, even in a discussion of an initial interview, to keep it in mind.

It also reminds us, at the societal level, to consider one other crucial system when planning treatment, namely, the mental health system itself. The clinician needs to be aware of the actual resources available for follow-up. It is useless to recommend behavioral therapy to a patient if there is no behavioral therapist available to the patient. Indeed, such "pie in the sky" thinking can frustrate patients, hanging false hopes before their eyes. Similarly, a common error at academic centers is the tendency to generate complex treatment plans for patients referred from community centers that these centers cannot implement when the patient returns to them. Such state-of-the-art treatment planning is in reality an example of poor assessment formulation, for its impracticality breeds frustration in the patient and anger in the treating clinician.

To finish our discussion of the societal system, an important mental health resource for Miss Baker was uncovered by further interviewing. An excellent day clinic had been providing intermittent support for Miss Baker over the past year or so. This community system suggested a future area for support.

The Existential System: The Framework for Meaning

On the seventh level, the interviewer examines the patient's framework for meaning. Although in actuality this system could be conceived of as part of the psychological system already discussed, it is so important that it is best viewed separately. To understand the patient more fully it becomes necessary to understand his or her religious beliefs, philosophical beliefs, and ethical standards. At times the patient's symptoms may be related to unrest within these basic existential areas. It is important to remember that in addition to religious beliefs, patients may find meaning in processes such as patriotism, community activity, and the care of their families. Information gained in this system may suggest the utility of individual psychotherapy slanted towards existential issues. A review of this system also serves to remind the clinician of the availability of clergy and pastoral counselors in the treatment of the patient.

In the initial interview this region was left relatively poorly explored in the case of Miss Baker. Later interviews revealed a paucity of religious and philosophical supports at this level, suggesting avenues for intervention such as augmenting the patient's participation in community or religious groups.

We have now concluded a brief survey of the seven levels used in a systems analysis. Although there exists some obvious overlap with the DSM-III-R, a systems analysis provides several new areas in which to deepen an understanding of the patient and suggests as well new areas of intervention. Systems analysis also provides a more realistic picture of the patient as one process inextricably woven among the other systems of the world at large.

ASSESSMENT OF CORE PAINS

I can see behind everyone's masks. Peacefully smiling faces, pale corpses who endlessly wend their tortuous way down the road that leads to the grave.
Edvard Munch, 19th century expressionist painter

Although Munch depicts a somewhat grim picture of human existence, he was a man keenly aware of the pains that all of us endure by our very nature of being human. His ability to intuitively sense underlying pain represents a gift that all clinicians hope to possess. Indeed this ability to understand pain provides a major gateway through which therapeutic trust is born.

Throughout this book an emphasis has been placed on combining intuition and analysis. Many times the clinician will be able to intuitively sense the pains of the interviewee, but this intuition is enhanced when guided by an increased awareness of underlying themes. One of the more fascinating themes is the coexistence of the complexity of human nature with the simplicity of that same nature. Nowhere is this curious juxtaposition more prominent than with the issue of psychological pain. Patients frequently present with complicated histories and concerns, sometimes even involving bizarre delusions and idiosyncratic perceptions. But the underlying pains that these patients are fleeing are few in number.

Skilled clinicians possess the knack of cutting through the complexities until the bare wounds, the core pains, are understood. An understanding of these core pains is a powerful clinical tool. This empathic understanding can suggest avenues for treatment planning. Even more importantly it can also guide the interviewer towards methods of navigating the resistances that develop during the interview itself, for the seeds of resistance are generally attempts to avoid these core pains by the patient. We have already had a glimpse of this process when we discussed methods of handling resistance in the opening phase of the interview in Chapter 2. Later we will use the same concepts as the cornerstone of our approach to resistance as explored in Chapter 10.

In any case, an understanding of core pains and the increased sensitivity such an understanding can bring provides an assessment perspective that complements both the DSM-III-R and systems analysis. It is based upon the principle that clinicians should intermittently ask themselves, "What are the core pains which are hurting this patient at this time?" Or as Edvard Munch would have it, what is behind the mask?

The relevance of the concept of core pains was made plain to me by a psychotic patient when I was least expecting it. The patient was a young woman in her mid twenties who presented violently and was riddled with terrifying delusions. During the initial interview she described her sincere belief that aliens were speaking directly into her mind, taunting her sanity. Her world was convulsed with a pricking sensation of paranoia. She had become convinced that the aliens were about to kidnap her to a distant world. Her affect was intense, and she spoke in a disorganized fashion with a loosening of associations.

At this point I asked her why she felt the aliens were coming for her. To my surprise she looked at me as if I had not been listening. Her affect calmed, her speech became coherent and she said, "Don't you understand? I am alone here. No one cares for me. I have no family, no friends. And I have no reason to be here. Wouldn't you want to leave this horrid place if you were me?" At which point she promptly popped back into her psychotic language and refuge.

In a sense she was right concerning my inadequate listening, for I had become overly involved in diagnosis and systems analysis. A balancing perspective was needed, a sense of her pathos on a human level. She provided me with a lesson that led me to think more carefully about the presence of core pains and methods of conceptualizing them more clearly even as the interview itself proceeds.

Towards this goal one can generate a list of core pains that singly or in combination appear to be driving any given individual. Each clinician may have a unique list; the following serve only as a platform for discussion. To me the core pains are as follows:

1. Fear of being alone
2. Fear of worthlessness
3. Fear of impending rejection

4. Fear of failure
5. Fear of loss of external control
6. Fear of loss of internal control
7. Fear of the unknown

With Miss Baker in mind one can survey these pains, examining their usefulness in both treatment planning and in understanding the dynamics of the interview itself.

The fear of being ultimately alone remains one of the most powerful and common pains. In the case of Miss Baker it appears to be surfacing in one of its frequent guises, intense dependency. As such it serves to remind the interviewer that some patients may seek an unhealthy dependency on the clinician even during the initial interview. Miss Baker would be one such person in whom this process could occur, as reflected by her intense feelings of abandonment when her lover goes to sleep.

Her dependency needs may be intimately related to the second core pain, the fear of worthlessness. Miss Baker may be convinced of her ultimate inability to cope with life. In this sense she probably avoids situations in which she could modestly succeed, thus depriving herself of the positive reinforcement needed to gain a sense of mastery. With these factors in mind the clinician might consider assigning Miss Baker small easily accomplished tasks, resulting in a gradually increasing sense of worth. A cognitive therapy approach might reveal that Miss Baker has a distorted self-image maintained by tendencies for negative thinking and inappropriate self-blame. In this light, techniques such as cognitive restructuring might be of use.

Like its predecessor this core pain appears to lead naturally into a discussion of the next core pain, an impending sense of rejection. This fear reared its head throughout the interviewing process. Miss Baker demonstrated poor eye contact and frequently commented, "That's a stupid thing for me to say." Such anxieties can hamper the progress of the initial interview as the patient expends inordinate amounts of attention attempting to please the interviewer. Alert to this situation, the interviewer may purposely reassure the patient. For instance, the clinician might choose to say to Miss Baker, "You are doing a very good job of discussing difficult material. It's really helping me to get a clearer picture of what has been going on." Even such a simple statement can make a patient such as Miss Baker feel considerably more comfortable, decreasing her fear of imminent rejection.

The fourth pain, the fear of failure, overlaps with a sense of worthlessness but has an intensity all its own. The initial interviewer needs to attend to this particular pain, since the patient may bring it into the initial interview itself. Specifically, the patient may predict an impending failure in therapy and consequently decide not to appear for follow-up. If left as a hidden issue, the risk of losing the patient is real. In the closing phase of the interview, the clinician may opt to bring this fear to the surface with questions such as, "Now that we have talked about possible therapies, I'm wondering what you think about their usefulness for you?" or "If you tried outpatient therapy, how do you think it would go?" The interviewer may be able to cite the patient's success in handling the initial interview as evidence that the patient has the needed abilities to succeed in therapy.

The fear of losing external control, the fifth pain, can be extremely frightening to patients, for suddenly it seems as if nothing they can do will alter their situation. This combination of fear and anger can present a fertile field for suicidal ideation. If one listens to the steelworker laid off indefinitely, the roar of this pain can certainly be heard. While interviewing elderly patients one should bear in mind that they may be dealing with a sense of the ultimate loss of external control, death itself. When this core pain appears particularly prominent, the initial interviewer can make an effort to consciously increase the patient's sense of control within the interview itself by using statements such as, "At this point what do you think would be the most important area we should focus our discussion on?" Such modest yet timely intervention can significantly return some feeling of control to the patient.

The sixth core pain, the fear of loss of internal control, surfaces in patients who are becoming increasingly frightened of their own impulses, such as drives towards suicide or violence. I doubt that this pain could be more vividly portrayed than in patients who are moving into progressively more psychotic or manic behavior. In Miss Baker's case her history of episodic violence, as evidenced by her throwing a picnic table through a picture window, suggests that this core pain may be a frequent motivator of her behaviors. Fortunately, in her initial interview she appeared to be in good control.

But in other situations the interviewer may find a patient who reports feeling imminently unstable. In such cases it is generally, if not always, sound to attend to these fears on the spot. If the interviewer chooses to ignore these feelings, the interviewer risks driving the patient into an act of violence. Ironically, the patient's own increasing fears of losing control may act to spur further anxiety, perhaps pushing the patient even closer to a loss of control. The clinician can gently probe to see what the patient is afraid may happen and ask the patient if indeed he or she feels in control. The appearance of this core pain may suggest the usefulness of an antipsychotic medication.

We now come to the last and seventh element in the assessment of core pains, the fear of the unknown. As described in Chapter 2, most patients are probably experiencing this pain during the interview itself, for they are frightened of what the results of the interview will be. As mentioned earlier a few minutes spent performing a sound introduction can greatly relieve the patient's unnecessary fears. In Miss Baker's case, her fear of the unknown may add to her dependent patterns, making her reluctant to try things on her own. With regard to treatment planning one sometimes finds that patients such as Miss Baker do not have the communication skills or the assertiveness to find out what the future may hold, thus locking them into the paralysis of the moment. Their lack of assertiveness may prevent them from asking appropriate questions even of the interviewer. The presence of this core pain should alert the clinician to the potential use of assertiveness training and social skills work as well as to the need to address unasked questions.

We have now reviewed our third assessment schema. I have not explored the use of this system in detail; we will do this in upcoming chapters. Instead I have tried to survey this assessment system, which provides a different avenue for generating treatment options. This particular schema provides more on-the-spot information pertinent to altering the course of the interview itself than either the DSM-III-R or systems analysis. Together, these three assessment perspectives complement each other, helping the interviewer change a potentially impotent mass of data into a crisp and practical formulation.

As the clinician becomes familiar with using these three systems, one of their most appealing aspects surfaces, their speed. Once familiar with their use the clinician can assess the known data base while generating a powerful list of treatment options in about five to ten minutes. This rapid integration of a large data base can be a godsend in a busy clinic or private practice. Furthermore the clinician can review the ongoing treatment plan quickly and with a fresh perspective as time passes.

Before wrapping up this chapter it may be gratifying to review the actual progress of Miss Baker in therapy, while also looking at the actual selections which were made from the lists of potential treatments generated by the above perspectives.

REVIEW OF THE CLINICAL COURSE OF MISS BAKER

In the first place, despite her chaotic history, Miss Baker brought to therapy a variety of healthy coping skills. Viewed in the light of Axis V concerning her best two months of functioning in the past year, she displayed motivation, intelligence, and a keen ability at self-reflection. She also possessed the often too rare quality of compassion. Indeed, it was her apparent inability to recognize and accept her strengths that stood as one of the major obstacles to her development. In a large measure, therapy consisted of an attempt to help Miss Baker develop the attributes hinted at during her moments of high functioning.

The rest of her eventual treatment plan evolved directly from the data gathered in the initial interview. On Axis I she did not fulfill the criteria for a major depression. She did appear to meet the criteria for dysthymia, which, as mentioned earlier, may respond to antidepressant medication. In her case I opted to forgo an antidepressant at first, hoping that psychotherapeutic measures would be more effective. In particular, because of her long-established pattern of self-debasement and a sense of worthlessness, I was concerned that she would immediately deny any credit for improvement if an antidepressant could be pointed to as the curative agent. If she had developed a major depression or if the chosen treatment track would have failed, I would most likely have promptly added an antidepressant. In the long run, the goal was to enable her to gain an increasing sense of self-worth and mastery over her environment.

Her problems with the development of a stable self were reflected by her primary Axis II diagnosis of a borderline personality disorder. She would probably have also met the criteria for a dependent personality. In any case, these diagnoses suggested the need to attend to her dependency issues quickly, a generalization extrapolated from the diagnosis and borne out by her long history of dependent relations. Consequently, in the closing phase of the initial interview, the issues of possible dependency upon me were discussed openly and mutually decided upon as a major concern to be avoided.

To sidestep a maladaptive dependency upon myself, she was seen only on a weekly basis. Moreover we agreed to adopt a long-term treatment plan built around the concept of meeting for three-month periods in which we focused upon a specific problem list generated by her. At the end of each three months we would break from therapy for progressively longer periods of time as she began functioning more and more independently.

During her three-month period of active therapy, specific tasks were assigned as homework, which she mastered easily, increasing her sense of worth. She also became adept at utilizing cognitive restructuring, which helped her to decrease her tendency for overgeneralization, splitting, and inappropriate self-blame. These cognitive techniques were implemented while simultaneously considering the psychodynamic issues of the development of her self.

Miss Baker began to make strides in her bewildering battle to discover her own identity. Her successes in this regard were poignantly illustrated by the fact that she began signing her real name to pieces of artwork instead of her fantasy name of "Paul." Furthermore, as therapy proceeded she stopped wearing her wristband with the false identity, a behavioral change paralleled by a significant decrease in her fantasy activity.

This treatment approach characterized by intermittent stretches of therapist-free time was only possible because of considerations made with regard to the societal system. Specifically, it was discovered that a day clinic was available that could offer appropriate support when needed, as she underwent the pangs of separating from me. Thus she received enough support to gain the added sense of independence offered by successfully navigating her loss of me. Only through the cooperation received by this agency of the mental health system could the treatment plan be made operational.

To help her with impulse control during her premenstrual unrest, small doses of the antianxiety agent Xanax were used as deemed necessary by Miss Baker and carefully monitored by me. A behavioral system, on which she played a major role in developing, was employed to help her to prevent suicidal and violent activity. The emphasis remained on her to help herself, using her decreased need for my "parenting" as reinforcing evidence of her ability to manage independently.

A further area for intervention appeared in the family assessment. To this end a session was arranged for Miss Baker and her partner. By explaining to her partner certain aspects of the overall plan for increasing Miss Baker's independence, her partner was better able to support progress. It was also discovered that her partner appeared to be a loving and dependable support system. This session also served to decrease her partner's anxieties concerning the therapy itself, thus decreasing the risk of resistance generated by her partner.

Two and one-half years later Miss Baker had been involved in three three-month therapy courses separated by increasingly large interludes. Her mood shifts have stabilized markedly as has her relationship with her partner. She has had only two minor suicidal gestures in this time period. She reports a significant sense of increased self-worth. Naturally much work lies ahead, but the progress so far has been very satisfying.

Conclusion

In this chapter we have looked at the process of effectively organizing the information gained from an initial interview. It has become apparent that the methods chosen for conceptualizing data can greatly affect the ultimate usefulness of the data. The three organizational methods discussed here provide a reliable method of generating a practical list of treatment options. These three assessment systems also establish a reliable method of noting pertinent gaps in the data base.

In the long run the major reason for performing an assessment interview remains the generation of a sound treatment plan. As we have seen this treatment plan arises from a thorough attempt to understand the patient and the systems of which the patient is an integral part. This understanding evolves directly from our abilities to sensibly organize data. At such times it almost seems as if the data speak for themselves. Our task becomes one of learning to listen.

References

1. American Psychiatric Association: *Diagnostic and Statistical Manual of Mental Disorders.* Third edition. Washington, D.C., APA, 1980.
2. American Psychiatric Association: *Diagnostic and Statistical Manual of Mental Disorders.* Third edition, revised. Washington, D.C., APA, 1987.
3. Fleck, S.: Family functioning and family psychopathology. *Psychiatric Annuals* 10:17–35, 1980.
4. Fleck, S.: A holistic approach to family typology and the axes of DSM-III. *Archives of General Psychiatry* 40:901–906, 1983.

II

The Interview and Psychopathology

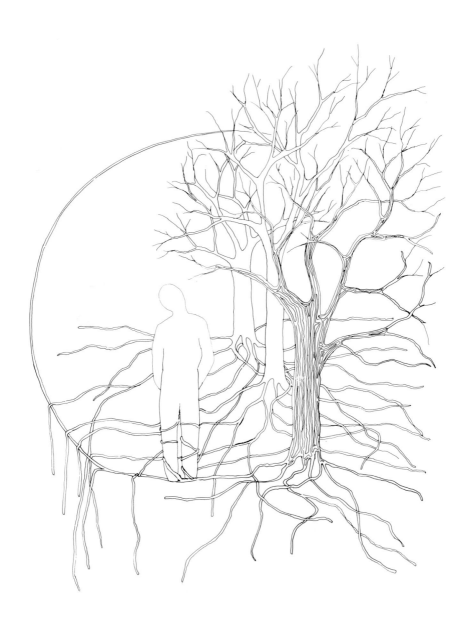

5

Interviewing Techniques in Depression and Other Mood Disorders

I wander thro' each charter'd street,
Near where the charter'd Thames does flow
And mark in every face I meet
Marks of weakness, marks of woe.
William Blake, London

In the early 1800's as Blake wandered the drab lanes of London, his eyes met the face of depression at every corner. Depression stalked among merchant, seaman, and prostitute alike, for depression impolitely ignored the proper boundaries of social class. Today, whether on Fifth Avenue in New York or at a community mental health center in rural Pennsylvania, mental health professionals encounter faces strongly reminiscent of those that William Blake described two centuries ago. As in Blake's time depression masquerades in many costumes and clinical presentations.

As an illustration of this diversity, I remember working with a woman of about forty, who had been a successful interior designer. In the economic depression of the early 1980's, she found herself jobless. Her confidence and self-esteem were affronted with each passing day. Her belief in herself insidiously weakened as if she were an invalid who decided there was no hope. Anxiety attacks punctuated her daily routine. Despite her pain she continued her frantic job search, terrified by each job interview. Her days became compacted cells of anxiety neatly delineated by bars of self-doubt.

How differently this woman's presentation appears when contrasted to a strikingly white-haired woman I met in North Carolina. Though only fifty years old, this woman's face was branded by thick wrinkles. She had been extremely dependent on her father, a carica-

213

ture of "daddy's little girl." Following his death four months earlier, she had felt as if her skin had emptied. She was no longer whole. His face could not comfort her. His touch could not reassure her. She was brought into the hospital on an involuntary commitment. According to the police she had been found wandering a local cemetery with a butcher knife in hand. She related that her father's voice was pleading with her to join him.

These people were obviously experiencing life very differently, yet both were suffering from depressive symptoms. I highlight this diversity of presentation to emphasize that depression is not a "thing." It is a constantly evolving process. As a process depression becomes a way of living. It is unique for each individual and for each environment the individual encounters. On the other hand, there are many similarities in the presentations of depression that enable the clinician to recognize depression despite atypical patterns. This dual capacity of depression to appear both foreign and familiar provides the interviewer with the first inkling that depression requires many levels of understanding. In the initial interview the interviewer attempts to integrate diagnosis and understanding with each question, continually probing deeper. Only when the patient feels this drive for understanding is it likely that the clinician's help will be accepted, whether it exists in the form of psychotherapy or medication.

In the two sections of this chapter two areas of major importance to the first interview will be explored: (1) diagnosis by DSM-III-R criteria and (2) understanding of the person and the personal ramifications of the depression.

These two processes occur simultaneously, but for clarity they will be discussed in separate sections. With regard to understanding the patient, one of the more expedient routes to understanding, systems analysis, has been described in chapter 4. In section two of this chapter we will study the ramifications of depression using this systems paradigm. It is beyond the scope of this chapter to be either a complete guide to the use of diagnosis or an all-encompassing review of the ramifications of depression. Instead I hope to offer a view of various ideas that may stimulate clinicians to develop their own methods of exploring depression in an initial interview. At this time I would like to describe four people who sought help for depression. These four presentations will provide a clinical base for entry into section one, The Diagnosis of Depression.

SECTION I: THE DIAGNOSIS OF DEPRESSION

Four Case Presentations

CASE ONE: MR. WHITE

Mr. White is a 61-year-old white single male who retired from a prestigious job at the police department one year ago. He is accompanied by his fiancée. With her help he hopes to open a bar in the next six months, if they can get a liquor license. Mr. White is well-groomed and dressed in a simple flannel work shirt and corduroy trousers. He appears very sad and relates, "It seems strange, but I can't really cry." He speaks softly and slowly, taking a while before answering questions as if thought required immense effort. On occasion, he tries to manage a smile. His eyes study the floor, seldom meeting the eyes of the interviewer. He complains of severe depression, of not being able to enjoy anything, sleep disturbance, loss of appetite and libido, and severe loss of energy. In the past three weeks he has held a loaded revolver to his head on several occasions. He spontaneously reports seeing no future. His fiancée, although obviously concerned, seems agitated and a bit cool. "He just won't help himself," she comments, "no matter how much I try to help him. Now I've got to meet with the Liquor Control Board agent alone next week."

CASE TWO: MR. WHITSTONE

Mr. Whitstone was admitted to a general hospital for evaluation of bizarre behavior described by his family as paranoid. He is a distinguished appearing 62-year-old white male who has been a prominent businessman. At the time of the interview he is refusing all hospital care, including intravenous lines and medication. The interviewer has been called in as an emergency consultant. During the interview Mr. Whitstone appears guarded, thoroughly grilling the interviewer about his training and his purpose. Outside of his suspiciousness Mr. Whitstone is cooperative. During the first ten minutes of the interview he appears tense, complaining, "I'm really having trouble with my thinking. I can't concentrate anymore. But they don't understand." When asked whether he feels depressed, he answers, "No, I don't feel particularly depressed." He reports problems with appetite and sleep. But of all his concerns, he is most upset about his business company, since he feels "someone in the company, and I'm not quite sure who, is out to get me." He has not returned to work since his triple bypass heart surgery in January, six months earlier. He is alert and oriented times three with a stable level of consciousness. Three members of his family are at bedside when the interviewer first enters the room.

CASE THREE: MS. WILKINS

Ms. Wilkins entered the outpatient office with hesitant steps. Her patterned blue dress was faded and wrinkled. She is a twenty-one-year-old white single woman who reports, "I feel horrible. I am so very depressed. Last night I was thinking of maybe (pause — tearfulness) killing myself." She reports numerous neurovegetative symptoms of depression such as sleep disturbance, decreased energy, decreased libido, and decreased appetite. She reports, "I've been depressed for years." She truly appears very sad. As the interview proceeds the interviewer feels a deepening desire to help as well as an increasing concern. There is also an angry quality to Ms. Wilkins as she relates, "My best friend is really a bastard. I can't believe I trusted her." Ms. Wilkins denies concrete suicidal or homicidal ideation at the time of the interview, stating, "I'm feeling in control now." She wishes to have both medication and psychotherapy.

CASE FOUR: MR. COLLIER

Mr. Collier and his wife presented at the psychiatric emergency room. Mr. Collier is a 26-year-old white male who is casually but nicely dressed. He has dark brown hair and a strong jaw. His voice is rich with a vigorous, almost aggressive tone. He answers quickly with authority. While he interacts with his wife the interviwer finds it easy to picture Mr. Collier giving his wife "the third degree." Mr. Collier complains bitterly of severe depression "ever since I was a teenager." He continues, "I remind myself of my father." He reports a tendency to sleep during the day and always feels tired. His appetite and libido are good. He complains of feeling worthless and lazy. He is upset that he has been sharp with his kids. In the week preceding their emergency room visit he slapped his ten-year-old daughter, Jackie, on the face. This incident frightened him and prompted the emergency room visit. He occasionally has fleeting suicidal ideation, remarking, "I'd jump in front of a car or bus . . . you know, to make sure my wife gets the insurance." He denies current suicidal ideation. He states "I'm the problem here. Help me and you'll help my family."

Discussion of Case Material

For the sake of discussion, let us assume that the above material had been elicited after roughly fifteen minutes of interviewing. As one reviews this material two points are obvious (1) all of these people are in significant psychological pain, and (2) all of them appear depressed. The next question facing the clinician deals with whether all of these people should be diagnosed as having a true major depression. The following case discussions will focus on the various lines of questioning that an interviewer might use to sort out this difficult differential.

In the first place, in order to diagnose accurately, the clinician needs to be thoroughly familiar with the basic criteria of DSM-III-R. This familiarization does not mean the clinician should obsessively memorize hundreds of criteria. On the contrary, this suggests a working knowledge of what material is necessary to clarify the major diagnoses. This diagnostic familiarization allows the clinician to focus upon the art of eliciting the necessary material while successfully engaging the interviewee. The establishment of therapeutic alliance, as usual, remains of paramount importance. The diagnostic criteria for two of the common affective disorders in the DSM-III-R are reviewed below. Before proceeding the reader might also find it useful to review the DSM-III-R criteria for other common mood disorders, such as bipolar disorder, cyclothymia, bipolor disorder not otherwise specified, and depressive disorder not otherwise specified. The DSM-III-R defines major depression and dysthymia as follows:

Major Depression Episode[1]

Note: A "Major Depressive Syndrome" is defined as criterion A below.

A. At least five of the following symptoms have been present during the same two-week period and represent a change from previous functioning; at least one of the symptoms is either (1) depressed mood, or (2) loss of interest or pleasure. (Do not include symptoms that are clearly due to a physical condition, mood-incongruent delusions or hallucinations, incoherence, or marked loosening of associations.)

(1) depressed mood (or can be irritable mood in children and adolescents) most of the day, nearly every day, as indicated either by subjective account or observation by others

(2) markedly diminished interest or pleasure in all, or almost all, activities most of the day, nearly every day, (as indicated either by subjective account or observation by others of apathy most of the time)

(3) significant weight loss or weight gain when not dieting (e.g., more than 5% of body weight in a month), or decrease or increase in appetite nearly every day (in children, consider failure to make expected weight gains)

(4) insomnia or hypersomnia nearly every day

(5) psychomotor agitation or retardation nearly every day (observable by others, not merely subjective feelings of restlessness or being slowed down)

(6) fatigue or loss of energy nearly every day

(7) feelings of worthlessness or excessive or inappropriate guilt (which may be delusional) nearly every day (not merely self-reproach or guilt about being sick)

(8) diminished ability to think or concentrate, or indecisiveness, nearly every day (either by subjective account or as observed by others)

(9) recurrent thoughts of death (not just fear of dying), recurrent suicidal ideation without specific plan, or a suicide attempt or a specific plan for committing suicide

B. (1) It cannot be established that an organic factor initiated and maintained the disturbance

(2) The disturbance is not a normal reaction to the death of a loved one (Uncomplicated Bereavment)

Note: Morbid preoccupation with worthlessness, suicidal ideation, marked functional impairment or psychomotor retardation, or prolonged duration suggest bereavement complicated by Major Depression.

C. At no time during the disturbance have there been delusions or hallucinations for as long as two weeks in the absence of prominent mood symptoms (i.e., before the mood symptoms developed or after they have remitted).

D. Not superimposed on Schizophrenia, Schizophreniform Disorder, Delusional Disorder, or Psychotic Disorder NOS.

Major Depressive Episode codes: fifth-digit code numbers and criteria for severity of current state of Bipolar Disorder, Depressed, or Major Depression:

1-Mild: Few, if any, symptoms in excess of those required to make the diagnosis, and symptoms result in only minor impairment in occupational functioning or in usual social activities or relationships with others.

2-Moderate: Symptoms or functional impairment between "mild" and "severe."

3-Severe, without Psychotic Features: Several symptoms in excess of those required to make the diagnosis, and symptoms markedly interfere with occupational functioning or with usual social activities or relationships with others.

4-With Psychotic Features: Delusions or hallucinations. If possible, specify whether the psychotic features are mood-congruent or mood-incongruent.

Mood-congruent psychotic features: Delusions or hallucinations whose content is entirely consistent with the typical depressive themes of personal inadequacy, guilt, disease, death, nihilism, or deserved punishment.

Mood-incongruent psychotic features: Delusions or hallucinations whose content does not involve typical depressive themes of personal inadequacy, guilt, disease, death, nihilism, or deserved punishment. Included here are such symptoms as persecutory delusions (not directly related to depressive themes), thought insertion, thought broadcasting, and delusions of control.

5-In Partial Remission: Intermediate between "In Full Remission" and "Mild," and no previous Dysthymia. (If Major Depressive Episode was superimposed on Dysthymia, the diagnosis of Dysthymia alone is given once the full criteria for a Major Depressive Episode are no longer met.)

6-In Full Remission: During the past six months no significant signs or symptoms of the disturbance.

0-Unspecified.

Specify chronic if current episode has lasted two consecutive years without a period of two months or longer during which there were no significant depressive symptoms.

Specify if current episode is Melancholic Type.

Dysthymia[2]

A. Depressed mood (or can be irritable mood in children and adolescents) for most of the day, more days than not, as indicated either by subjective account or observation by others, for at least two years (one year for children and adolescents)

B. Presence, while depressed, of at least two of the following:
   (1) poor appetite or overeating
   (2) insomnia or hypersomnia
   (3) low energy or fatigue

(4) low self-esteem

(5) poor concentration or difficulty making decisions

(6) feelings of hopelessness

C. During a two-year period (one-year for children and adolescents) of the disturbance, never without the symptoms in A for more than two months at a time.

D. No evidence of an unequivocal Major Depressive Episode during the first two years (one year for children and adolescents) of the disturbance.

Note: There may have been a previous Major Depressive Episode, provided there was a full remission (no significant signs or symptoms for six months) before development of the Dysthymia. In addition, after these two years (one year in children or adolescents) of Dysthymia, there may be superimposed episodes of Major Depression, in which case both diagnoses are given.

E. Has never had a Manic Episode or an unequivocal Hypomanic Episode.

F. Not superimposed on a chronic psychotic disorder, such as Schizophrenia or Delusional Disorder.

G. It cannot be established that an organic factor initiated and maintained the disturbance, e.g., prolonged administration of an antihypertensive medication.

Specify Primary or Secondary Type:

Primary type: the mood disturbance is not related to preexisting, chronic, nonmood, Axis I or Axis III disorder, e.g., Anorexia Nervosa, Somatization Disorder, a Psychoactive Substance Dependence Disorder, an Anxiety Disorder, or rheumatoid arthritis.

Secondary type: the mood disturbance is apparently related to a preexisting, chronic, nonmood Axis I or Axis III disorder.

Specify Early Onset or Late Onset:

Early onset: onset of the disturbance before age 21.

Late onset: onset of the disturbance at age 21 or later.

DISCUSSION OF MR. WHITE

Mr. White was the sixty-one-year-old retired police officer who had held a loaded revolver to his head. Of all the cases presented, Mr. White appears to be showing some of the most classic symptoms of a major depression. The craft of eliciting such symptoms deserves further examination. In the first place, Mr. White states clearly he has a persistently dysphoric mood, thus fulfilling one of the first two symptoms of criterion A needed for a diagnosis of major depression in the DSM-III-R. It is important to note that one does not need to feel "depressed" to fulfill criterion A, for one needs the presence of either symptom 1 or symptom 2 before making a diagnosis of a major depression. Symptom 2 reads "markedly diminished interest or pleasure in all, or almost all, activities most of the day, nearly every day." Symptom 2 is essentially an undeclared definition of anhedonia. The word "anhedonia" is a derivative of the Greek word "hēdonē," referring to pleasure, as also seen in the English "hedonism." In anhedonia, one demonstrates a decreased ability to experience pleasure or to develop interest. This alteration in the experience of pleasure is a common symptom of depression warranting a careful search in the initial interview.

One of the ways in which to explore anhedonia smoothly is to discover first what types of activities the interviewee enjoys in general. Questions such as the following may be fruitful for setting up such an exploration:

a. What kinds of things do you like to do when you're away from work?
b. In the past, have you generally enjoyed your work?
c. Do you have any types of hobbies or sports you enjoy?
d. Do you enjoy reading or watching television?
e. In the past have you enjoyed socializing?

Oftentimes I will spend considerable time exploring these interests further, for they can provide important insights to the clinician about the person's viewpoints and psychological integration, as seen, for instance, in the following:

Clin: Do you enjoy reading or listening to music?
Pt.: I used to enjoy reading quite a bit . . . sort of odd stuff . . . (tiny smile) . . . like St. Augustine, Thomas Aquinas, and other theological books.
Clin.: Sounds like pretty heavy reading?
Pt.: Yeah, it is. But I used to enjoy it (pause) I used to be fairly religious . . . used to be (said with a trailing off of the voice)

From this dialogue it appears that religious themes may be important issues for this patient, perhaps contributing to his depressive anxiety. This questioning has not only laid the groundwork for a discussion of anhedonia, it has also served the dual function of gathering pertinent intrapsychic material while further engaging the patient. At this point one may continue the search for anhedonia with questions referring to the groundwork laid above.

   a. Over the past several weeks have you felt like doing these activities?
   b. Do you find it as enjoyable to do these things as you used to, or has there been a change?
   c. Have you been feeling interested in your hobbies over the past several weeks?

At times interpersonal questions can uncover anhedonic complaints, as evidenced by the following:

Clin.: You mentioned your grandchildren. Do you have a good time when you're around them now?

Pt.: (sigh) Sort of . . . Don't get me wrong, I love my grandchildren, but I just can't seem to enjoy anything anymore, even them.

Along with anhedonia, Mr. White appears to be suffering from many of the neurovegetative symptoms of depression. Although it is difficult to find a standard definition of neurovegetative symptoms, I view them as symptoms suggesting that basic regulatory physiology has been disturbed. With such a definition in mind, the neurovegetative symptoms can be listed as follows: change in appetite, change in weight, sleep disturbance, change in energy, change in libido, altered concentration, and retarded or agitated motor activity. Although not always labeled as neurovegetative symptoms other common physiologic correlates of depression exist, including constipation, dry mouth, and cold extremities.

Sleep disturbance warrants a more thorough discussion. Part of the lore of psychiatry has been that people suffering from major depressions often display early morning awakening. The exact frequency of this phenomenon is not entirely clear yet, although there is good evidence that feeling worse in the morning is a reasonably reliable indicator of a major depression. In any case it seems expedient to understand the extent and pattern of the sleep disturbance in the patient for the following reasons.

Thorough questioning of such a topic conveys to the patient that the interviewer is sensitively interested in the day-to-day disturbances of the patient's life caused by the depression. Furthermore, sleep disturbances can also provide early clues to other diagnostic possibilities. For instance, sleep continuity disturbances (e.g., waking up during the night) are common in depression, psychosis, drug and alcohol abuse, and in the elderly. Difficulty falling asleep can also be seen in a variety of disturbances, including depression, anxiety disorders, adjustment disorders, and various psychotic processes. Besides decreased sleep, one should also search for evidence of increased sleep or a tendency for daytime sleeping. A reversed diurnal pattern of sleep, whereby the patient sleeps during the day and remains awake at night, can be seen in entities such as depression, bipolar disorder, and schizophrenia. By eliciting a detailed sleep history, one may also stumble upon an unsuspected primary sleep disturbance such as sleep apnea, narcolepsy, or nocturnal myoclonus.

With regard to neurovegetative symptoms, such as decreased energy, mention should also be made concerning the investigation of libido. At times interviewers feel shy about asking about libido. Seldom should this present a problem in engaging a patient if approached appropriately. In the first place, the topic should be broached smoothly while in a natural context. For example, if the clinician has been discussing the neurovegetative symptoms at length one might ask:

a. It sounds like your depression has really upset your system. Do you think it has also affected your sexual drive?

Alternatively, if the patient has been talking at length about the disruption of a romantic relationship one might query:

a. From what you are saying, it sounds as if there has been a lot of tension between you and your husband. Do you think it has also affected your sexual relationship?

I would like to add several points about questions concerning libido. I have found many patients relieved to know that decreased libido is a common feature of depression. Consequently, after asking about libido, I might add, "I ask about sexual drive because basic drives such as appetite and sexual desire are commonly decreased by depression." To such a statement, patients sometimes respond with sentiments such as "Thank god. I thought my loss of desire was just another one of my failures."

Another important issue remains tone of voice. If interviewers ask their questions matter-of-factly, without hesitation, it greatly decreases the risk that the patient will feel put off. In a different light, if the patient does react unusually strongly, then one may have incidentally learned something about the patient's views on sex or their bodies or their views on what is proper for them to disclose. Such information is grist for the mill in later sessions. As a final note, some people confuse sexual drive with actual intercourse. It sometimes helps to clarify this issue with remarks such as "By sexual drive, I mean your interest in having sex, not whether you are actually having it or not." If this point is not clarified, a patient who is not dating may quickly state that libido is absent, "since I'm not seeing anyone," when in actuality a strong libido may be present.

The neurovegetative symptoms are classic hallmarks of a major depression, fulfilling many of the criteria of the A section of the DSM-III-R. If they are not elicited spontaneously, they should always be actively sought. When done properly, such questioning powerfully engages the interviewee. It shows the interviewee two reassuring characteristics: (1) that the interviewer is interested in him/her as a person whose depression affects every aspect of their lives, and (2) that the interviewer is knowledgeable as witnessed by the fact that the questions seem right on the mark.

Questions dealing with neurovegetative symptoms should seldom be asked in a checklist fashion with statements such as, "I need to ask a few questions now," or "Let me just go over a few things here." Instead, they should be imperceptibly woven into the fabric of the conversation, as shown below:

> **Pt.:** I don't know how to keep coping with all this strain, what with my unemployment and now my wife on my back.
>
> **Clin:** You're going through some tough times. Is this affecting your sleep at all?
>
> **Pt:** Hell, yes. I can't sleep at all.
>
> **Clin.:** Tell me more about it?
>
> **Pt.:** I'm waking up a couple of times a night. I just toss and turn thinking about Janet and whether she'll leave me. I don't know why she stays, except I think she needs the money.
>
> **Clin.:** How many times do you think you actually wake up?
>
> **Pt.:** Maybe four or five, it's really bad. I feel horrible in the morning, no rest.
>
> **Clin.:** Roughly what time are you waking up in the morning?
>
> **Pt.:** Around 5:00 A.M.
>
> **Clin.:** Do you wake up naturally or are you sort of jolted out of your sleep by worries?
>
> **Pt.:** Oh no, I feel horrible. I can't get back to sleep no matter how hard I try. It ruins the whole rest of my day.
>
> **Clin.:** It sounds like mornings are really a rough time for you. Are you having any problems falling asleep too?
>
> **Pt.:** Nope, and I never have. Oh, maybe a little bit years ago, but not much now.

Clin.: Well, it sounds like your sleep has been pretty disturbed. I'm wondering whether all the loss of sleep has affected your energy at all?

Pt.: None. Everything is an effort. Just getting up is an effort. Trying to cut the grass is like trying to swim the English Channel. I have no energy, no desire to do anything.

Clin.: What about your golf, or your dancing?

Pt.: Sometimes I get a little satisfaction, but I really just don't enjoy them anymore. I haven't golfed in four weeks, and I used to golf three times a week. When I was a young man, I golfed five times a week.

Clin.: That must be an upsetting feeling, not wanting to do anything.

Pt.: Yes it is (pause) everybody just thinks I'm lazy . . . who knows.

Clin.: It's not uncommon for people with depression to lose their interest in things. Sometimes it even affects their appetite. Have you noticed any change in your appetite?

Pt.: As a matter of fact, food doesn't taste very good. I only eat two meals a day, and sometimes I don't even eat at all.

Clin.: Have you lost any weight?

Pt.: A little, I think.

Clin.: Are your clothes getting too big or loose?

Pt.: Actually, they are. I probably lost at least five pounds.

Clin.: Over how long a time did it take to lose that weight?

Pt.: Oh, about two months.

Clin.: So your appetite has decreased, your energy is low, and your interest in things has decreased. What about your concentration? [And so on].

In summary, anhedonia and the neurovegetative symptoms are critical areas to explore when considering any affective syndrome such as a major depression or dysthymia. Furthermore, by asking such questions, one can gain a vivid picture of what depression feels like to the interviewee. To the interviewee the interviewer will appear one step closer to understanding.

At this point I would like to look at some further, revealing dialogue with Mr. White.

Clin.: Mr. White, you've been explaining how very depressed you feel. I'm wondering if there has been a time in your life when you felt just the opposite?

Pt.: I'm not sure I know what you mean.

Clin.: Well, has there ever been several days or even weeks when you felt really super energized?

> **Pt.:** (very faint smile) Hmm, yeah, about fifteen years ago, I was really on the go.
>
> **Clin.:** Tell me a little about that time.
>
> **Pt.:** I was working real hard and suddenly it all became so easy. It seemed like I just didn't need sleep. I went for days with only a couple of hours of sleep. I was like Mighty Mouse.
>
> **Clin.:** Did you start to speak rapidly or did any of your friends remark that you were talking too fast?
>
> **Pt.:** Yeah. They began calling me motor mouth. At first I thought that was funny. God, it all seems so foreign to me now. I'd give my right arm for one tenth of that energy right now.
>
> **Clin.:** Certainly it would be nice for you to have some of that energy now, but do you think that you might have had too much energy back then?
>
> **Pt.:** Oh yeah, things got crazy back then.
>
> **Clin.:** How do you mean?
>
> **Pt.:** Well I didn't really know what I was doing. I couldn't get anything done well. Oh I started plenty of stuff, but I didn't finish anything.
>
> **Clin.:** Did you start to do anything you were embarrassed about, like spending too much money or giving your money away?
>
> **Pt.:** Yes I did. I wanted to help everybody. I wanted to help the prisoners. That's why I tried to let a couple of them go . . . (pause) and that's when the Chief called me in and told me I needed a rest, and they put me in a hospital.
>
> **Clin.:** So things got so upsetting you needed a hospital?
>
> **Pt.:** Oh yeah.
>
> **Clin.:** What hospital was that?
>
> **Pt.:** Saint Anthony's. It was a tolerable place.
>
> **Clin.:** Have you ever had any other episodes like that one?
>
> **Pt.:** Yeah, one other time but just for a couple of days. I didn't think anything of it.

The above dialogue strongly suggests that Mr. White is not suffering only from a major depression. To the contrary he is probably best viewed as having bipolar disorder in a depressed phase. He illustrates one of the easiest traps to fall prey to when interviewing a severely depressed person. As both the interviewer and the interviewee become empathically absorbed by the depression, contextual clues suggesting mania do not appear. Without such clues the interviewer may forget to ask about current or past manic behavior. The depressed patient may be too preoccupied with depressive thought content to spontaneously bring up manic history if not asked. Therefore, one should always inquire about manic symptoms. The DSM-III-R criteria for mania are as follows:

Manic Episode[3]

Note: A "Manic Syndrome" is defined as including criteria A, B, and C below. A "Hypomanic Syndrome" is defined as including criteria A and B, but not C, i.e., no marked impairment

A. A distinct period of abnormally and persistently elevated, expansive, or irritable mood.

B. During the period of mood disturbance, at least three of the following symptoms have persisted (four if the mood is only irritable) and have been present to a significant degree:

(1) inflated self-esteem or grandiosity
(2) decreased need for sleep, e.g., feels rested after only three hours of sleep
(3) more talkative than usual or pressure to keep talking
(4) flight of ideas or subjective experience that thoughts are racing
(5) distractibility, i.e., attention too easily drawn to unimportant or irrelevant external stimuli
(6) increase in goal-directed activity (either socially, at work or school, or sexually) or psychomotor agitation
(7) excessive involvement in pleasurable activities which have a high potential for painful consequences, e.g., the person engages in unrestrained buying sprees, sexual indiscretions, or foolish business investments

C. Mood disturbance sufficiently severe to cause marked impairment in occupational functioning or in usual social activities or relationships with others, or to necessitate hospitalization to prevent harm to self or others.

D. At no time during the disturbance have there been delusions or hallucinations for as long as two weeks in the absence of prominent mood symptoms (i.e., before the mood symptoms developed or after they have remitted).

E. Not superimposed on Schizophrenia, Schizophreniform Disorder, Delusional Disorder, or Psychotic Disorder NOS.

F. It cannot be established that an organic factor initiated and maintained the disturbance. Note: Somatic antidepressant treatment (e.g., drugs, ECT) that apparently precipitates a mood disturbance should not be considered an etiologic organic factor.

Manic Episode codes: fifth-digit code numbers and criteria for severity of current state of Bipolar Disorder, Manic or Mixed:

1-Mild: Meets minimum symptom criteria for a Manic Episode (or almost meets symptom criteria if there has been a previous Manic Episode).

2-Moderate: Extreme increase in activity or impairment in judgment.

3-Severe, without Psychotic Features: Almost continual supervision required in order to prevent physical harm to self or others.

4-With Psychotic Features: Delusions, hallucinations, or catatonic symptoms. If possible, specify whether the psychotic features are *mood-congruent* or *mood incongruent.*

Mood-congruent psychotic features: Delusions or hallucinations whose content is entirely consistent with the typical manic themes of inflated worth, power, knowledge, identity, or special relationship to a deity or famous person.

Mood-incongruent psychotic features: Either (*a*) or (*b*):

(*a*) Delusions or hallucinations whose content does *not* involve the typical manic themes of inflated worth, power, knowledge, identity, or special relationship to a deity or famous person. Included are such symptoms as persecutory delusions of being controlled.

(*b*) Catatonic symptoms, e.g., stupor, mutism, negativism, posturing.

5-In Partial Remission: Full criteria were previously, but are not currently, met; some signs or symptoms of the disturbance have persisted.

6-In Full Remission: Full criteria were previously met, but there have been no significant signs or symptoms of the disturbance for at least six months.

0-Unspecified.

Another important issue to remember about bipolar disorders concerns the fact that they may demonstrate a mixed presentation. "Mixed presentation" suggests that simultaneously (or in extremely rapid alternation) the person exhibits the full symptomatic picture of both mania and depression. The first time I encountered this phenomenon, I was stunned by its apparent oddness. The patient, an x-ray technician, was in his mid-thirties. He had a scraggly beard and a pair of wild eyes. He could barely sit still. He kept leaning forward as if about ready to bolt from his chair. His speech was extremely rapid and pressured with a tangential quality, suggesting mania. Yet the content of his speech was markedly depressive, with guilty ruminations, self-derogatory exclamations, and suicidal ideation. Within a split second his eyes would fill with tears, which would soon transform into laughter. Such incongruities of behavior, affect, and thought content should alert the interviewer to a possible mixed state.

Mr. White's case also underscores another important point. Past psychiatric history may be very valuable. In particular, the following material should be actively elicited:

a. Previous hospitalizations (names and dates of hospitalizations).

b. Previous outpatient treatment (including names of mental health professionals).

c. Previous medications (names, dosages, and length of time on medications). I also often ask if the patient liked the drugs, or if they had side effects.

d. Previous psychotherapy (name of clinician and when). I often ask their opinion of the psychotherapy as well as a brief description of what they did in therapy.

e. Any history of ECT.

f. Past diagnosis.

g. Current therapy.

h. Periods of time when they feel they could have benefited from mental health care but did not seek it.

The information from the first ten minutes of Mr. White's interview highlights another important issue. He relates that he hopes to open a bar with his fiancée. Further questioning revealed that Mr. White had had severe problems with drinking in the past, including evidence of both dependence and significant social dysfuntion. He has not been drinking for over one year. Drinking, drug abuse, and depression often go hand in hand. Drinking itself can actually be an organic cause of depression. According to Renner, most alcoholics complain of depression and anxiety.[4] In most cases these depressive symptoms clear after detoxification. But depressive symptoms can continue up to two months after detoxification, with sleep disturbances lasting as long as six months. Consequently, when heavy drinking appears, the validity of the diagnosis of a major depression is somewhat suspect, and may best be viewed as a tentative diagnosis or a rule-out diagnosis. Many clinicians would wait to see if the depressive symptoms remained after detoxification, before considering the use of antidepressants. In actuality, depressive symptoms, triggered by the alcohol abuse, could actually remain for many months after detoxification.

As opposed to being caused by the drinking, the depression may antecede the drinking or coincide. In a sense these patients may be self-medicating with either alcohol or drugs as opposed to antidepressants. A true major depression is more likely if there is clear-cut evidence of depressive symptoms before the onset of sustained drinking. In any case no survey of depressive symptoms is complete until a thorough drug and alcohol history has been taken.

With regard to Mr. White, a summary of his diagnostic formulation seems in order. There was no evidence of a personality disorder upon further interviewing. Concerning Axis III and physical disorders, Mr. White complained of chronic and painful osteoarthritis in his knees. His formulation might appear as follows:

Axis I: Bipolar Disorder, Depressed 296.53
Alcohol Dependence (in remission) 303.90
Axis II: None V71.09
Axis III: Chronic Osteoarthritis

Before leaving the discussion of Mr. White, some key points are worth reiterating.

1. A major depression may present with anhedonia as the major complaint instead of a dysphoric mood.

2. Neurovegetative symptoms should be artfully woven into the fabric of the interview and seldom used in a checklist fashion.

3. Manic symptoms should always be actively sought.

4. Past psychiatric history may not be spontaneously stated and should always be elicited.

5. Alcohol and drug abuse are commonly associated with depression. What may appear as a major depression may actually be primarily related to alcohol or street drugs.

DISCUSSION OF MR. WHITSTONE

Mr. Whitstone was the distinguished appearing 62-year-old man admitted to the medical hospital because of paranoia. He had had heart surgery six months earlier. Currently he was refusing all medical help. One of the curious facets of Mr. Whitstone's presentation remains the fact that when asked directly about depression he stated, "No, I don't feel particularly depressed." Further questioning suggested differently. Since his bypass surgery in January, he had been experiencing many neurovegetative symptoms of depression, including difficulty falling asleep, sleep continuity disturbance, loss of appetite, weight loss, poor concentration, and anhedonia. Collaborative information from his wife and children pointed towards depression. They felt he appeared withdrawn, sad, and not himself. Mr. Whitstone appeared to be depressed, and yet denied it. Such a denial of depression is common. Donald Klein estimates that roughly 30 percent of people fulfilling the criteria of major depression will deny being depressed.[5] Consequently the following series of questions may be useful in determining whether dysphoric mood may be present:

a. How would you describe your mood over the past several weeks?
b. Tell me a little bit about how you've been feeling recently.
c. Would you say that you've been feeling depressed?

If they deny depression, the interviewer can then switch to a different word than "depressed," which, for whatever reason, patients may identify with more, such as:

a. Have you been feeling sad at all?
b. Have you been feeling unhappy?

It is not uncommon for a person suffering from depression to deny depression while admitting to sadness. Another useful question for uncovering dysphoric mood remains, "When was the last time you felt like crying?" The phrasing of this question automatically conveys that the interviewer feels it is both normal and acceptable to cry. Certain patients, especially males, feel hesitant to admit tearfulness. This question helps to skirt this resistance by asking only if they felt like crying. Such sensitive phrasing allows the self-conscious patient many avenues for saving face. The direct question, "Have you been crying?" may yield false negatives, since it does not offer any avenue for the patient except denial or admission of tearfulness.

Finally, if the patient denies both depression and sadness (Mr. Whitstone actually vigorously denied both), the following question may unearth material suggesting dysphoric mood:

a. Have you been feeling yourself recently? or,
b. Have you been feeling up to par over the past several weeks?

Upon such questioning, Mr. Whitstone pensively yet openly discussed his concerns over inadequacy and his fears about his thinking:

Clin.: In what ways haven't you felt yourself?
Pt.: My concentration is shot. It's been very upsetting, let me tell you. I'm a fairly intelligent man, I've gone far. But

about a month ago, I called my secretary to dictate a memo. I had to hang up, because I couldn't do it. (Mr. Whitstone was dismally nodding his head from side to side). It took me two days to write that memo (pause). I could normally do it in twenty minutes.

Other useful questions concerning cognitive processes include:

a. Have you noticed if your thinking appears to have speeded up or slowed down?
b. Are you finding it more difficult to make decisons recently?
c. Do you find yourself feeling frustrated when you are trying to make a decision?
d. Does it ever seem like your thoughts are getting disconnected or confused?
e. Has it been difficult for you to hold a train of thought?
f. Are you finding it difficult to read or to follow people as they talk?

The above discussion illustrates that a seriously depressed person may not always complain of depression. In line with this thinking, the possibility of an atypical depression naturally comes to mind. With regard to atypical depressions (referred to as depressive syndromes not otherwise specified in the DSM-III-R), two other common presentations of dysphoric mood are pertinent: (1) irritability and anger and (2) pain (or somatic complaints). When either of these symptoms is in the forefront of the patient's presentation, the clinician should vigorously pursue the possibility of depression. Oftentimes the interviewer will uncover the patient's hidden depression by subsequently eliciting neurovegetative symptoms.

Mr. Whitstone's case also emphasizes the critical importance of sources of information other than the patient. A hallmark of shrewd interviewers remains the ability to know when their interview was inadequate. In the case of Mr. Whitstone, both his wife and other family members felt that he had been pervasively depressed for at least two months.

Mr. Whitstone also demonstrates that psychotic process often emerges in severely depressed patients. The DSM-III-R refers to such psychotic material as either mood-congruent or mood-incongruent. Mood-congruent material concerns itself with depressive ideation or themes of decay. According to the DSM-III-R such themes include "personal inadequacy, guilt, disease, death, nihilism, or deserved punishment." Mood-incongruent delusions or hallucinations do not revolve about the above themes. They are more bizarre or peculiar and include such phenomena as paranoid delusions, thought insertion, delusions of control, and other themes not necessarily related to depressive ideation. Mr. Whitstone would fulfill the criteria for mood-incongruent psychotic features.

Finally, I have saved perhaps the most important point for last. When confronted with an affective presentation, one should always "think organic." Further investigation revealed that Mr. Whitstone had qualities suggestive of delirium, including auditory hallucinations, rapid fluctuations in affect, and a fluctuating level of consciousness according to the nursing notes. Besides the standard clues hinting at an organic state, Mr. Whitstone's history was suggestive of an organic etiology for several reasons. (a) He had not seemed normal since his bypass surgery. (b) He had been on anticoagulants, raising the possibility of emboli (blood clots) having been previously dislodged from his heart and passed to his brain or of a hemorrhage in his brain related to his anticoagulants. (c) He was significantly dehydrated.

In relation to organic precipitants of depression, it is important to stress the need for asking questions about both over-the-counter medications and prescription medications. A brief list of medications that commonly affect mood includes cimetidine, propranolol, methyldopa, reserpine, amantadine, steroids, birth control pills, and opiates. Even thiazide diuretics can cause depression by altering electrolyte balance.[6] In considering an organic cause of depression, besides medications and intracranial disease, one should keep in mind extracranial diseases such as hypothyroidism, hyperparathyroidism, lupus, hepatitis, and carcinoma. Pancreatic carcinoma is notorious for initially presenting with depressive complaints. Looked at more systematically, Anderson has separated the organic causes of depression into six categories, including (1) drugs and poisons, (2) metabolic and endocrine disturbances, (3) infectious diseases, (4) degenerative diseases such as multiple sclerosis, (5) neoplasm, and (6) miscellaneous conditions such as chronic pyelonephritis or Meniere's disease.[7] It is well beyond the scope of this chapter to discuss a thorough differential of the organic causes of depression, but I heartily urge the reader to review this material.

Naturally, even the best clinician will sometimes miss organic causes of depression despite a search for them. This failure is to be expected. But in the last analysis, there is probably no excuse for not having thought of looking for an organic cause of depression. In particular, one situation presents itself in which I unfortunately find it very easy to forget about possible organic factors. This situation arises when the patient presents complaining of a significant life stress such as unemployment, housing problems, divorce, or a death in the family. In such instances it is easy to assume psychological causality, but this assumption is patently misleading. Simply because a person has ample reason to be depressed does not mean that a depression does not also have a concurrent organic cause. Quite to the contrary, physical and psychological disability often go hand in hand. For instance, Schmale has reported a high incidence of separation events preceding the onset of medical illnesses.[8] The clinician should think holistically, checking for both psychological and physiological roots of depression. One can often be fooled by what appears obvious. Thus, apparent adjustment reactions may be hiding something more ominous. On the other hand, the obvious endogenous depression may actually be triggered or sustained by some not so obvious psychological factor or family dynamic.

In closing the discussion of Mr. Whitstone, let me diagnostically summarize his situation at the end of the initial interview.

Axis I: Organic delusional disorder (provisional) 293.81
Rule out delirium 293.00
Rule out major depression with mood incongruent psychotic features 296.24

Axis II: Deferred
Possible paranoid or compulsive traits (derived from data elicited from the family)

Axis III: Significant dehydration
Status post bypass cardiac surgery
Rule out embolism to brain or hemorrhage

By way of follow-up, a rigorous organic evaluation, including dementia chemistry screen, EEG, CT scan of head, lumbar puncture, and echocardiogram (checking for clots in the heart which could have embolized to the brain), was without abnormality. Moreover, once Mr. Whitstone was rehydrated he continued to be symptomatic. Apparently he was most likely suffering from a major depression with psychotic features.

At this point I would like to summarize the major issues underscored by Mr. Whitstone's interview:

1. People suffering from depression often deny they have depression.
2. Specific questions should be asked in an effort to uncover dysphoric mood not readily described by the patient.
3. Atypical depression often presents with complaints or irritability (anger) or pain (somatic complaints).
4. Outside information from family and significant others may be needed to delineate the diagnosis.
5. Even mood incongruent psychotic features such as paranoia or thought insertion can occur during severe depression.
6. It is imperative to ask questions that help rule out possible organic causes of depression.

DISCUSSION OF MS. WILKINS

Ms. Wilkins was the tearful, twenty-one-year-old woman recently contemplating suicide who remarked, "My best friend is really a bastard." She was requesting medication and psychotherapy. Despite her sad affect, further questioning revealed some intriguing differences when comparing her with both previous individuals:

> *Pt.:* I'm really feeling horrible. My whole world is collapsing. I don't know who to trust.
>
> *Clin.:* How long have you been feeling this way?
>
> *Pt.:* Years, for years. I can't think of a time when my life went smoothly. It's all a big mess.
>
> *Clin.:* When you say "for years" do you mean your depression never lifts?
>
> *Pt.:* Well, not really, I mean, I have my good days. Even a bad apple has its good parts . . . so . . . sometimes I feel fine.
>
> *Clin.:* When looking back over the past several weeks, did you have some of those good days?
>
> *Pt.:* Oh, I actually had a couple of good days last week, right before the big blow-up with Janet, but I knew Janet would blow it.
>
> *Clin.:* Tell me how you felt on those days.
>
> *Pt.:* Fine. In fact, I was having a great day on Friday until Janet had to open her mouth.
>
> *Clin.:* You say you've been feeling depressed for years, but it sounds like your mood changes a lot. Have you ever had a period of at least two weeks, where for the entire two weeks, you felt down and depressed?
>
> *Pt.:* That's a little hard to answer. I haven't felt that way for a long time . . . back home though, yeah, back home I was about 19, I was depressed for almost four months straight.
>
> *Clin.:* Tell me more about it.

From this dialogue it becomes apparent that Ms. Wilkins is probably not experiencing a sustained depression. Without a sustained alteration in mood or marked anhedonia lasting for two weeks, she will not fulfill criteria for a major depression. On the other hand, she appears to have undergone a four-month major depression in her teens. Further interviewing revealed that this episode was accompanied by persistent neurovegetative symptoms. From her history she appears to have had a major depression, which is currently in remission. This previous depression had responded to imipramine successfully. Her history of fluctuating depressive symptoms for years also suggests the possibility of dysthymia.

The above dialogue emphasizes two points. One, a detailed history of the present illness should be carefully elicited. In this explanation, the interviewer pays particular attention to both the time course and the duration of the symptoms. The foundation of a good diagnostic interview remains a good history of present illness. Two, one should rigorously evaluate whether the depressive symptoms are sustained or whether they fluctuate towards normal. Many people whose depressed feelings come and go will describe their symptoms as unrelenting unless questioned carefully, perhaps related to the fact that most depressive feelings tend to be experienced as intolerable, thus overshadowing the moments of normal mood. The DSM-III-R criteria suggest that the depressive symptoms need to have each been present nearly every day for a period of at least two weeks. Consequently if the interviewer uncovers significant fluctuation of symptoms, then they must look elsewhere than a major depression for a diagnosis.

Incidentally, I have found that statements such as, "I've been depressed for years," are, curiously enough, often indications that a major depression is not present. When questioned in more detail such people usually do not describe a sustained depression. Instead, they relate histories of depressive moods that fluctuate in response to environmental rewards or pleasures as is commonly seen in some personality disorders or in dysthymia. The following questions may be of value concerning the exploration of mood fluctuation:

    a. Do you find that your mood can shift during a single day?
    b. Would you describe yourself as a moody person?
    c. When you are feeling down, do you ever find that a friend or "something to do" can perk you up quickly?

If the patient answers "yes," then the interviewer asks them to describe some examples of such experiences.

The lack of a sustained mood disorder suggests other diagnoses such as a dysthymia, cyclothymia, certain personality disorders, or drug abuse. Upon further interviewing, Ms. Wilkins described a longstanding history of angry outbursts (such as throwing a hammer through a window), severe loneliness, intense feelings of boredom and emptiness, confusion over homosexual versus heterosexual relationships, and a series of overdoses. Ms. Wilkins fulfills many criteria of a borderline personality disorder. Her presentation emphasizes the following simple but easily forgotten principle: no matter how severely depressed a person looks, the diagnosis is not always a major depression. In fact, when it comes to looking severely upset, individuals with borderline personality disorder have a knack for such a dramatic presentation. With these ideas in mind, when the interviewee complains of sadness or depression, the following diagnoses should be considered in addition to a major depression or a bipolar disorder:

a. borderline personality disorder
b. other personality disorders such as the histrionic personality, the dependent personality, or the compulsive personality
c. dysthymia
d. cyclothymia
e. alcohol or drug abuse
f. adjustment disorders with depressed mood
g. organic etiologies of depression such as an organic affective disorder
h. V codes such as marital problem or a phase of life problem

Far from being a complete differential, this list represents the common entities that are often misdiagnosed as a major depression. As opposed to a major depression, these entities tend to show significant fluctuation in both mood and symptomatology. To mislabel these disorders as a major depression can lead to rather serious errors in triage or medication prescription. For instance, it could be a fatal mistake to prematurely prescribe antidepressants for Ms. Wilkins because one has mistakenly diagnosed her as having a major depression. Indeed, Ms. Wilkin's psychiatric trail is littered with empty bottles signifying her suicidal gestures by overdosage.

Delineating the history of the present illness and determining the consistency of the symptoms are not tasks as easily accomplished as one might think. The process is greatly complicated by a variety of factors, including (1) patient difficulties with memory, (2) unconscious distortion of the facts by the patient, (3) conscious and/or histrionic distortions by the patient, and (4) misunderstandings by the patient of the questions asked. These problems are only compounded when the clinician becomes lost in the facts and has no general approach to eliciting the history of the present illness.

Consequently it is worth spending some time examining some approaches to the history of the present illness. This history can be broken down into three contiguous phases: the early phase, the mid-phase, and the recent phase of the illness (the two months directly preceding the interview). All three phases are important, but because of the time constraints facing the intake clinician, an emphasis should be placed on the early phase and the recent phase.

The early phase may provide critical diagnostic information, for it allows the clinician to see the natural unfolding of the pathologic process. A patient may present with striking hallucinations while also reporting depressive feelings. If the patient has a major depression, then the early phase will generally demonstrate the appearance of depressed symptoms first, subsequently followed by psychotic symptoms. On the other hand, the schizophrenic patient will generally demonstrate psychotic symptoms and agitation first with depressive symptoms appearing later. Unless the clinician asks the patient or collaborative sources for this information, it can easily remain buried in the history.

A careful delineation of the recent history is an absolute must, for it provides the information needed to determine the patient's immediate level of functioning and the present diagnostic reality of the patient. This immediate diagnostic picture can be confusing if the patient is currently on medications, for the patient's symptom picture may be incomplete, since partial remission may be present. As obvious as this point may seem, it is surprisingly easy in a busy clinic setting to be trapped into thinking that a patient does not have a major depression when, in actuality, it is hiding beneath the facade created by partial treatment. In such circumstances it is important to explore the symptom picture at the time directly preceding the use of medications.

With the understanding that it may be of value to emphasize the early phase and the recent phase, two rather different approaches can be utilized in eliciting the history of the present illness. Both are effective. Clinicians must learn which seems best suited to their styles and the needs of the specific patient.

In the first technique, as the patient discusses the history of the present illness, an effort is made to quickly direct them to the early phase of the illness. The history is then taken chronologically from past to present with less emphasis upon the middle phase. Stressors and responses to stressors are frequently elicited as the history naturally unfolds. The strength of this approach is the detailed and well-ordered history that results. The weakness is the fact that because patient histories are frequently both complex and fascinating the clinician can easily spend too much time on the early and middle phase, coming away with a hazier picture of the immediate problems and current presentation.

A brief piece of dialogue will demonstrate two important features concerning the delineation of the onset of the illness.

> **Clin.:** When did this depression first begin for you?
> **Pt.:** Uh . . . a couple weeks after Thanksgiving . . . yeah, after Thanksgiving everything began to fall apart.
> **Clin.:** Think carefully, in the months before Thanksgiving were you feeling totally normal or were you already feeling not quite yourself?
> **Pt.:** Huh . . . actually I had been feeling somewhat de-

> pressed shortly after Patty, my daughter, went away to college.
>
> **Clin.:** What were the first symptoms you noticed?
>
> **Pt.:** I felt tearful at times and unusually tired, yes, yes I remember being struck at how little I wanted to get out of bed in the morning. But I'm not really certain when that feeling began . . . no, now that I think of it, that might have happened much later, I'm just not certain (looking frustrated).
>
> **Clin.:** It's hard to remember details like this and you're doing an excellent job. Let's focus upon Thanksgiving. Did you have a hard time getting out of bed then?
>
> **Pt.:** Oh yes, that I do remember. I didn't want to clean the house either or even cook the turkey.
>
> **Clin.:** What was your appetite like over Thanksgiving?
>
> **Pt.:** Very poor.

As illustrated in the preceding, when first asked to date the onset of the illness, patients frequently give an inaccurately late date, for it is easiest to remember when they began to feel really bad, a period after several weeks or months of the illness. Consequently they should be gently pushed by asking a second time, as shown in the example. Another useful method of increasing the validity of the data, as illustrated in the dialogue, is to prime the memory of the patient by giving specific holidays or personal events that can function as a trigger for increased memory production.[9]

The second approach to eliciting the history of the present illness consists of focusing the patient upon the recent and current phase of the illness first. The clinician then skips to the early phase and delineates the remainder of the history chronologically, with less emphasis upon the middle phase. This method provides the clinician with a sound understanding of current symptoms, stresses, and level of functioning, ensuring that these critical areas do not get short shrift because of time constraints. Patients also frequently like talking about recent symptoms first. Generally, this method also provides the early generation of a good diagnostic differential, which can help guide the subsequent questioning concerning the earlier phases of the history of the present illness.

When delineating the recent history, it is often useful to frame the time period with comments such as, "Let's look for a moment at just the last three weeks. All of the following questions deal only with the last three weeks. During that time how has your energy been?" Because patients have been coping with large amounts of psychological pain and confusion, even with the above framing, it is easy for them to eventually begin discussing earlier symptoms without letting the clinician know that this is the case. Consequently, it is useful to remind them several times of the time frame with statements such as, "Once again, just looking at the past three weeks, what has your sleep been like?"

Let us now return to the presentation of Ms. Wilkins, for her history provides one more practical interviewing point.

With further questioning she denied the recent death of any close friends or family. This point is mentioned because her initial symptoms would have been consistent with an uncomplicated bereavement. In fact, the full major depressive syndrome often appears in an uncomplicated bereavement. If the full major depressive syndrome appears during grief, it is labeled simply as an uncomplicated bereavement. On the other hand, if the depression lasts for too long a time (the DSM-III-R is unclear as to the actual time cut-off here, but I tend to use about 3 to 6 months as an upper limit; this time may vary considerably from culture to culture), then the diagnosis of a major depression should be made instead of an uncomplicated bereavement. In a similar light, if the bereavement begins to present with atypical qualities, then a diagnosis of major depression should be made. Atypical qualities include morbid preoccupation with worthlessness, prolonged and marked functional impairment, marked psychomotor retardation, or any psychotic features.

As a final note, like an uncomplicated bereavement, an adjustment disorder can present some confusion with regard to the diagnosis of a major depression. For purposes of clarification, an adjustment disorder must have a clear-cut psychosocial stressor within three months of the depression. But even if there is a clear-cut stressor, once the criteria for a major depression are fulfilled, then the diagnosis adjustment disorder is no longer applicable. If the criteria for a major depression are present, then the diagnosis should be a major depression and the diagnosis of an adjustment disorder should be dropped. As we close, a diagnostic summary for Ms. Wilkins seems in order.

Axis I: Rule out dysthymia   300.40
           Rule out major depression, single episode, in remission
           296.26
Axis II: Borderline personality (principal diagnosis)   301.83
Axis III: None

By way of summary Ms. Wilkins's presentation illustrates the following points:

1. A careful history of present illness is the foundation of a diagnostic interview.

2. The duration of the depressive mood should be thoroughly

discussed. To fulfill a major depression it must last at least two weeks with little fluctuation in symptoms.

3. Many other diagnoses may present with depression. In particular, one should be careful to check for a borderline personality disorder, dysthymia, drug or alcohol abuse, or an adjustment disorder.

4. The clinician should develop a well thought out approach to the history of the present illness. Otherwise, it is easy to become lost in the data base.

5. Patients frequently date the onset of their illness later than it was in reality. Once a date is given, ask them to carefully consider whether they had felt completely normal in the month or two before that date.

6. One can prime the patient's memory by referring to holidays or special events in the patient's life.

7. When gathering the recent history, it is useful to frame the time period for patients and intermittently remind them of the time frame being discussed.

8. Uncomplicated bereavement may fulfill the criteria for a major depression. If this occurs, the process is still labeled an uncomplicated bereavement. The diagnosis of a major depression is not made.

DISCUSSION OF MR. COLLIER

Mr. Collier was the twenty-six-year-old man with dark brown hair and a strong jaw. He had an authoritarian air and had recently slapped his ten-year-old daughter. In some respects, Mr. Collier's interview sounds reminiscent of Ms. Wilkins's presentation. Further questioning revealed that, like Ms. Wilkins, his mood tends to fluctuate. He has never had a period of pervasively depressed mood lasting for two weeks or more. Questions pertaining to the history of the present illness revealed that he had felt intermittently depressed for over six years. He has had no periods of good mood lasting consistently longer than a month or two. Mr. Collier did not relate further symptoms consistent with a borderline personality or any other personality disorder. The above information suggests a diagnosis of dysthymia a relatively common psychiatric syndrome.

Mr. Collier's comment that "I remind myself of my father," warrants further follow-up. This statement may be the first indication that affective disorders run in his family. The clinician should carefully probe for evidence of such a genetic predisposition when dealing with a depressed or manic patient. Genetic studies by Rudin indicated that the incidence of manic depressive psychosis is twenty-five times as high among the siblings of bipolar patients when compared with the normal population. Furthermore, monozygotic twins will be affected in more than half the cases.[10] In a similar fashion, patients with a major depression show a higher prevalence of relatives with major depression and depressive personalities. Other studies have suggested some correlation between affective disorders and alcoholism. For instance, Winokur studied 259 alcoholics and 507 of their relatives. In this study, female relatives appeared to have an increased incidence of unipolar depression.[11] In any case, such material emphasizes the importance of taking a thorough family history.

Elaborating a valid family history in the first fifty minutes is no easy task. A variety of variables can get in the way, including (1) the patient's lack of information about his family history, (2) the patient's decreased concentration and other cognitive impairments, decreasing the accuracy of his statements, (3) the patient's protection of other family members, and (4) the interviewer's ineffective exploration of the patient's family history. This last variable is the only one we have direct control over.

Frequently, vague questions, such as "Does anyone in your family have a mental illness?" lead to blanket negatives. The interviewee may have no idea that the interviewer is including blood relatives such as aunts, uncles, or cousins in such a question. Along the same lines, the interviewee may have no idea that the interviewer is including alcoholism as a mental illness. To anticipate these problems, it may be of value to help the patient understand the reason for obtaining a family history. Such an approach also "focuses" patients, increasing their willingness to jog their memories. Just one of many lead-ins is illustrated below:

> *Clin.:* Carl, you mentioned earlier that you sometimes remind yourself of your father. In what ways is this true?
> *Pt.:* Hmm . . . Well, my father often seemed upset to me as a kid. He got irritable and would yell at us, all of us, even Annie, the baby. He just seemed troubled.
> *Clin.:* Do you think he was depressed?
> *Pt.:* Yeah, I do.
> *Clin.:* Had he ever received help from a therapist or psychiatrist?
> *Pt.:* Oh, no! He would never do that. He didn't believe in that sort of thing; even so, I think he needed help.
> *Clin.:* While we are talking about your father's depression, I would like to touch upon other family members. Sometimes we can gain clues from psychiatric problems in relatives, that may give us better ideas of how to help you.

Following such an introduction to the topic, the clinician can proceed to discuss each member of Carl's nuclear family, inquiring specifically about drinking, schizophrenia, and other affective disorders. With regard to more distant family members, it is important to state whom you are interested in.

> **Clin.:** The rest of these questions concern any of your blood relatives, including grandparents, aunts, uncles, and cousins. Have any of your father's blood relatives had depression or schizophrenia? (Repeat questions later from other side of family.)
>
> **Pt.:** Well, I'm not really sure. I had an aunt who was sort of crazy.
>
> **Clin.:** How do you mean?
>
> **Pt.:** They put her away for a while because she had a nervous breakdown.

The preceding exchange illustrates several points. First, one needs to be careful of technical words like "schizophrenia" or "manic depression." Many patients do not know what these terms mean and will consequently deny their presence. A brief definition may help clarify the issue. Second, it can be of use to ask the question, "Has anybody in your family been hospitalized or institutionalized for a mental disorder?" People may remember a concrete hospitalization concerning a distant relative much easier than a nebulous process like depression. Third, terms such as "bad nerves" or "nervous breakdown" are common labels for serious disorders such as schizophrenia or an agitated depression. Such terms warrant further inquiry. Another helpful question is simple and to the point, "Has anybody in your family ever tried to hurt themselves or actually kill themselves?" Surprisingly, after having denied any serious psychiatric illnesses in their family, interviewees will suddenly recall a suicide following this question. This phenomenon parallels the finding that later interviewing will often reveal positive family history that the initial interview missed.

Before leaving the issue of family history, I would like to add a few points. The family history may provide even more information than indicated by the genetic findings of such an inquiry. The tone of voice and the manner in which the patient talks about family members may provide subtle clues concerning family relations themselves. At times it pays to take a brief excursion into interpersonal and dynamic issues during this part of the interview, as illustrated below.

> **Clin.:** Do you feel your brother had problems with depression or drugs?
>
> **Pt.:** Him (said with an astonished and sarcastic tone)! No. He's lily white. He's never had any problems.

> **Clin.:** You sound almost surprised by my question.
> **Pt.:** Oh, it's just that he has always been everybody's favorite.
> **Clin.:** How have you noticed that?
> **Pt.:** He always made better grades. Report card day was a real pain in the ass for me. I used to . . .

In this example, "family history" has taken on a richer meaning.

Mr. Collier's presentation also raises some issues concerning medication. One wonders whether certain symptoms suggest responsiveness to antidepressants. It is not entirely clear yet which symptoms specifically predict tricyclic response. It was hoped that the symptoms in the DSM-III-R subcategory of melancholia would be indicators of an "endogenous" depression implying drug responsiveness. Evidence seems to support this relationship. With regard to anhedonia, Donald Klein feels that persistent anhedonia (as well as autonomous depressive symptoms) may indicate drug responsiveness. By "autonomous mood" he refers to the idea that a biochemical depression will not abate even if good or pleasant stimuli occur to the person. The underlying pathophysiology prevents the normal responsiveness to pleasurable stimuli such as friends or changes in luck.[12] Aesthetically this idea appears pleasing but is not yet fully substantiated. A review article by Nelson and Charney addresses some of these issues directly.[13]

Nelson and Charney reviewed 13 research papers that performed factor analytic studies of depressed patients. The studies were searching for evidence of symptom clusters suggestive of an endogenous or drug responsive depression. According to Nelson and Charney motor retardation remains the most valid indication of treatment response. Other moderate indicators were agitation, severe depressed mood, depressive delusions, self-reproach, and loss of interest. They also feel there is some indication — but with less supporting evidence — that endogenous depressions are associated with a distinct quality of mood, diurnal morning worsening, and difficulty concentrating. Some symptoms commonly assumed to indicate an endogenous depression were also supported but not as strongly, such as early morning awakening, other sleep difficulties, and appetite and weight loss. Obviously the answers are not completely available at present. In the meantime, the first two clusters of symptoms mentioned, as well as the presence of other neurovegetative symptoms, should arouse the clinician's suspicion of possible medication responsiveness.

Mr. Collier demonstrated several of these symptoms, including motor retardation, intermittently depressed mood, self-reproach, and a sporadic loss of interest. A growing body of evidence reviewed by Hagop Akiskal suggests that certain forms of dysthymia may respond to antidepressants.[14] It is beyond the scope of this chapter to discuss this material thoroughly. But I feel it is important for the initial interviewer to keep in mind the symptoms suggesting drug responsiveness. Such diligence may result in more appropriate triage.

At this juncture, a diagnostic summary of Mr. Collier's presentation seems in order. Two points should be added. First, with regard to medical problems, Mr. Collier related having bronchitis secondary to smoking. Second, on an interpersonal level, further interviewing indicated significant marital distress. Couples therapy was recommended. This interpersonal problem represented a core issue with regard to Mr. Collier's depression. The next part of this chapter will more fully investigate the importance of such issues in the initial interview. Mr. Collier's diagnostic summary is as follows:

Axis I: Dysthymia 300.40 (Primary Type — early onset)
Marital problems V61.10
Axis II: None V71.09
Axis III: Chronic bronchitis secondary to smoking

In conclusion Mr. Collier's presentation emphasizes several points:

1. Individuals with dysthymia commonly experience many neurovegetative symptoms of depression, but the symptoms do not last in a sustained manner for over two weeks.

2. The depressive symptoms of a dysthymia can often rapidly shift towards normal if there is something "fun" to do.

3. Family history should be an integral component of any interview where depression is suspected.

4. Blanket questions such as "Does anybody in your family have a mental illness?" will often yield false negatives.

5. A detailed family history provides a nice take-off point for exploring family dynamics.

6. Certain syndromes, such as various subtypes of dysthymia, may respond to tricyclics.

7. Certain symptoms such as motor retardation, agitation, severely depressed mood, depressive delusions, self-reproach, and loss of interest may be positively correlated with medication responsiveness.

The above four case discussions are not intended to be an exhaustive review of the diagnostic subtleties associated with affective disorders. I have attempted to present a sound introduction to the process of diagnostic evaluation during an initial interview. The "art of diagnosis," of learning about the person as one delineates the diagnosis, will always present the clinician with a challenge. In the next section of this chapter, an attempt will be made to explore some of the phenomena that help the interviewer reach a deeper understanding of depression as a human experience, for this understanding is the path to compassion.

SECTION II: THE UNDERSTANDING OF DEPRESSION

When the low heavy sky weighs like a lid
Upon the spirit aching for the light,
And all the wide horizon's line is hid
By a black day sadder than any night; . . .

When like grim prison bars stretch down the thin,
Straight, rigid pillars of the endless rain,
And the dumb throngs of infamous spiders spin
Their meshes in the cavern of the brain, . . .

Charles Baudelaire, Spleen

Diagnosis represents a powerful and rigorous instrument for conceptualizing depression, often laying the critical foundation for effective treatment planning. But, as shown in the previous section, the search for a diagnosis provides even more. It represents one step in the process of understanding the person in the manner in which that individual experiences the world. In this section, emphasis will be upon the search for an understanding of depressive phenomena, exploring more fully the impact of such a search on the initial interview.

To begin with, depression is not a static thing that occurs in isolated items called people. Depression is a process. As a process, it constantly unfolds, manifesting itself in phenomena that affect numerous systems outside the individual identified as depressed. Depression exists as an impact that can be identified, and perhaps treated, through any number of systems. The more the interviewer understands this concept, the more open the interviewer becomes to the subtle clues suggesting depression and the harsh realities of the destruction left in its wake. From this understanding, interviewers enhance their sensitivity, their clinical acumen, and their ultimate engagement with patients. The interview is, at once, both more human and more clarifying.

In Section II an effort will be made to explore the ramifications of depression throughout various systems. The discussion will begin with the very smallest system of interaction, physiological, and move outwards, through progressively larger systems, as was discussed in Chapter 4.

To understand depression more fully in the initial interview, the clinician must understand its reflection in each system. Ultimately, the knowledge gathered may suggest possible interventions within that system, as described in detail in Chapter 4. A good interview immediately suggests possible avenues of intervention. By understanding the depressive process, treatment planning suggests itself.

At another level, the following approach emphasizes the fact that interviewers, whether they want to or not, will by their very presence become a subsystem touched by the patient's depression. The interviewer will both affect and be affected by the depressive processes explored. Awareness of this fact can lead to important insights in intervention. Blindness to this fact can lead to dismally short-sighted conclusions and mislaid interventions. With these ideas in mind the exploration begins. At its conclusion we will have a better understanding of what it is like to be at a place where:

> . . . all the wide horizon is hid
> By a black day sadder than any night.

Fields of Interaction

I: THE PHYSIOLOGICAL SYSTEM

As one enters the room occupied by a person experiencing depression, the physiological ravages of the process are often disturbingly apparent. In a severely depressed person the initial glance may reveal unkempt hair, ragged or mismatched clothes, dirty nails, untied shoes, and a vacant look to the eyes. More striking may be the slowness of movement and the person's lack of responsiveness. It may take a few seconds or much longer for the depressed person to acknowledge the interviewer, if such acknowledgment occurs at all. In a similar manner, more subtle decrements in responsiveness may be the first clues of a milder depressive state. Thus, the interview begins with the first look, before any words are uttered.

The slowness of movement probably parallels the disquieting sensation of heaviness often reported by depressed people. Depression, as Baudelaire suggested with his line "When the low heavy sky weighs like a lid . . . ," often feels like a heavy shawl descending on leaden shoulders. The arms and limbs may literally feel weighted down. This abnormal sensation may be related to the powerfully intense sense of inertia that can accompany depression. It becomes distressing for the depressed person to initiate movement; it seems so much easier to simply rest. A young woman with a dsythymia vividly describes this phenomenon:

It is so strange. Depression is exhausting in a physical sense. You know, most people have chores they have to do just to keep their lives going. And if the chores are waiting for you, and you sit there and look at them, they just seem overwhelming. And I could easily sit for two hours in a chair just looking at some clothes I left on the bedroom floor and not be able to motivate myself to pick them up. My body just feels heavy, as if it wouldn't want to respond unless I absolutely forced it to . . . Hmm . . . You know it is actually almost as if your brain lost half of its ability to control your body in the sense that even making a decision to pick something up required so much energy that you don't want to make it. You feel like it couldn't possibly be worth it. I just want to vegetate.

This sensitive excerpt brings up another important point with the opening comment, "It is so strange." Depressed patients, at times, present a peculiar dichotomy in the manner in which they cognitively and affectively experience their profound condition. On a cognitive level, they often feel they are the root of their problem, their speech becoming an entangled web of self-recrimination and belittlement. They cognitively experience their depression as being actively caused by their own flaws. Simultaneously, they affectively experience the depression as coming on them or over them from an outside source. In a sense, they feel invaded and violated. They feel they are the passive recipients of a phenomenon they do not understand or control. This incipient "loss of control" presents a terrifying threat to their sense of ideal self. Karl Jaspers with a single word captures the pith of this process when he describes depressed patients as experiencing a physical and emotional "ossification."[15]

At present the etiologic meaning of such radical changes in movement and body perception remains unclear. Such changes may represent psychological defenses, biological attempts to withdraw a malfunctioning organism from a potentially dangerous environment, social indicators that an organism needs help, or direct results of primary biochemical imbalance. Any combination of the preceding is possible. No matter what the etiology of these phenomena, they can create a frightening experience for the depressed person. In essence, even their bodies become strangers to them, one more step toward their intense sense of isolation.

The other neurovegetative symptoms also represent an array of physiological markers of depression. Baseline energy withers. Appetite and libido dry up, as if parched by the intensity of the process. These feelings of altered functioning can become immensely disturbing to patients, sometimes being perceived as further evidence of their personal failure. With these phenomena in mind, questions such as the following may add depth to the interview:

a. What has your body felt like to you recently?
b. What does it feel like to you to have lost your energy and drive?
c. You mention that you have lost your energy, your appetite, and

your ability to sleep. How have all these changes made you feel about yourself?

As well as allowing patients the chance to ventilate, these questions emphasize that the interviewer is interested in them as unique people whose depression they alone can explain.

Before leaving the physiological field, I would like to briefly describe some of the biologic ramifications of an agitated depression. Here too there exists a peculiar dichotomy, as described by an elderly male patient in response to a question about losing energy, "I don't know exactly what you mean, but yeah, I've got energy all over the place, driving me constantly, but no, I don't have any sustained energy to do anything." In the agitated state there exists a nagging need to move. The energy is unbridled and disobedient. Consequently, the body tends to assume an incessant display of "bad nerves." Hands wring each other in a frenzy of confusion. Fingers pick at the body or pluck the clothes. Sitting becomes an act of will power. From deep inside the legs, there erupts a need to move. Pacing becomes a necessary method of release as natural as breathing. In many instances, this agitated state appears worse in the morning. In the interview it can be revealing to ask, "What part of the day seems worse to you?" It is important to remind oneself that a relatively calm patient interviewed at 4:00 P.M. may have looked remarkably more agitated at 8:00 A.M. Depression nags the body with an intermittent voice.

II: THE PSYCHOLOGICAL SYSTEM

Depression has a calling card. This calling card consists of a distinct set of changes that occur within the mind of those experiencing the depression. Not all depressed people experience these feelings, but many do in one combination or another. Four broad areas are touched by depression and will be the focus of this discussion: (1) perception of the world, (2) cognitive processes, (3) thought content, and (4) psychodynamic defenses. An understanding of the above processes can increase the ability of the interviewer to recognize the subtle clues of depression and can increase empathic abilities, as well.

Concerning the perception of the world, depression alters both the sense of time and the size of the world actively engaged. To the depressed person the concept of current or future change appears conspicuously absent. A mantle of flatness suffocates spontaneity. Moment-by-moment existence seems void of any chance of alteration. Without this feeling of possible change, time passes arrogantly slowly. In a literal sense time passes painfully. Such a state of psychic monotony can have a curious effect on the interviewee's perception of the future. In effect, if change does not exist, then the future is essentially meaningless. All days are merely replicas. Our sense of the future is partially dependent upon our sense that the future may be different. To the depressed interviewee, the future is draped in a radically bland light. This perception may be one reason that depressed people often appear unmotivated. Without a perceived future why should they attempt change? This phenomenon has been described by the phenomenologist Eugene Minkowski as a "blocking of the future."[16]

The second alteration in world perception does not involve time. It revolves about space. The "active world" of the depressed person undergoes a profound alteration. By active world I refer to the area of the environment that a person remains interested in engaging. In depression the active world shrinks. The patient's sense of space gradually vanishes, creating a cataract of the mind. This shrinking of the active world can powerfully short circuit environmental reinforcement and reward. The depressed person becomes a behavioral isolate. The dysthymic woman quoted before elegantly depicts this process.

I'm so focused inward . . . When I feel depressed it is such a great pain, and I am paying so much attention to it trying to control it, that I walk down the street and really don't see much at all . . . I screen out other people because I don't want to interact with others . . . I probably miss a lot. Even in the sense that I can walk down the street where I work and there can be roses blooming. And if I am really depressed, I don't even see them. And I love roses. Whereas, if I am feeling better, even despite the smell of the buses running around, I will still smell the roses. And I will admire them. . . .

It can come as quite a shock to the interviewer to realize that the interviewer may not be a feature of the interviewee's active world. To engage such patients, the clinician needs to enter their world as best as possible. Consequently, the interview with a severely depressed patient may require a change in style. At times the clinician must be more active while also accepting, with patience, the interviewee's difficulty in responding.

A second broad area of alteration concerns changes in the cognitive processes of the depressed person. In a retarded depression, the thought process slows as if the stream of thought were frozen by an unexpected drop in temperature. In contrast, in an agitated depression thought races as if the same stream had sustained a turbulent boil. In both cases, the thought process becomes disjointed. Concentration becomes annoyingly elusive.

Besides these alterations in the speed and flow of thought, depression creates an ideational caging. The term "caging" suggests that the mind becomes trapped within a small network of limiting themes.

Such depressive rumination can lock the depressed person into worries about the past, the present, or the future. Once within the cage, the depressed patient has great difficulty attending to new and perhaps therapeutic influences. In the interview, caging may demonstrate itself as a frustrating tendency for the patient to return to a specific topic. Or the patient may, alternatively, repeatedly ask the same question, despite the interviewer's reasonable reassurances. Such caging can seriously block an interview. One method of trying to circumvent it consists of attempting to acknowledge it while simultaneously refocusing the patient, as illustrated below. In this interview more than enough time had been spent helping the patient to ventilate. When more direct questions were asked, the patient would not move on.

> ***Clin.:*** Mrs. Jones, can you tell me a little bit about the effect of all these troubles on your sleep?
>
> ***Pt.:*** Sleep, can't sleep . . . (pause) can't sleep because of the bills. I just know we won't be able to pay the bills. Oh God, my children, we'll be ruined.
>
> ***Clin.:*** I understand your concern, Mrs. Jones, but I need to know about your sleep, it will help me to understand your depression. For instance, how long has it been taking you to fall asleep?
>
> ***Pt.:*** I don't know, all I think about are the bills. I know that somehow I'm to blame. What will we do? What will we do! Somebody has got to help.
>
> ***Clin.:*** Mrs. Jones, it seems very hard for you to stop talking about your finances. I understand your concern, but in order to help you, I must learn more about what has happened to you. I will ask you some important questions and if you get side-tracked, I will pull you back to the question. I want to help, but I need your help as well. Once again think carefully, how long is it taking you to fall asleep? (The preceding is said with a calm but firmer tone.)

With proper timing, such an intervention may open a cage. At other times, the caging of the patient will not yield despite the interviewer's best intentions.

Aaron Beck, one of the founders of cognitive psychotherapy, has delineated many specific cognitive impairments in depression. Beck has pointed out that depressed patients may overgeneralize with statements such as "Everything has fallen apart" or "No one cares about me." They can exaggerate, in essence creating the proverbial mountain out of a mole hill with a statement such as, "My boss Mr. Henry looked angry. He's dissatisfied with me. I'm sure it is only a matter of time until I'm fired." They also have a tendency to ignore the positive. For instance, a businesswoman confused me with the following statement which illustrates this principle, "It's the best Christmas season we've ever had. We're really selling books all over the place. I set myself a remarkably high quota. If we don't meet it, I will have failed miserably as a manager."

Beck has also described a trio of distortions, the cognitive triad, that frequently appear in depression.[17] The patient relates a negative view of the world, a negative concept of the self, and a negative appraisal of the future. This negative view of the world is partially generated by the tendency of the depressed patient to continually validate their depression. They speak as if they had placed a negative filter over their eyes, as witnessed by the following taped comments:

When I'm really depressed every negative, every unpleasant thing that I could possibly think of that might be happening to another person like someone being hit by a car or someone getting cancer or a dog being injured will trigger personal fear and worry that the world is bad. And so the depression has no justification to ever lift because everything about life is horrible. It's all just proof that depression is reality just looking itself in the face . . .

With regard to negative self-concept, the tendency to assume self-blame may be a major contributing factor. I do not think I have ever seen this quality as strikingly portrayed as in the original Bob Newhart Show. In this show, Newhart plays a psychologist with a client named Mr. Herd who epitomizes the self-blamer. A typical exchange might be as follows:

> *Newhart:* (after entering the office) I can't believe it, I left my wallet at home.
> *Mr. Herd:* I did it . . . You were worried about me and forgot your wallet over me . . . I'm sorry, I'm really sorry. I won't let it happen again.

Although funny in the Newhart Show, the process of self-blame stands as a vicious cognitive trap. In a sense, it may represent a milder variant of the much more ominous symptom known as delusional guilt.

Another jarring twist in cognitive process comes to mind at this point. Depressed patients sometimes exhibit a trait I prefer to call "an immunity to logic" that can be very frustrating to family, therapist, or initial interviewer. This immunity to logic was brilliantly depicted by Eugene Minkowski while at the same time he illustrated the blocking of the future mentioned earlier. Minkowski spent several months living with a man experiencing a psychotic depression. The following excerpt refers to Minkowski's vain efforts to convince him that he would not be horribly mutilated and subsequently executed:

> From the first day of my life with the patient, my attention was drawn to the following point. When I arrived, he stated that his execution would certainly take place that night; in his terror, unable to sleep, he also kept me awake all that night. I comforted myself with the thought that, come the morning, he would see that all his fears had been in vain. However, the same scene was repeated the next day and the next, until after three or four days I had given up hope, whereas his attitude had not budged one iota. What had happened? It was simply that I, as a normal human being, had rapidly drawn from the observed facts my conclusions about the future. He, on the other hand, had let the same facts go by him, totally unable to draw any profit from them for relating himself to the same future. I now knew that he would continue to go on, day after day, swearing that he was to be tortured to death that night, and so he did, giving no thought to the present or the past. Our thinking is essentially empirical; we are interested in facts only in so far as we can use them as basis for planning the future. This carry-over from past and present into the future was completely lacking in him; he did not show the slightest tendency to generalize or to arrive at any empirical rules.[18]

Although this is a description of a psychotically depressed man, a similar, albeit milder, process commonly accompanies nonpsychotic depression.

All of these disturbances in cognitive process may be encountered by the initial interviewer. By training themselves to listen for such abnormalities, interviewers may increase their ability to detect depression. For instance, people with atypical depressions may initially betray their underlying depression by the use of such pathological processes. Of course, the presence of such processes, in a less severely disturbed patient, may also alert the interviewer to the possible use of cognitive psychotherapy as a future treatment modality. At this juncture, I would like to turn attention to the third major psychological area affected by depression, thought content itself.

The distinction between cognitive process and cognitive content is sometimes a blurred one, but I would like to focus briefly on four content themes: loneliness, self-loathing, helplessness, and hopelessness. These factors blend with one another, reinforcing their mutual perpetuation. The loneliness of the depressed person can become practically insurmountable. As shown earlier, processes such as caging and the shrinking of the active world separate depressed patients from friends, family, and even the clinician. Their loneliness reaches such a magnitude of intensity that it may begin to assume a qualitative difference from the more common loneliness encountered in daily living. Put differently, they are not only lonely, they feel alone. The loneliness assumes an irrefutable realization that they are isolated, somehow cut off permanently from others. Such isolation does indeed diminish social reinforcement and therapeutic intervention.

Coupled with this alienation from others, depressed patients may encounter a profound alienation from and hatred of their selves. Such a self-loathing only itensifies their feeling of loneliness for they are repulsed by their own company. To the seriously depressed patient, it seems as if they lack any real existence or purpose at all, except for their pain. These feelings can shift imperceptibly into the potentially lethal thought that, "I am truly a burden to those I love." These ideas may emerge in the interview in a more oblique fashion as in, "Don't bother with me. Talk with someone you can help." The initial interviewer needs to probe beneath such comments, hunting for the more dangerous logic that "others would be better off if I were dead."

From their social isolation and their repugnance toward their selves, feelings of helplessness emerge naturally. This profound sense of helplessness can contribute to the inertia that effectively prevents therapeutic encounters. Phrased succinctly, they wonder "why bother?" The interviewer can easily estimate the role of this factor by simply asking, "Have you been feeling helpless?" A more sophisticated gauge may emerge with the question, "At this time, what kinds of ways of getting help do you see for yourself?" A blank negative or dismal shake of the head in response to this question should alert the interviewer to the potential seriousness of the depression.

Finally, all of the above depressive themes may lead to hopelessness. Beck has demonstrated that hopelessness represents a more specific and sensitive predictor of suicide potential than depressive mood itself.[19] As such, the interviewer should always try to measure the degree of hopelessness with either oblique questions, such as "What do you see for yourself in the future?," or more simply, "Are you feeling hopeless?"

The above discussion has examined the critical role of depressive thought content in the initial interview. It is time to examine the fourth major area of psychological disturbance in depression, dynamic defenses.

I have found the discussion by MacKinnon and Michels in their book, *The Psychiatric Interview in Clinical Practice*[20] to be particularly illuminating in this area. I shall summarize some of these points, focusing upon those defenses that can most easily confuse the interviewer.

In the first place, some people seem incapable of admitting depression into cognitive awareness. They tend to verbally deny depression. In fact, they may be truly unaware that they are depressed. Such an ironic state may be the result of dynamic defenses such as denial and repression. Despite these defenses careful questioning will often uncover the depression by eliciting neurovegetative symptoms or evidence of depressive cognitive functioning such as caging or generalization. Other common defenses include isolation and rationalization. The patient may isolate all their depressive rumination onto one symptom complex. They too may deny depression, as illustrated by "I've got no real problems other than the fact that I can't sleep at night and I've got daily headaches."

The patient's anger can provide the interviewer with the first glimpse of the depressive phenomena. Analytic theorists such as Abraham and Freud have stressed the idea that depression may represent anger turned inward.[21] This anger may originate in a variety of situations, including perceived abandonment, rejection, frustration, direct or indirect attacks on oneself, or feelings of betrayal or injustice. In line with this thinking, anger often pierces the sadness of the person experiencing an agitated depression. Thus a patient who quickly verbally attacks the interviewer may be betraying their depression to that same interviewer. I have even been surprised to see anger unexpectedly shooting through the apathy of the supposed "retarded depression," as evidenced by vicious diatribes against past doctors or relatives. Anger also routinely disrupts the existence of people displaying borderline personality disorders or dysthymia. Anger and depression can form a damaging positive feedback loop, as follows. The patient lashes out at a close friend. From this angry display, the patient develops guilt for having such inappropriate feelings. This guilt triggers further depression. As the depression deepens, the patient becomes increasingly irritable. Soon enough, the patient lashes out again, thus completing and fueling the cycle.

A third confusing clinical picture, resulting from dynamic defenses, involves the defense of projection with resultant paranoia. MacKinnon emphasizes that depression and paranoia may alternate with each other. The person's intense self-incrimination can become too painful. Deflection of this pain occurs through projection. Instead of hating themselves, they find that "other people hate me," or "others want to punish me." This last statement demonstrates the projection of suicidal ideation outwards. The need to consider paranoia as a defense against depression dramatically demonstrates itself in the following vignette provided by a colleague of mine.

Apparently he had consulted on a patient who presented as psychotically paranoid in a medical hospital. This patient denied all suicidal ideation. Furthermore he related few neurovegetative symptoms. Transfer to the psychiatric hospital was recommended in the morning. The patient was checked throughout the night but was not placed on a one-to-one observation. During a period of nonsurveillance, the patient quickly and efficiently hung himself. Little more need be said.

A final dynamic mechanism that can easily fool the interviewer exhibits itself in the process of hypomanic or manic defenses against depression. One needs to be wary of anybody who appears "too happy" while describing numerous unsettling stressors. If watched carefully, the surprisingly buoyant person may betray sadness by a minute quivering of the chin or a hesitancy to the voice. At these moments a quiet statement, such as "You know, as you are talking you seem sort of sad to me" may open a floodgate of tears. This hypomanic defense is very apparent in bipolar patients with a mixed presentation. In fact, in my own experience I have seldom found a purely elated mania. Usually, patients with mania have some elements of anger or sadness that linger just beneath the surface of their laughter.

Perhaps it is best to end the exploration of the psychological field at this time. Much more could be said, but it seems an opportune time to move to the next larger system in which depression manifests itself, the realm of the interpersonal system.

III: THE DYADIC SYSTEM

When two people interact, a dyadic system is born. Depression often first shows itself through its impact on the flow of communication and affection within this dyadic system. In this sense depression exists as an interpersonal phenomenon, seldom, if ever, restricted to the world of a single individual. Perhaps the following description by a patient will illustrate the power of depression to alter the interpersonal field:

It makes it harder to interact with people. It decreases your motivation for talking . . . first of all because you are so acutely aware of how depressed you are that you are convinced that other people are going to recognize it immediately, and it is very embarrassing to think that. So it makes you feel as if any interaction with other people will make you feel as if you will need to put on a front. It requires a lot of energy to do that. And that makes you very tired. It is sort of circular motion . . . you see how much energy it will take to relate so you avoid doing it. I have even noticed that if I enter a store or say a Burger King and I want coffee I tend to speak softer and not really smile like I normally do. When I am depressed I want to limit the interaction as much as possible so I don't smile and I don't really look at them. I just want to get it over with and pretend it is all over . . . .

This excerpt illustrates several subtle facets of interpersonal disruption. At one level, the depressed person feels withdrawn and consequently attempts to decrease interaction. This decrease in interaction robs the depressed person of the chance to gain positive reinforcement from others, as mentioned earlier. But, perhaps more importantly, depression decreases the quality of the remaining interactions as evidenced in the above excerpt. The decreased smiling, decreased spontaneity, and curtness of interaction displayed by the patient can be perceived by others as coolness or aloofness. Once perceived in this manner people may treat the depressed person with increased reserve. For instance, a hamburger-stand attendant may snap at them, thus further creating a hostile environment. Like a self-fulfilling prophecy, the patient creates a hostile world, a world lacking rewards for interactions with others.

This destructive cycle can be one of the forerunners of the learned helplessness sometimes seen in depression and postulated by Seligman as an etiology of depression.[22] Seligman discovered that if you experimentally expose an animal, such as a dog, to nonescapable aversive stimuli, it will eventually stop attempting escape. The animal appears to give up. It does not attempt to find new ways of coping. Once this learned helplessness has occurred, exploration ceases. With the cessation of exploration, the chance for new learning and positive reinforcement vanishes. In a sense, the depression has insured its own survival. A very similar process may occur in humans, perhaps, made even more damaging by the uncanny ability of the human being to cognitively reframe such interactions into self-derogatory beliefs such as, "Obviously, nobody likes me," or "I don't even know why I bother."

The interviewer can search for evidence of interpersonal dysfunction and learned helplessness with questions such as the following:

a. Do you find yourself going out as frequently as you used to?
b. Tell me what it is like for you when you are around people at work?
c. When you talk with people what kinds of feelings do you have, like if you meet a friend on the street?
d. How do people seem to be treating you?
e. Do you find yourself easily irritated or "flying off the handle" recently?
f. Does it require much energy to be around people such as your friends?

At this point one of the more fascinating elements of interviewing presents itself. I am referring to the fact that not only are the friends and family of the patient affected by the patient's depression, but the interviewer cannot escape the process. It benefits clinicians to periodically look within themselves at their own emotional responses. In the first place, such intuitive responses may be the tip-off that one has encountered a depression or a depressive equivalent. In the second place, both negative feelings generated in the interviewer or overly empathic feelings can seriously damage engagement. The interviewer may inadvertently distance the interviewee by tone of voice or nonverbal cue. Put differently, the interviewer needs to adjust to the needs of the patient in a continuous, adaptive creativity. To accomplish this process, interviewers must be aware of the impact of patients on themselves and vice versa.

There exist several emotions commonly felt by interviewers besides generally acknowledged reactions such as sympathy, empathy, or a desire to help. For instance, the depressed patient's slowness of movement and speech, caging, and hesitancy to answer questions can create a sense of frustration in the interviewer. Questions may have to be asked repeatedly. Answers may be vague. The interview may loom as a long and tedious process. Such feelings of frustration may be useful indicators that the clinician should be on the lookout diagnostically for depression while being wary of countertransference. In a similar fashion, the patient's depressive manner of interaction may create anger in the interviewer as well as frustration. At times interviewers may subsequently feel guilt because they suddenly catch themselves being "noncaring." This resulting guilt may provide the initial clue to a diagnosis of depression. This guilt also provides the interviewer with a vivid, experiential glimpse into the world of family members and friends who interact with a depressed patient on a daily basis. Occasionally, the first suggestion that one has encountered an atypical depression may be a growing sense of unexpected sadness within the interviewer.

The preceding interactions also emphasize the need for interviewers to adjust both their pace and their expectations. The interview with the depressed patient requires both a calm and a calming style. Indeed, any suggestions of haste or irritation may be interpreted in a highly disengaging fashion by the depressed patient. A frustrated interviewer may be perceived as, "Just like everyone else, you find me irritating." Such an interaction hardly sets an ideal platform for a therapeutic alliance.

So far I have been describing the impact of the patient on the therapist, generating feelings such as sadness, annoyance, or guilt. Flipping the coin, one finds that the therapist can unwittingly affect the patient's presentation. With regard to depression, this phenomenon occurs most frequently with dysthymia and in characterological depression. People with these disorders are often highly responsive to the immediate surroundings. A patient with dysthymia or a histrionic personality can sometimes be cheered up deceptively rapidly, if the patient feels that someone is showing an interest. Therefore, an overly warm or extroverted interviewer can unknowingly shift the patient's affect.

To such an interviewer the presentation of the patient may not seem very sad or depressed. Such an initial impression might mislead the interviewer into downplaying the significance of the depressive complaints. It should also be remembered that "happy people" are often very annoying to depressed people, being perceived as incapable of understanding how miserable they feel. The interviewer best approaches the patient from the calming middle ground of gentle warmth and interested listening.

While interviewing depressed patients, the clinician will undoubtedly encounter tearful patients. The first time a patient cries in an interview, it is generally comforting to allow the patient to cry for a brief period. If the patient is on the brink of tears, statements such as, "You seem sad right now," or as MacKinnon and Michels suggest, "Are you trying not to cry?" may be very helpful. Said with a soft tone, they will offer the patient a chance to ventilate, thus decreasing a sense of discomfort. Many patients feel embarrassed or vulnerable at such moments. I generally address this unstated issue with a statement such as, "It's all right to cry. We all cry at times. It's our body's way of telling us we are hurting; (after a brief pause) maybe you can tell me a little more about what is hurting you."

I generally will also ask, "Would you like a tissue?" while simultaneously offering one in my outstretched hand. Such an interaction has many metacommunications. The clinician is conveying an acceptance of crying as a normal aspect of sadness. Simultaneously, respect is given to the patient's current needs. Rather than just giving the patient a tissue, the clinician asks if one is needed. By the process of asking, the clinician conveys confidence that the patient is still in control, fully capable of making decisions. Generally, such an interaction usually results in the end of tearfulness in about a minute or two.

As the tearfulness subsides, the interviewer has an ideal chance to learn about the core pains of the patient. Tearfulness tends to decrease the use of defenses. At such a point, pertinent and startling information may emerge. If the clinician had prevented the tearfulness by cutting it off abruptly or by changing topics, then valuable information might have been lost.

Of course, at times, one might find a patient whose uncontrollable crying prevents progress. To further the interview, statements said reassuringly but firmly such as the following may be effective, "Mr. Jones this is obviously very upsetting and would be to anybody. Take a moment to collect yourself. It's important for us to talk more about what is bothering you."

But, generally speaking, if anything, interviewers tend to prematurely shut down crying perhaps because it is disturbing to feel another person's pain. Another emotion may also contribute to this premature shut down, for the patient's tearfulness can make the interviewer feel awkardly helpless. On a deeper level, it remains important for interviewers to understand their spontaneous feelings when someone cries. In this regard part of the interviewer's basic training should be a search for answers to questions such as the following:

   a. What do I feel when someone cries?
   b. Do I ever perceive crying people as weak or ineffectual?
   c. How often do I cry and how do I feel about myself when I do?
   d. Have I ever seen my parents, family, or friends cry, and how did I feel then?

By exploring such questions, the interviewer decreases the risk that countertransference issues will adversely affect the ability to deal with a crying patient. In the last analysis, many a powerful therapeutic alliance has been forged by a clinician's calming and mature response to a patient's first tears.

A final feeling that an interviewer may experience while interviewing a depressed patient stems from both the withdrawal of the patient and the shrinking of the patient's active world. In short, as the patient introverts, the interviewer may feel ineffectual or out of touch. Such feelings are to be expected. They do not necessarily suggest that the interview is going poorly.

IV: THE FAMILY SYSTEM AND OTHER GROUP SYSTEMS

Sometimes depression seems to possess a life of its own, independent of the person labeled as depressed. It is within the family that this phenomenon comes most vividly to mind. To understand a depression fully, one must understand its role in the family. Family interaction may be the primary root of the depression, as in a hateful sibling rivalry. At other times the depression may have its roots in a biochemical process, yet the ramifications of this process will reverberate throughout the family. A case in point would be a spouse laid off from work secondary to a severe endogenous depression. Surely, all members of the family will feel the pains of this depressive process, almost as if the biochemical imbalance were in their own neurochemistry. Finally, the family pathology may feed a depression already caused by another system, such as the biochemical or psychological system. In this section the focus will be specifically upon the impact of depression on other family members as it pertains to the initial interview.

I will introduce this topic by describing an interview I supervised in person. The interviewer was talking with the identified patient, whom I shall refer to as Mrs. Ella Thomas. In the same room the husband and son of Mrs. Thomas were also present. Mrs. Thomas was a gray-haired woman with angry eyes that seemed resentful of all seventy of her years. She fidgeted and cried throughout the interview. At times she would suddenly change topics, whining out such statements to her husband as, "You've got to help me, Leonard! I can't go on. The pain! The pain!" She complained about the hospital and warned that, "I had better get my sleeping pills or I'll leave."

As the interview proceeded, an atmosphere of increasing tension pervaded the room. Her husband had refused to have a chair brought for himself. Consequently, he stood throughout the interview, stationed reservedly behind the interviewer. As the interview proceeded, he tightly rolled his lips upon each other, while his arms closed over his chest. Mrs. Thomas' son sat down, his body turned sideways to his mother. He occasionally tossed a glance at her when his eyes were not staring at his shoes or the floor. Later in the interview, with an angry tone plucking each word, he challenged the clinician, "Why can't she have those meds?" I felt a growing sense of discomfort inside me. The poor interviewer was nervously breaking eye contact with Mrs. Thomas, while he sheepishly performed a mental status.

I can safely say that no one in that room was comfortable. That room represented a classic reflection of the impact of depression on the family system, and even on the hospital system itself. Diagnostically, Mrs. Thomas had an agitated major depression. In reality, this entire family was experiencing the depressive process. But it did not stop at the boundary of her age-spotted skin. Depression is often reflected in the actions and words of family members. Her husband and son demonstrated the frustration and anger often generated in those who love the patient. These people experience a sense of helplessness, fearing that nothing will change, despite their best efforts. Not personally experiencing the patient's anhedonia and loss of energy, they cannot understand why the patient does not help himself or herself. They also find their own daily activities continuously interrupted by the complaints and actions of the depressed person. Occasionally, secondary to such frustration, they will develop a depression of their own. In a sense, the depression will have replicated itself. As illustrated above, their anger may not only be expressed towards the patient, but also towards the interviewer. Unfortunately, as described earlier in the section on dyadic process, the negative feelings generated by Mrs. Thomas may backfire upon her, creating a hostile environment even within the hospital.

If the interviewer meets family members, their statements and nonverbal messages may be the first clue that depression is the diagnosis. At a different level, the interviewer should keep in mind that other family members may need help. The problem is not "just Ella's problem." Viewed at an even more sophisticated level, the family system may in some way need Mrs. Thomas' depression as a stabilizing force, as theorists such as Bowen or Minuchin have discussed.[23] All of these points emphasize the need for the interviewer to carefully explore the family in order to understand the depression.

Within the individual interview, family tensions may be spontaneously brought up by the patient. But at other times questioning may be needed to illuminate the issues. Questions such as the following represent some good jumping off points:

a. Who in your family seems to understand you?
b. Who in your family are you concerned about right now?
c. How do you think your family members view your depression?
d. What kinds of suggestions have your family members been making to you about how to feel better?
e. What kind of pressures has your spouse been coping with recently?

Questions such as the above will often yield information about the state of the family. They may elicit interpersonal tensions towards specific family members, where more direct questioning might have elicited denial. For instance, when answering the question about pressures on the spouse, the patient may relate feelings of guilt for being a burden, feelings of anger towards the spouse for perceived neglect, or disgust at the spouse's overattention to work or other family members, or may seem detached and uninterested in the spouse. From such a question one may also learn valuable information about situational stressors in the family system as well.

Fields of interaction other than the family can experience depression. On a direct level, reflections of depression will be seen in systems such as the job environment, church groups, and social organizations. From a different perspective, such systems may act as the major stressors triggering the depression in the first place. On the other hand they may act as important supports, buffering the patients from their depression. Society itself can be an integral system involved in depression. Careful questioning might reveal that the husband of Mrs. Thomas had been forced to retire secondary to economic lay offs. Or perhaps her family had recently relocated because of increasing taxes in their former state. Likewise the hospitalization of Mrs. Thomas will ultimately affect the Medicaid and Social Security systems.

Thus depression leaves its mark throughout all these interlocking systems. The sensitive interviewer understands these inter-relationships and attempts to make a reconnaissance of each system during the initial interview. Through this diligent search the puzzle of depression may become clearer, and avenues of therapeutic intervention more apparent.

V: THE FRAMEWORK FOR MEANING

During an initial interview one can become so involved in the diagnosis that issues of major concern to the patient may be overlooked. In particular one should attempt to understand how patients view their problems, their life, and their beliefs. Such views represent the patient's framework for meaning as described in Chapter 4. In an initial interview, one will seldom have the time to explore this framework in any depth, but even a few minutes of discussion may provide clues for engagement or for future therapeutic discussion. Such questioning may also further convey interest in the interviewee as a person, not as a "case." Failure to have evolved a framework for meaning or a sudden breakdown in a pre-existing framework can function as triggers or perpetuators of the patient's depression, representing an existential crisis.

To investigate these areas of existential framework, several regions of information may be of value. At times demographic questions concerning religious background may act as springboards for further inquiry. Significant information may present itself following questions such as, "What role does religion play in your life?" If asked with a nonjudgmental tone, people generally respond naturally and specifically. Very quickly, the interviewer will register the role of religious doubt or ambivalence in the current crisis.

Religion is not the only axis upon which a framework for meaning is built. Other areas include family, job, community, charities, patriotism, and subcultures such as those associated with sports and rock music.

Ignorance of these factors can result in markedly disrupted engagement. Moreover, these systems can have a very powerful influence on whether the patient will comply with treatment recommendations. Consequently, it remains critical for the initial interviewer to understand these factors, as illustrated below:

Clin.: What kinds of things do you like to do in your spare time?

Pt.: When I felt better, I used to love to sing.

Clin.: Oh . . . (with an increased interest in tone of voice) What kinds of music did you like to sing?

Pt.: All types, but I really loved gospel music. What a beautiful way to bring God to people . . . I think if you put all of your trust in God, he will help you. Man is not the answer. Man provides artificial answers.

Clin.: Have you been praying recently in an attempt to gain some guidance?

Pt.: Yes I have. Every day. It helps, but I wonder if maybe I ask for too much. Perhaps I am to blame.

This vignette provides a wealth of information for the clinician. In the first place, religion obviously plays a major role in this person's life. The interviewer may want to further examine the possible therapeutic supports that religion could provide, such as meetings with a minister or choral church activities. On the other hand, religion may be feeding some guilty ruminations that are part of the depressive process itself. Perhaps, even more importantly, the clinician has some clues concerning where engagement could go wrong. In particular, the patient's statement, "Man is not the answer. Man provides artificial answers," serves as a warning to the clinician. Specifically, the patient may find treatment modalities such as psychotherapy or medication as clearly "artificial answers." Premature reference in the interview to such treatments could easily rupture engagement. The clinician will need to proceed cautiously, trying to gently find out what this particular patient wants in the way of help.

It is beyond the scope of this chapter to discuss the numerous ramifications that the search for meaning may play in depression. I refer the reader to authors such as Viktor Frankl[23] and Irvin Yalom[25] who discuss these issues in the detail they deserve. In closing, I am reminded of another example in which understanding the patient's framework for meaning helped in the initial interview of a patient with depressive complaints. I had been asked to see this patient as a psychiatric consultant in a medical ward.

Mr. Kulp (as I shall refer to him) was a fifty-five-year-old alcoholic suffering from moderately severe Parkinson's disease (a progressive form of muscular rigidity). He had been admitted with suicidal ideation following a drunken spree. He had many stressors, not the least of which was a markedly battered self-image created by the stiffening of his body from Parkinson's disease. Mr. Kulp had always prided himself on being an energetic bread winner for his family. He viewed himself as a tough, former Marine. This latter role affiliation surfaced when I asked him if he liked to read. He mentioned that he loved to read, pointing to his books. When I asked if I could see them, he enthusiastically showed them to me. All of them concerned Marines and various war heroes, which led to a discussion of his former Marine days, including his boot camp experiences. At the time I did not exactly know what to make of this information. Later its usefulness became apparent.

By way of understatement, Mr. Kulp did not respond positively to my recommendations that he needed to enter a local alcoholic rehabilitation center. As the discussion proceeded, I felt he would decide against entering the program. He balked, stating that it would be too big of a time commitment and too tough. At which point I made a comment to the effect, "Well Mr. Kulp I guess you're right. It's a tough commitment, but not your first. It's sort of like boot camp was a tough commitment. But you needed boot camp. It made a good soldier of you. Maybe you and your family need this program." This statement appeared to affect Mr. Kulp. He eventually decided to enter the rehabilitation program. Perhaps he would have entered anyway, but the understanding of his framework for meaning certainly seemed to help. Suddenly the rehabilitation program was not viewed as a foreign entity; it was akin to his familiar and respected boot camp. Mr. Kulp had been given a chance to be a soldier again.

References

1. American Psychiatric Association: Diagnostic and Statistical Manual of Mental Disorders, Third edition, revised. Washington, D.C., APA, 1987, pp. 222–223.
2. DSM-III-R, 1987, pp. 232–233.
3. DSM-III-R, 1987, p. 217.
4. Renner, J. A.: Alcoholism. In *Inpatient Psychiatry, Diagnosis and Treatment,* edited by Lloyd I. Sederer. Baltimore, Williams and Wilkins, 1983, p. 185.
5. Klein, D., Gittelman, R., Quitkin, F., and Rifkin, A.: *Diagnosis and Drug Treatment of Psychiatric Disorders.* Baltimore, Williams and Wilkins, 1980, p. 226.
6. Bernstein, J. G.: Medical psychiatric drug interaction. In *Massachusetts General Hospital Handbook of General Hospital Psychiatry,* edited by T. Hackett and Ned Cassam. Saint Louis, The C. V. Mosby Company, 1978, p. 502.
7. Anderson, W. H.: Depression. In *Outpatient Psychiatry: Diagnosis and Treatment,* edited by A. Lazarre. Baltimore, Williams and Wilkins, 1979, p. 259.
8. Akiskal, H., and McKinney, W.: Research in depression. In *Major Psychiatric Disorders, Overview and Selected Readings,* edited by F. Guggenheim and C. Nadelson, New York, Elsevier Science Publishing Co., 1982, p. 77.
9. Cohen, R. L.: History taking. In *Basic Handbook of Child Psychiatry. Vol. 1,* New York, Basic Books, Inc. 1979, p. 495.
10. Kolb, L., and Brodie, H. K.: *Modern Clinical Psychiatry.* Philadelphia, W.B. Saunders Company, 1982, p. 408.
11. Renner, J. A., 1983, p. 188.
12. Klein, D. et al., 1980, p. 225.
13. Nelson, J., and Charney, D.S.: The symptoms of major depressive illness. *American Journal of Psychiatry* 138:1-13, 1981.
14. Akiskal, H. S.: Dysthymic disorder: Psychopathology of proposed chronic depressive subtypes. *American Journal of Psychiatry.* 140:11–20, 1983.
15. Jaspers K.: Symptom complexes of abnormal affective states. In *General Psychopathology.* Manchester University Press, 1923, p. 598.
16. Minkowski, E.: Findings in a case of 'schizophrenic' depression. In *Existence,* edited by Rollo May. New York, A Touchstone Book, 1958, p. 133.
17. Beck, A. T.: *Cognitive Therapy and the Emotional Disorders.* New York, The American Library, 1976, p. 105.
18. Minkowski, 1958, p. 132.
19. Beck, A. T., Kovacs, M., and Weissman, A.: Hopelessness and suicidal behavior. *Journal of the American Medical Association* 234:1146–1149, 1975.
20. MacKinnon, R., and Michels, R.: *The Psychiatric Interview in Clinical Practice.* Philadelphia, W.B. Saunders Co., 1971.
21. Akiskal, H., and McKinney, W., 1982, p. 73.
22. Akiskal, H., and McKinney, W., 1982, p. 74.
23. Gurman, A. S., and Kniskern, D. P. (editor): *Handbook of Family Therapy.* New York, Brunner/Mazel Publisher, 1981.
24. Frankl, V. W.: *The Doctor and the Soul.* New York, Vintage Books, 1973.
25. Yalom, I.: *Existential Psychotherapy.* New York, Basic Books Inc., 1980.

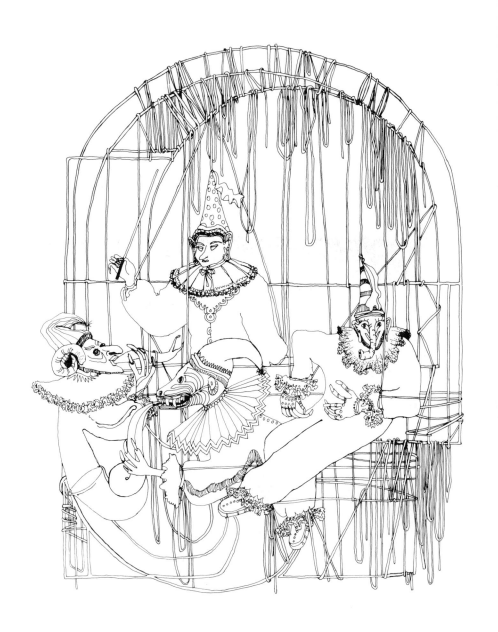

6

Interviewing Techniques While Exploring Psychosis

And then a Plank in Reason, broke,
And I dropped down, and down —
and hit a World, at every plunge,
And finished knowing — then — . . .
Emily Dickinson

One wonders what the world is like when a plank in reason splinters, as Emily Dickinson describes the slip into psychotic process. To the degree that the clinician possesses a feeling for this world, it becomes easier to uncover subtle psychotic states. As intuitive understanding increases it also becomes easier to understand the needs of the patient, an understanding that leads directly into a more compassionate interview.

To begin our exploration we will turn to Gérard De Nerval, a poet of extreme talent, who had the misfortune of falling through a plank in reason sometime during the middle of the Victorian Era. De Nerval was a gifted Symbolist poet, who was also a world traveler and a man deeply interested in philosophy, blessed with a childlike awe of nature. In 1841 he experienced his first psychotic break. Eventually, some fourteen years later, psychotic process would lead him on a cold winter night to an iron gate bordering an alley near the Boulevard St-Michel. He would be found in the morning hanging from a railing with his neck fatally embraced by an apron string.[1]

On the morning after his suicide, fragments of a work entitled "le Rêve et la Vie" were found in his pocket. It is this piece that provides us with our first glimpse into the world of psychosis.

First of all I imagined that the persons collected in the garden (of the madhouse) all had some influence on the stars, and that the one who always walked round and round in a circle regulated the course of the sun. An old man, who was brought there at certain hours of the day, and who made knots as he consulted his watch, seemed to me to be charged with the notation of the course of the hours . . .

I attributed a mystical signification to the conversations of the warders and of my companions. It seemed to me that they were the representatives for all the races of the earth, and that we had undertaken between us to re-arrange the course of the stars, and to give a wider development to the system. An error, in my opinion, had crept into the general combination of numbers, and thence came all the ills of humanity. . . .

I seemed to myself a hero living under the very eyes of the gods; everything in nature assumed new aspects, and secret voices came to me from the plants, the trees, animals, the meanest insects, to warn and to encourage me. The words of my companions had mysterious messages, the sense of which I alone understood.[2]

In some respects, it is De Nerval's last statement that provides one of the most telling clues as to the nature of psychotic process. As psychotic process becomes more intense, the patient's world becomes progressively more unique to the patient, receding further from the experience of the world as witnessed by others. In this sense, psychosis can be defined in simple terms as a breakdown of perceptual, cognitive, or rationalizing functions of the mind, to the point that the individual experiences reality very differently than other people within the same culture.

De Nerval's world became filled with a maelstrom of curious and disturbing sensations. His words sensitively depict a variety of classic symptoms of psychosis, including delusions, ideas of reference, and hallucinations. It also demonstrates the fact that some aspects of psychotic process may be exciting and even beautiful. But, and this is an important but, psychosis is almost invariably ultimately accompanied by an intensely painful collection of fears. The patient senses impending catastrophe. For instance, De Nerval states, "An error, in my opinion, had crept into the general combination of numbers, and thence came all the ills of humanity." Such paranoid perception can create a tremendous sense of urgency and responsibility in those experiencing psychotic process. Perhaps for De Nerval it was the realization that he could not correct this heinous error in the universe that led him to believe that his life should be ended, for he had failed both god and humanity.

There are many aspects of psychotic process that, in my mind, demarcate it from the innovative workings of eccentric men and women, whose thought is clearly at variance with the world view of most people but is not a psychotic process. Creative thinking may bear a resemblance to psychotic process, but it is not identical to it. We shall see that it is not so much the content of the psychotic thinking that is pathological, but more the way in which the thinking occurs that marks the process as psychotic.

Now that we have arrived at a working definition of psychosis, an important point needs to be emphasized. The word "psychosis" is not a diagnosis. Psychosis is a syndrome that can result from any number of psychiatric disorders delineated in the DSM-III-R. It is never enough to simply state that the patient appears to be psychotic, for one must proceed to determine what diagnostic entity is causing the psychotic process.

The following chapter, like the preceding chapter; is divided into two sections. In The Diagnosis of Psychotic States, we will look at seven case vignettes, which illustrate the diversity of agents that may be responsible for a psychotic presentation. Once again, the emphasis will be upon a discussion of practical points that help the initial clinician to both uncover and diagnose psychotic states. In The Understanding of Psychosis, systems analysis will be used to expand an understanding of psychosis as a uniquely human process. To begin our discussion let us meet some people who have had the misfortune of falling through a plank in reason.

SECTION I: DIAGNOSIS OF PSYCHOTIC STATES

Case Presentations

CASE ONE: MR. WILLIAMS

Mr. Williams presents to the Emergency Room accompanied by three police officers. His behavior has not put the officers in particularly good spirits. As one officer states it, "This guy is wacko. Every once in awhile he tries to bolt as if something was after him." The officer has no idea what the "thing" is that appears so disturbing to Mr. Williams. In the interview, Mr. Williams presents as a thirty-three-year-old male, who initially appears relatively calm despite the beads of perspiration on his forehead. He is just finishing supper from his dinner tray and is neatly wiping his mouth with a napkin. His pants are torn and soiled; obviously, they are not strangers to the harshness of street life. He appears oriented to person, place, and time. As he begins to talk he becomes more animated, displaying tangential speech with occasional glimpses of a loosening of his associations. He denies any recent drinking or drug use, but his story is vague, concerned primarily with the appearance of some creature that has been following him. Suddenly, in the middle of the interview, his eyes widen as he stares down at his feet. He cannot attend to the interview, as his attention is riveted to the floor. He begins kicking at some invisible object and angrily looks at the clinician, yelling, "Get rid of that thing!"

CASE TWO: MR. WALKER

Mr. Walker is a twenty-year-old male. He is thin and his clothes tend to hang on his gaunt frame. Beneath his black hair a rather handsome face sits quietly darkening with a day's worth of beard. As the interviewer enters the room, Mr. Walker acknowledges him with a slight nod of his head. His speech is soft and mildly slowed. He appears almost shy. As he speaks, there is barely a hint of facial expression, his voice painted gray by a conspicuous lack of highlights. All seems bland. Mr. Walker proceeds to describe a chaotic situation at home. He is being avidly pursued by three filthy women who enter his house at night. They attempt to force sex on him. When asked if he knows who these women are, he nods, stating that one is "that devil Miss Brown." He proceeds to describe a recent party he attended, where sex games were played. He relates that he had been tricked into going. As he entered the kitchen three men tied him to a chair and stripped him. When asked what happened, he pauses and proceeds to say, "They violated my anus." As he says these words a slight smile steals across his face. His speech is without any evidence of loosening of associations, tangential thought, thought blocking, or illogical thought. He is alert and well oriented. Both he and his family deny that he has used any street drugs. During the interview the clinician feels uncomfortable and somewhat frightened.

CASE THREE: MS. HASTINGS

Ms. Hastings walks into the clinic with a disgruntled look on her face. She is fifty years old and appears a bit bedraggled. The first words out of her mouth are, "Can you help me with my husband?" Her speech is fluent, without any evidence of loose associations, illogical thought, or bizarre ideation. In actuality she is somewhat eloquent but clearly upset. When asked to elaborate, she responds with an indignant snort, "It's the divorce game, that's all!" She proceeds to relate an elaborate tale of infidelity on the part of her husband. At the present time, she says, he has hired a variety of men to harrass her into a state of insanity. Her craziness will provide grounds for his sought after divorce. The men are using "conventional spy tools," and she is beginning to feel that her own mother may be in on the plot. Her story is literally illustrated by a journal filled with drawings and time schedules she has compiled on the activities of her husband and "his goons next door." She denies hallucinations or a previous psychiatric history. She also denies most depressive symptoms except, "I'm edgy of course, wouldn't you be?"

CASE FOUR: MISS FAY

Miss Fay is a twenty-three-year-old divorced woman who presents to the Assessment Center for the second time in two weeks. She is casually dressed in jeans and a yellow blouse that tends to overshadow her curly, dull blonde hair. She has come alone to the Center and relates, "I just had to talk to someone again, I'm a nervous wreck." Indeed, she appears somewhat of a nervous wreck, in that she wriggles uneasily about in her chair while incessantly picking at her nails. It seems difficult for her to maintain eye contact. She states to the male clinician, "You make me nervous. These are hard questions." She relates that things are terrible at home, where she lives with her mother and her two children. She never gets a moment's rest and reports significant problems falling asleep, as well as a general inability to relax. Her speech is mildly pressured and characterized by an evasive style, which clearly frustrates the interviewer. She bluntly denies any delusions or hallucinations, but seems greatly concerned with an incident of sexual abuse from her distant past, which she prefers not to discuss at the moment. As the interviewer proceeds she becomes intermittently more anxious and coyly giggles at times, perhaps out of nervousness. One senses that if she could burrow beneath her chair to escape scrutiny, she would most surely do so. At the time of her first evaluation, she was diagnosed as having a relatively severe generalized anxiety disorder.

CASE FIVE: MR. LAWRENCE

Mr. Lawrence is a good looking man of about thirty. Despite his good looks he is not particularly attractive at the moment, for he is in the midst of a rage. He was found in his apartment smashing a typewriter through the bedroom window. He had trashed the apartment, madly throwing white paint over his furniture. The landlord found him screaming. Mr. Lawrence has a longstanding history of paranoid schizophrenia. He has been violent at times in the past. Tonight he refuses hospitalization, and the crisis worker has to involuntarily commit him, for he apparently seems to be in the midst of yet another acute psychotic relapse. It took two policemen to bring Mr. Lawrence into the emergency room, and on the way in he managed to creatively coin a few new obscenities.

CASE SIX: KATE

The moment that one sees the look of concern on the faces of this young girl's parents, one feels that something is very wrong. Kate is fourteen years old. She is slightly overweight. Her blond hair drops in a tangle down her back. Her parents relate that they feel she is very depressed, having become more depressed over the past two months. Things had reached a crisis when five days earlier Kate had thrown a slumber party. No one came. Since then she has been acting oddly, talking about "reality" and wandering about the house. The most bizarre incident occurred two nights ago, when Kate knocked at her parents bedroom door at two in the morning. When they opened the door, Kate stood topless, stating in a dull monotone that she felt a need to talk. At no time had Kate been delusional or heard voices. Kate's parents had taken her to two emergency rooms in the past week. At both places her parents were told that she was hysterical. Referrals were made for outpatient therapy.

CASE SEVEN: MISS FLAGSTONE

Miss Flagstone walks into the clinic dressed in a stylish fashion, sporting a cigarette in hand, waving it about like a baton of sorts. During the interview, her affect changes periodically, as she relates a longstanding history of "just not going anywhere in my life." At times she is tearful but is able to quickly pull herself together. She is very dissatisfied with her poor relationships with men, despite her good looks and thick black hair. Her speech rate and volume are within normal limits. Although mildly tangential at times, she does not display any loosening of associations or thought blocking. She is well oriented and denies any history of delusions. When asked about hallucinations she denies any except for one episode two years earlier. She continues as follows. "I've really never told anyone this story, but it has had a profound affect on me. At the time I was extremely upset. Everything was horrible in my life. Fortunately, I was not taking any drugs or else I might not have found God. I was in my kitchen doing the dishes when a sudden light filled the room. I just knew it was a message from God. He had come to bring me back to the His flock. From inside the light I heard the angel Gabriel speak. He said, 'Janet, you are with child.' I knew this was a test from God and I showed strength by accepting the mission. He talked with me, and I convinced him of my great love of God. At that point the angel told me that all was well and that I was back with God, my father. A blinding light moved in and out of the room many times. The whole thing only lasted about fifteen minutes, but my life has never been the same since." This episode is the only time that she has ever heard a voice, and she denies that she has any special mission for God other than to be a good Christian.

Discussion of Case Material

As with the last chapter it is assumed, for the sake of discussion, that the, preceding clinical material was obtained during an initial assessment interview. Before proceding with this case material, it may be of value to review the DSM-III-R criteria for schizophrenia, for schizophrenia may very well represent the classic example of a psychotic illness. One could say that one of the main goals in the approach to any psychotic patient remains the determination of whether or not schizophrenia is present. To this end the DSM-III-R criteria are as follows:

Schizophrenia[3]

A. Presence of characteristic psychotic symptoms in the active phase: either (1), (2), or (3) for at least one week (unless the symptoms are successfully treated):

(1) two of the following:
(a) delusions
(b) prominent hallucinations (throughout the day for several days or several times a week for several weeks, each hallucinatory experience not being limited to a few brief moments)
(c) incoherence or marked loosening of associations
(d) catatonic behavior
(e) flat or grossly inappropriate affect
(2) bizarre delusions (i.e., involving a phenomenon that the person's culture would regard as totally implausible, e.g., thought broadcasting, being controlled by a dead person)
(3) prominent hallucinations [as defined in (1)(b) above] of a voice with content having no apparent relation to depression or elation, or a voice keeping up a running commentary on the individual's behavior or thoughts, or two or more voices conversing with each other

B. During the course of the disturbance, functioning in such areas as work, social relations, and self-care is markedly below the highest level achieved before onset of the disturbance (or when the onset is in childhood or adolescence, failure to achieve expected level of social development).

C. Schizoaffective Disorder and Mood Disorder with Psychotic Features have been ruled out, if a Major Depressive or Manic Syndrome has ever been present during an active phase of the disturbance, the total duration of all episodes of a mood syndrome has been brief relative to the total duration of the active and residual phases of the disturbance.

D. Continuous signs of the disturbance for at least six months. The six-month period must include an active phase (of at least one week, or less if symptoms have been successfully treated) during which there were psychotic symptoms characteristic of Schizophrenia (symptoms in A), with or without a prodromal or residual phase, as defined below.

Prodromal phase: A clear deterioration in functioning before the active phase of the disturbance that is not due to a disturbance in mood or to a Psychoactive Substance Use Disorder and that involves at least two of the symptoms listed below.

Residual phase: Following the active phase of the disturbance, persistence of at least two of the symptoms noted below, these not being due to a disturbance in mood or a Psychoactive Substance Use Disorder.

Prodromal or Residual Symptoms

(1) marked social isolation or withdrawal
(2) marked impairment in role functioning as wage-earner, student, or homemaker
(3) markedly peculiar behavior (e.g., collecting garbage, talking to self in public, hoarding food)
(4) marked impairment in personal hygiene and grooming
(5) blunted or inappropriate affect
(6) digressive, vague, overelaborate, or circumstantial speech, or poverty of speech, or poverty of content of speech
(7) odd beliefs or magical thinking, influencing behavior and inconsistent with cultural norms, e.g., superstitiousness, belief in clairvoyance, telepathy, "sixth sense," "others can feel my feelings," overvalued ideas, ideas of reference
(8) unusual perceptual experiences, e.g., recurrent illusions, sensing the presence of a force or person not actually present
(9) marked lack of initiative, interests, or energy

Examples: Six months of prodromal symptoms with one week of symptoms from A; no prodromal symptoms with six months of symptoms from A; no prodromal symptoms with one week of symptoms from A and six months of residual symptoms.

E. It cannot be established that an organic factor initiated and maintained the disturbance.

F. If there is a history of Autistic Disorder, the additional diagnosis of Schizophrenia is made only if prominent delusions or hallucinations are also present.

It should be noted that there also exists a diagnosis, schizophreniform disorder, that is applied when a patient meets criteria A and C of schizophrenia but the symptoms do not last for six months nor necessarily result in a marked decline in functioning. In the schizophreniform disorder the symptoms (including prodromal, active, and residual phases) must last less than six months. Many patients who have received this diagnosis provisionally will eventually receive the diagnosis of schizophrenia if their symptoms last longer than six months. The diagnosis schizophreniform disorder is not used if the psychosis is caused directly by a stressor, as seen in a brief reactive psychosis.

Now that we have examined the criteria for schizophrenia, let us begin our discussion of the case material.

DISCUSSION OF MR. WILLIAMS

Mr. Williams was the wild-eyed male brought in by the police. While with the police he appeared to be responding to visual hallucinations, a process that reappeared during the interview itself. And herein lies the first clue to the diagnostic entity causing his immediate psychosis, for the presence of visual hallucinations should alert the clinician to the possibility that an organic etiologic agent may be at work. Schizophrenia may cause visual hallucinations, but auditory hallucinations are more frequent. On the other hand, organic causes of psychosis frequently present with extremely vivid visual hallucinations.

Fish has suggested that the quality of the visual hallucination may tend to vary depending on whether schizophrenia or an organic process is present,[4] but no specific characteristic clearly differentiate the visual hallucinations seen with organic states from those seen with more functional psychoses such as schizophrenia or bipoplar disorder. On the other hand, some characteristics seem to be more common in each category and may provide clues to etiology. Visual hallucinations in organic patients, presenting with delirium, tend to vary from the non-organic psychoses by preferentially occurring at night, by being briefer in duration, and by being more frequently perceived as moving. They may also have little personal significance to the patient. For example, the schizophrenic patient may hallucinate a recently deceased relative while the delirious patient may see snakes.[5]

With organic patients the hallucinations may appear more frequently and more vividly when the patient is in a darkened room or has his eyes shut. This is not the case with schizophrenics, who tend to see their hallucinations with eyes open or who experience little change whether the eyes are open or closed.[6,7] In this sense it is of value to ask patients, "When you see your hallucinations, do they go away when you close your eyes?" With a hospitalized patient it is of value to check with the nursing staff concerning whether the patient is hallucinating more at night.

With schizophrenic patients visual hallucinations seldom occur by themselves. They usually present with auditory hallucinations or hallucinations from some other sensory modality.[8] Also of interest to the interviewer is the fact that schizophrenic hallucinations are frequently superimposed on an otherwise normal appearing enviroment or may even appear with the surrounding enviroment absent. In hallucinogenic drug-induced psychoses the entire enviroment frequently seems distorted with numerous illusions and hallucinations.[9] In a similar vein the visual hallucinations of schizophrenia tend to appear suddenly without preceding visual illusions or less formed visual hallucinations. Organic visual hallucinations tend to have a prodrome of visual illusions, simple geometric figures, and alterations of color, size, shape, and movement.[9]

Schizophrenic patients tend to see concrete things such as faces, body parts, or complete figures as opposed to geometric patterns or poorly formed images. On the other hand, once organic patients begin seeing concrete images, it has been my experience that the images frequently appear extremely real to the patients. The delirious patient may look on with terror pointing towards the hallucination, eyeing it warily or moving away from it as it appears to approach. Occasionally the patient's affective response may be pleasurable, as experienced with hallucinations of miniature people, so-called Lilliputian hallucinations, sometimes seen in the early stages of delirium tremens and other organic states.[10]

In Mr. Williams's case the interviewer asked him if he could point more closely to the creature in question. Mr. Williams hesitantly obliged by cautiously moving his hand towards the open space in front of his feet. Abruptly he halted, "I ain't getting no closer!" It became even more apparent that the hallucination was vivid and quite real. At times these types of hallucinations can create a peculiar sensation in the interviewer, for the actions of the patient, like the movements of a mime, create the feeling that one ought to be seeing something.

Sometimes the terms "hallucination" and "illusion" are misunderstood. Mr. Williams presents with a true hallucination, for his perceptual image is arising from an open space and is not being triggered by an enviromental stimulus. With illusions the image is triggered by some actual object or stimulus in the room. For instance, one patient vividly described watching the face of a man standing beside him on the bus. He saw the man's face begin to twist in a grotesque fashion and saw his eyeballs shatter and begin to bleed. This experience represents a visual illusion and also emphasizes that such illusions may be as striking and terrifying as true hallucinations. We have seen that the appearance of vivid visual hallucinations ought to arouse suspicion that an organic agent may be at work. Mr. Williams represents one of the more typical organic causes of psychosis that the initial interviewer must constantly keep in mind, abuse and withdrawal from street drugs and/or medications. It is important to realize that there exist two different manners in which drugs may precipitate a psychosis; acute intoxication or withdrawal. First, let us look at the issue of withdrawal, for Mr. Williams is suffering from an alcohol withdrawal delirium, also known as delirium tremens (DTs for short).

This book is not intended to represent a thorough review of drug abuse, and the reader should study these states elsewhere in detail. But there are some basic facts with which all assessment clinicians should be familiar. With regard to withdrawal states, alcohol and sedative/hypnotic drugs are the most likely to present with psychotic features. They are also the most likely to result in death if not recognized and treated. Withdrawal from these drugs is significantly more dangerous than withdrawal from drugs such as heroin or amphetamines. Some estimates of the mortality rate of patients in definite delirium tremens from alcohol, who have been hospitalized, have been as high as 15 percent, although with good management this number should be markedly lower.[11]

As people begin to withdraw from alcohol and sedative hypnotics, they generally move from mild symptoms of withdrawal towards progressively more severe states such as delirium tremens. As withdrawal occurs, patients frequently experience sleep disturbances, nausea, anxiety, overalertness, tremulousness, and a peculiar intensification of their sensory modalities.[12] Even if patients such as Mr. Williams deny recent drug abuse, they may willingly admit to these symptoms if asked matter of factly and without the suggestion that they have "a personal problem." In this regard, questions such as the following may be useful:

    a. Have you been noticing problems with your sleep?
    b. Have you been feeling edgy over the past couple of days, you know, just can't seem to relax?

    c. Over the past couple of days have you been feeling sick in your stomach?

    d. Do you find yourself being startled by noises or upset by people moving or talking around you?

To develop delirium tremens, the patient must use alcohol for long periods of time. It typically does not occur under the age of thirty, although it clearly can, and it usually requires consistent use of large amounts of alcohol for several years.[13] This chronic use of alcohol sets up a complex set of compensatory physiologic changes in autonomic bodily regulation. When the alcohol is abruptly stopped, these compensatory changes go unchecked, resulting in such abnormalities as increased pulse, increased temperature, normal or elevated blood pressure, rapid breathing, muscle twitching, and sweating. As the syndrome becomes more serious, the patient may become so tremulous that walking appears to be difficult.[14]

In interviewing the psychotic patient, the clinician should do a quick survey to see if any of these physiologic signs of withdrawal are present. With Mr. Williams, he was noted to appear sweaty. The clinician also knew that his pulse rate was elevated at 100 with a mild increase in temperature. This emphasizes an important point. In general, a patient presenting with an acute psychosis should have his vital signs taken before the clinical interview, thus alerting the clinician that an organic process may be at work.

Mr. Williams proceeded to become more agitated, claiming that some kind of bug was crawling on him and that some "wires are running around on the floor. They're shocking the hell out of me, man!" It is not uncommon for people with delirium tremens to hallucinate small animals and sometimes large objects such as trains or the proverbial pink elephant. Tactile hallucinations or illusions such as mice or lice crawling about one's skin also occur, as seen with Mr. Williams.[14]

The clinician astutely cut this interview short, proceeding rapidly with a physical examination and appropriate medical management, which raises another important point. These people need prompt medical attention. If one is not a physician, then one must quickly have such a patient seen. An appointment for "later in the day or tomorrow" is totally inappropriate.

Before leaving the topic of delirium tremens, a few more points seem worth mentioning. Seizures ("rum fits") sometimes precede delirium tremens, usually occurring the first two days of the cessation of drinking. More than one out of three patients who have withdrawal seizures will go on to develop delirium tremens. Delirium tremens usually begin 24 to 72 hours after the cessation of drinking but can appear much later, even as long as seven or more days later.[14] Moreover, while performing an initial assessment on a psychotic patient in the hospital a few points are worth considering.

Some patients may have a temporary drug source, such as a friend, who eventually stops bringing drugs. In these cases, delirium tremens may not appear until much longer into the hospitalization. Keep in mind that higher income patients may purposely lie about alcohol consumption and may consequently develop withdrawal problems only as the hospitalization proceeds. Curiously, surgery may delay the appearance of delirium tremens as well. All these facts considered, clinicians should be alert to the possibility of drug withdrawal in any patient who develops a psychosis at any time during a hospital stay, especially if vital signs are abnormally elevated.

Thus far the material gained from the actual interview of Mr. Williams has been the focus of discussion. But in addition, one of the most important interviews to perform when a patient is brought to the emergency room by the police is with the officers, and there is an art to this process. The first trick is training oneself to take the time to perform this interview. Both the police and the clinician are frequently harried, but nevertheless this interview can provide invaluable information. In particular one wants to establish the following: (1) What were the circumstances in which the patient was found? (2) Is the patient a known alcoholic or drug abuser? (3) Do the officers know the patient's family and have they been contacted? (4) Did the patient appear disoriented or demonstrate any signs of psychosis? (5) Has the patient appeared drowsy or been unconscious? (6) Has the patient been in a fight involving a possible head blow?

This last question raises an important aspect of interviewing the police. The clinician should always consider whether an officer may have delivered a head blow either justly or unjustly. Uncovering a history of a physical confrontation can help alert the clinician to the possibility of a subdural hematoma or an intracranial bleed as the source of the psychosis, especially in older patients who have been struck. It may also help the clinician understand and perhaps decrease the patient's fear that more violence may follow.

A savvy clinician approaches these topics in a manner that puts the officers at ease and decreases any sense that the clinician is antagonistic towards the officers. It is important to remember that most officers would resort to violence only when necessary. Angry countertransference feelings directed towards the police can only get in the way of gaining valid information from them. The following type of approach may be useful:

> **Clin.:** It really looks like you had your hands full with this guy.
> **Police:** You can say that again, that guy's nuts. It took three of us to get him down.

Clin.: Yeah, he's wound up, maybe he's on something. Listen, did any of your officers get hurt? We'd be glad to take a look at them and check them over.

Police: No, don't worry about it, thanks anyway.

Clin.: By the way when you were wrestling this guy down, did he accidentally get struck on the head?

Police: No, can't say that he did.

Clin.: The reason I ask is that if he got a blow on the head we need to make sure he didn't get a small fracture or something like that?

Police: Hmmm . . . Well, you might want to take a look, this guy was wild, someone might have used a stick on him. He was out of control.

Clin.: O.K., thanks a lot for all your help. We'll take a look at him. I hope the rest of your night goes better than this.

This matter-of-fact type of inquiry tends to yield accurate answers while unobtrusively reminding the officers of the dangers of a head blow.

Violently psychotic patients, frequently brought in by the police, serve as a bridge to the next topic, patients who are acutely intoxicated by a psychosis-producing agent. This list is extensive, and includes common agents such as speed, LSD and other hallucinogens, marijuana, cocaine, crack and PCP. For a concise and practical discussion the reader is referred to articles by Goldfrank and Lydiard.[15,16]

By way of example I will briefly describe some of the more typical aspects of a patient intoxicated on PCP, a drug originally developed in the 1950's as an anesthetic-analgesic agent. These patients frequently present as markedly psychotic, although they can present without any psychotic features. In addition they can be extremely violent. In this regard any violent patient should alert the clinician to the possibility of PCP abuse. Even at low doses this drug can produce the three A's of PCP use: analgesia, amnesia, and ataxia (problems with gait). The analgesia can result in self-mutilatory behaviors such as eye gouging. If PCP use is even remotely suspected, the initial interviewer should have safety officers informed and immediately available during the interview.

On a behavioral level, the psychotic features of these patients may be quite bizarre, such as running naked in public or crawling around on all fours like an animal. They may develop paranoia, disorientation, auditory hallucinations, and visual hallucinations.

The physical exam may provide important clues, such as the various types of nystagmus (abnormal eye jerks) and hypertension reported as occuring in 57 percent of these patients.[17] These patients generally show miosis (smaller than normal pupils) but may also present with mydriasis (larger than normal pupils), especially if they also ingested an anticholinergic agent. Increased muscle tone and increased salivation are also common. Rather than presenting as agitated, these patients may present lethargically or in a coma if on high doses of the drug.

Returning in a more general sense to psychosis as precipitated by drugs, a few more points are worth mentioning. The rapid appearance of a full-blown psychosis in a matter of hours should make the clinician very suspicious of a drug-induced psychosis. Processes such as schizophrenia tend to develop more slowly. Some patients may not know that they have been given a drug; it may have been slipped to them or sprinkled on a joint. In this regard it is always worthwhile checking with friends who may know more about the actual circumstances surrounding the drug ingestion. One should always be on the look out for two possibilities when faced with drug-intoxicated, psychotic patients:

1. Is the patient actually under the influence of more than one street drug?

2. Has the patient possibly ingested not a street drug but a medication which is precipitating the psychosis?

I am reminded of a young woman with a chronic history of paranoid schizophrenia. She had been doing very well in the hospital and was consequently sent home on a pass. Within a few hours of returning from her pass, she began to appear agitated and reported feeling apprehensive. In another thirty minutes she became grossly psychotic, reporting that small dragons were chasing her. Indeed she was seen racing down the hall as if pursued by a bevy of such monsters. Physical examination revealed dilated and poorly responsive pupils, a dry mouth, and an elevated pulse. It was discovered that she had taken "a few extra" Cogentin (benztropine mesylate) tablets while at her apartment. Cogentin is a commonly prescribed anticholinergic agent that helps to alleviate some of the side effects of antipsychotic medications.

If taken in excess, these anticholinergic agents can quickly precipitate a delirium, as was the case with this patient. Elderly patients appear to be particularly susceptible to such anticholinergic deliriums. It is therefore important to inquire about both prescription and nonprescription medications. Keep in mind that specific medications may have a mild anticholinergic effect but that when given together these medications may have an additive effect strong enough to precipitate a delirium.

Classes of medications that may have some anticholinergic property include some over the counter hypnotics and "cold medicines," certain antidepressants, some antipsychotics, certain anti-Parkinsonian medications, some medications for peptic ulcer disease, and even antihistamines.[18] A classic story of medication-induced delirium would begin with an elderly patient being treated with an antidepressant such as Elavil (amitriptyline hydrochloride), who becomes mildly psychotic related to the depression. The patient would then be placed on Mellaril (thioridazine hydrochloride), an antipsychotic. This medication would relieve the patient's psychosis but could also create a significant parkinsonian syndrome. To relieve this side effect the clinician might add Cogentin. By now the patient would be on three different medications with anticholinergic effect, Elavil, Mellaril, and Cogentin. Such a patient might soon be delirious and plagued by impish demons, compliments of the treating clinician. The clinician must always carefully elicit a medication history from both the patient and the patient's family.

The clinician should also keep in mind one other broad category of agents that could precipitate a drug-induced psychosis, namely, herbs and other natural agents. A naturally occurring source of anticholinergic agents is a family of plants known as the Solanaceae. Such an innocuous sounding name actually houses a variety of not so innocuous plants, including *Atropa belladonna* (commonly called deadly nightshade), jimson weed, mandrake, and henbane. Historically, ointments and potions made from such agents may have resulted in the psychotic states that, at least partially, functioned as the source of the wild phenomena reported by the witches of the Middle Ages. In the present, it remains important to consider the ingestion of herbs and other "natural foods" while evaluating an unexplained presentation of psychosis.

Perhaps at this time it is best to return to the presentation of Mr. Williams. An interview with the police revealed that Mr. Williams had a long history of alcohol dependence, although he did not appear intoxicated presently. They also thought that he had a history of "stuffing his face with any drug he could get his hands on." Further interviewing with Mr. Williams revealed that he had a history of DTs. Physical exam and lab work revealed no other probable cause for the psychotic presentation. He was felt to be in the early stages of DTs and was begun on Valium (diazepam). In a matter of several hours he calmed, and all psychotic symptoms vanished. His case would be summarized as follows:

Axis I: Alcohol withdrawal delirium   291.00
Alcohol dependence (unspecified)   303.90
rule out Psychoactive substance abuse not otherwise specified   305.90

Axis II: Deferred V71.09

Axis III: Rule out a variety of alcohol-related diseases such as hepatitis, gastritis, and pancreatitis

As we leave the discussion of Mr. Williams, several key points are worth summarizing.

1. The presence of visual hallucinations, especially if they appear to be particularly vivid and real to the patient, are frequently seen in psychoses caused by physiological insults to the brain, including drugs and medical disease.

2. Despite the fact that such organic psychoses may tend to have some features that distinguish them from entities such as schizophrenia, all psychoses can present in a similar fashion. Consequently, any patient presenting for the first time with psychotic features should be promptly medically evaluated.

3. One of the most frequent organic causes of psychotic symptoms is the use of street drugs and/or alcohol.

4. Withdrawal from alcohol, in heavy drinkers, may lead to an alcohol withdrawal delirium (commonly called delirium tremens.) Delirium tremens can be fatal if not treated promptly.

5. The onset of a marked psychosis in a matter of hours, in a previously normal individual, is strongly suggestive of a drug-related etiology.

6. Both over-the-counter and under-the-counter medications may cause psychotic states, especially in the elderly. Anticholinergic medications are notorious for precipitating deliria.

7. If police bring in the patient, they should be questioned thoroughly.

8. Any patient who presents violently should be thoroughly evaluated for evidence of psychotic process and the possible use of PCP.

DISCUSSION OF MR. WALKER

Mr. Walker was the young male who was being harrassed by abusive women like "that devil Miss Brown." He also described brutal scenes of sexual abuse with a peculiar blandness. This blandness represents an important diagnostic clue, for Mr. Walker is suffering from schizophrenia. Criterion A-1e from the DSM III-R states that patients with schizophrenia may present with flat or inappropriate affects. This type of peculiar affect can be seen in other psychotic states, but it is very common in schizophrenia.

A useful interviewing habit consists of asking oneself if the patient seems to be appropriately disturbed while describing traumatic incidents. In the case of Mr. Walker, as he related his rape, there was little display of fear, anxiety, or anger. His affect changed very little. When present to a moderate degree, this type of unresponsive affect is usually called blunted. If the patient demonstrates essentially no change in affect, it is usually referred to as a flat affect. Mr. Walker also nicely demonstrates the concept of an inappropriate affect. Rape victims do not generally smile as they describe their assaults. This peculiar combination of flattened affect and inappropriate affect is not infrequent in schizophrenia. It is one of the qualities that can create an unsetting emotional response in a clinician, as it did in this case.

An important point to remember concerning blunted affect remains the ironic and sometimes confusing fact that antipsychotic medications frequently also cause a blunting of affect as a side effect. The wary clinician keeps this point in mind, for a patient inappropriately labeled as schizophrenic by a previous clinician may present with a blunted or flat affect related to current medication. This blunted affect may be misinterpreted by the new clinician as further "proof" that the patient has schizophrenia, resulting in a perpetuation of the first diagnostic error.

Perhaps even more striking than Mr. Walker's blunted affect is the fact that he is clearly delusional. The appearance of delusions of any kind should always alert the clinician to the possibility of schizophrenia.

These delusions are frequently bizarre in the sense that they are patently absurd and have no possible basis in fact. The patient may feel that forces are controlling his or her body or that thoughts are being inserted or withdrawn from his or her body. Other delusions tend to be concerned with magical, grandiose, or intensely religious themes. In this light, a patient may believe that God wants the patient to cut off a finger and sprinkle the blood over the earth in order to bring flowers into bloom. In paranoid schizophrenia, the patient may present with delusions of persecution or jealousy, as did Mr. Walker.

But this point raises an important diagnostic issue, for how does one separate paranoid schizophrenia from a different class of psychopathological states collectively called the paranoid disorders? The distinction is actually somewhat easier to make than one might assume, if one keeps the following guideline in mind.

In paranoid schizophrenia, the paranoid delusions are only part of the pathological process. Other aspects of psychotic process are invariably present in addition to the disorder in the patient's belief system. In paranoid schizophrenia, as delineated by the DSM III-R, the paranoid delusions are either accompanied by some type of prominent hallucination, by evidence of a severe formal thought disorder, catatonic behavior, or a flat or grossly inappropriate affect, as seen with Mr. Walker. The thought disorder may manifest itself as incoherence or as a marked loosening of associations.

With these ideas in mind, Mr. Walker's presentation becomes even more clearly typical of schizophrenia following an interview with his mother.

Clin.: What does your son do down in his room all day long?

Moth.: That is what is so peculiar. He talks with her.

Clin.: How do you mean?

Moth.: He talks with this devil woman. I'll hear voices that sound like a woman's voice coming up out of the basement. It is really weird. Late at night I can hear him arguing with her, swearing at her, and sometimes it sounds like holy hell is breaking out down there. I'm terrified, I never go down there.

Clin.: When he is with you, does it ever look like he is hearing voices?

Moth.: Oh yes, he's always mumbling to himself like he's answering someone. But the strange thing is that he's not always like this. Sometimes he seems so calm and almost normal and other times he's in a frenzy. Just last night he came screaming up out of that basement with a butcher knife in his hand. He kept screaming at me that I'd better make them stop. I couldn't take it anymore so I brought him in.

From the above it is apparent that Mr. Walker is hearing voices and clearly fulfills the criteria for schizophrenia. It also serves to stress the importance of carefully interviewing family members or other significant others. For whatever reasons, psychotic patients may withhold information critical to the diagnosis, and the family may gratefully provide the missing pieces.

Mr. Walker also illustrates the fluctuating nature of psychotic process even in schizophrenia. The severity of the psychotic process may vary substantially. Many an interviewer has been lulled into a belief that a patient is not psychotic during the interview. In such cases it is always wise to listen carefully to the family, for the interviewer may simply be catching the patient at a period of decreased psychotic process. Moreover, patients with psychotic process may not be too eager to tell the "shrink" that they are plagued by voices. Their more rational sides warn them that such talk may provide a quick ticket to the "looney bin." We may not agree with such a choice of words, but the truth of the matter remains that the patient is right.

At this point it may be useful to turn our attention to one of the exclusion criteria for schizophrenia as delineated by the DSM III-R. Exclusion C directly addresses the issue of affective symptoms. Several points are worth remembering here. In the preceding chapter we noted that a major depression may eventually manifest psychotic symptoms, representing an important diagnosis to rule out when psychosis is suspected. The particular psychotic symptoms may be either mood congruent or mood incongruent. It is important to note that in a major depression with psychotic features, the psychotic symptoms generally appear a considerable time period after the onset of the affective syndrome. It is almost as if the depressive or manic process builds with a slow crescendo that culminates with the blooming of psychotic process.

Guze reports that most schizophrenics experience affective syndromes at some time during the course of their illness.[19] Moreover, anhedonia is frequently seen in schizophrenia.[20] But in contrast to the time course of psychotic features in a major depression, the psychotic symptoms in schizophrenia tend to appear early in the process, usually predating any striking affective symptoms. While interviewing it becomes critical to spend considerable time attempting to delineate the actual history of the present illness, as discussed in Chapter 5.

Two points are worth emphasizing here. First, family members and the records of other mental health professionals can be invaluable in gaining a clear history of which came first, the psychotic symptoms or the affective symptoms. Second, it is always important when evaluating a patient who has had numerous psychotic breaks to return to the first break in an attempt to determine the role of depression in the chronology of the illness. Sometimes patients are mislabeled as schizophrenic who in actuality have a bipolar disorder or major depression. These people might benefit from lithium or antidepressants. American psychiatrists have tended to overdiagnose schizophrenia while underdiagnosing bipolar disorder.[21] With chronic patients whose initial diagnosis may have been made twenty or thirty years ago, bipolar disorder may not have been considered as strongly, for lithium was not available.

The role of the timing of affective versus psychotic symptoms is also important in the differential between bipolar disorder (manic phase) and schizophrenia. A patient can be manic without being psychotic. The mania itself is manifested by excessive energy, unstable mood, agitation, decreased need for sleep, pressured speech and other classic manic symptoms. The mania does not become psychotic unless reality contact is disturbed, as manifested by the presence of delusions, hallucinations, or other psychotic symptoms such as grossly disorganized thought. It has been estimated that about 50 to 70 percent of manic patients display psychotic symptoms.[22] As with depression, psychotic symptoms in mania tend to appear significantly later than the affective symptoms. This point once again helps to ease the difficulty of distinguishing between schizophrenia and mania with psychotic process.

We can now look at a curious diagnostic dilemma. We have seen that in schizophrenia the psychotic symptoms usually predate marked affective symptoms. And in the affective disorders the psychotic symptoms generally appear later in the process, after the affective symptoms have been around for a while. But what diagnosis is appropriate when the psychotic symptoms appear at or near the same time as the affective symptoms? Here the reader's guess is about as good as the opinions of the numerous writers on the subject. The issue is controversial. Most of the controversy focuses around a proposed diagnosis, which probably has some validity, called schizoaffective disorder.

This diagnosis is supposed to fill the diagnostic gap just described. The DSM III-R defines schizoaffective disorder as follows:

Schizoaffective Disorder[23]

A. A disturbance during which at some time, there is either a Major Depressive or a Manic Syndrome concurrent with symptoms from the A criterion of Schizophrenia.

B. During an episode of the disturbance, there have been delusions or hallucinations for at least two weeks but no prominent affective symptoms.

C. Schizophnenia has been ruled out, i.e., the duration of all episodes of a mood syndrome has not been brief relative to the total duration of the psychotic disturbance.

D. It cannot be established that an organic factor initiated and maintained the disturbance.

Specify: bipolar type (current or previous Manic Syndrome) or depressive type (no current or previous Manic Syndrome)

The vagueness of this definition certainly would be at home in the campaign speech of any presidential candidate. But then at this stage of current diagnostic knowledge, this degree of vagueness may be appropriate. It serves to remind us that diagnostic categories are not necessarily real-life entities but represent our labels for observed behaviors sometimes arbitrarily forced to confirm diagnostic labels.

Clinicians vary on what they really feel that the schizoaffective disorder will prove to be. For instance, Tsuang feels that this diagnosis represents a heterogeneous category with two probable subtypes, an affective subtype and a schizophrenic subtype. According to this theory it does not really represent a genetically distinct category.[24]

The DSM-III-R definition represents a definite step forwards when compared with the DSM-III definition, which was extremely vague. Despite the advances with the DSM III-R criteria, the concept of the schizoaffective disorder will probably require years of refinement. In my own practice I utilize a definition of schizoaffective that is somewhat more specific than the definition above and attempts to define the process with an ear towards phenomena that may separate it from other disorders. I include it as an example of a slightly different approach to the schizoaffective disorder than utilized in the DSM-III-R:

1. The patient's history suggests that during the initial onset of the illness, striking psychotic features appeared at essentially the same time as symptoms fulfilling the criteria of either a major depression or a manic episode.

2. The psychotic symptoms are generally not those typically seen in either a major depression or a manic episode. For instance, if delusions are present, they are mood incongruent, such as a depressed patient reporting that aliens are invading the earth. Unusual psychotic thought processes such as marked loosening of associations or strikingly illogical thought would also make one think of the schizoaffective disorder.

3. The later course of the illness continues to predominantly demonstrate this mixture of affective and severe psychotic symptoms, especially as each new episode begins.

4. If the psychotic symptoms are typical of an affective disorder then an affective diagnosis is given, even if the psychotic symptoms appear a short time before the full affective symptoms appear.

To me these guidelines make the distinction among the diagnoses of schizophrenia, schizoaffective disorder, and affective disorders somewhat easier.

On a practical level there exists some relevance to making these distinctions. If one labels the patient as demonstrating schizophrenia, this tends to bias subsequent clinicians to not think of the use of antidepressants or lithium. The diagnosis of schizoaffective disorder serves to remind clinicians that the patient may have an affective component to the illness, suggesting medications such as those just mentioned. The diagnosis may also have some prognostic importance, for some authors feel that schizoaffective disorders have a significantly better prognosis than schizophrenia.[25]

Concerning Mr. Walker, a diagnostic summary seems in order. No history suggestive of a personality disorder or a medical problem was found upon further interviewing. Apparently he had been displaying a downhill course for almost a year, thus fulfilling the time criteria for schizophrenia. His family reported that he appears intermittently depressed, and they were not entirely clear about the time course of the interplay between depressive symptoms and the psychotic process, but they did not feel that Mr. Walker had been consistently depressed. Once within the hospital, lab tests and other medical examinations would need to be ordered to rule out an organic cause for his psychosis, but his history does not particularly suggest such an entity. Consequently, the working diagnostic formulation would probably look as follows:

Axis I: Schizophrenia, paranoid type (provisional) 295.30
Rule out schizoaffective disorder
Axis II: None V71.09
Axis III: None

Before leaving the discussion of Mr. Walker, several key points are worth summarizing:

1. A blunted or flat affect is frequently seen in schizophrenia.
2. Antipsychotic medications can cause a blunted or flat affect. Consequently, when a patient is on an antipsychotic, it is difficult to determine whether the unusual affect is secondary to the medication or a psychopathological process.
3. In order for a patient presenting with paranoid delusions or other nonbizarre delusions to fulfill the criteria for schizophrenia, the patient must also demonstrate one of the following: hallucinations, evidence of a severe formal thought disorder, catatonic behavior, or flat or grossly inappropriate affect.
4. Psychotic process frequently fluctuates. The interviewer should keep in mind that the patient may not be strikingly psychotic during the interview itself.
5. Collateral interviews with family members may provide invaluable diagnostic information.

Mr. Walker has provided a good example of the paranoid process that frequently appears in paranoid schizophrenia. It should be noted that the DSM-III-R recognizes five major types of schizophrenia: disorganized type, catatonic type, paranoid type, undifferentiated type, and the residual type. It is not infrequent for a patient to fluctuate among these types over the course of years. At present it remains unclear as to how valuable these subclassifications will be with regard to prognosis and treatment planning, but in any case, the clinician should be aware of their various presentations.

The concept of schizophrenia, residual type, is used when the patient has a history of schizophrenia but does not appear grossly psychotic in the near past or the present. These patients do not demonstrate psychotic symptoms such as hallucinations, a moderate or severe formal thought disorder, or delusions, but they do show residual signs of schizophrenia such as a blunted or inappropriate affect, a mild loosening of associations, eccentric behavior, or social withdrawal. This category emphasizes the point that one can be suffering from schizophrenia without being actively psychotic all the time. Many patients treated with antipsychotic medications eventually move into a prolonged remission and may be labeled as schizophrenia, residual type.

At this point it is worthwhile moving to the next case history, for it adds a new twist to the diagnostic issues arising when a patient presents with paranoid symptoms.

DISCUSSION OF MS. HASTINGS

Ms. Hastings was the fifty-year-old woman who presented with the chief complaint of, "Can you help me with my husband?" She then proceeded to describe an elaborate delusional system, which she alluded to as the "divorce game."

Unlike Mr. Walker, Ms. Hastings did not present with a blunted or odd affect. To the contrary, she seemed convincingly quite normal. Her affect was appropriately upset for someone believing that she was the object of foul play. She did not complain of any hallucinations, and subsequent interviewing revealed that she had none. There was no evidence of a formal thought disorder or the other psychotic symptoms frequently seen in schizophrenia. Furthermore, she had no evidence of any psychotic disorder before the age of fifty.

The only psychopathology that she displayed was a concrete delusional system. Such a delusional system alone does not fulfill the criteria for schizophrenia unless the delusion is extremely bizarre. Instead, Ms. Hastings brings us to a curious collection of disorders referred to as the delusional paranoid disorders. In the DSM-III-R these disorders include six types: persecutory type, jealous type, erotomanic type, somatic type, grandiose type, and other type. All six of these disorders share the following criteria of a paranoid disorder:

Delusional (Paranoid) Disorder[26]

A. Non-bizarre delusions(s) (i.e., involving situations that occur in real life, such as being followed, poisoned, infected, loved at a distance, having a disease, being deceived by one's spouse) of at least one month's duration.

B. Auditory or visual hallucinations, if present, are not prominent [as defined in Schizophrenia, A(1) (b)].

C. Apart from the delusion(s) or its ramifications, behavior is not obviously odd or bizarre.

D. If a Major Depressive or Manic Syndrome has been presented during the delusional disturbance, the total duration of all episodes of the mood syndrome has been brief relative to the total duration of the delusional disturbance.

E. Has never met criterion A for Schizophrenia, and it cannot be established that an organic factor initiated and maintained the disturbance.

Ms. Hastings demonstrates many of the classic findings seen in an interview with a patient suffering from a typical paranoid disorder. These patients frequently appear surprisingly normal. One would hardly suspect any psychopathology until one uncovers the topics engulfed by the delusional system, at which point, these patients often describe elaborate ramifications and subplots that would gratify the needs of any soap opera buff. Their delusions are generally unshakeable. They simply do not believe that there is anything wrong with them, as evidenced by the fact that Ms. James did not seek help for herself but for the problem she was having with her husband. In the long run this striking lack of insight can make these patients frustratingly resistant to therapy.

Their delusions are frequently of a persecutory nature, but other variants exist. One such variant has been referred to as "the Othello syndrome," in which the patient becomes convinced that his or her spouse is having a sexual affair, referred to as the jealous type in DSM-III-R.[27] In erotomania, sometimes referred to as Clerambault's syndrome, the patient, usually a woman, comes to believe that a man has fallen madly in love with her. She may proceed to pursue him across the country or into the bedroom. One can imagine that such patients are seldom popular with the wives of the men they so diligently pursue.

Another type of paranoid disorder consists of an unshakeable belief that one has a serious medical illness, the so-called hypochondriacal paranoia or somatic type of delusional disorder. These patients differ from the person suffering from simple hypochondriasis by the fact that the belief has reached a truly delusional proportion and is essentially unshakeable. These patients may also believe that a plot has evolved to hide the truth from them.

The somatic type of delusional disorder may also present with the belief that the patient is deformed, infected, ugly, or smells badly, referred to in the literature as a monosymptomatic hypochondriacal psychosis. One of our patients was convinced that "my muscles of mastication are disordered." He had carefully produced a beautifully drawn anatomic atlas illustrating the problems with his jaw. At the interview he just happened to bring along a human skull, which he used to demonstrate in a disturbingly convincing fashion his specific anatomic defects. Sometimes these patients proceed to develop schizophrenia.

The subtype of delusional disorder referred to as "other type" is used for disorders that do not fit any previous categories, such as persecutory and grandiose themes without either theme predominating.

Brief mention should also be made of the shared paranoid disorder referred to as the induced psychotic disorder in the DSM-III-R. In this relatively rare condition, sometimes poetically referred to as "folie á deux," two patients share the same delusion. One of the patients develops the delusion after the other patient has evidenced it for some time, and in this sense, the other patient is said to be induced into a delusional system. Frequently one of the patients is a dominant and powerful personality while the second patient tends to be dependent and suggestible. The second patient's delusion may even crumble if not in the presence of the dominant figure.[28]

Diagnostically, if a patient presents with a paranoid disorder, it is critical to rule out an organic delusional disorder. This is particularly true in patients who first develop paranoid symptoms over the age of forty. There exist numerous medical illnesses that can present as paranoia. Perhaps at the top of the list one should consider a brain tumor, for these tumors tend to occur in adult life. Indeed, malignant gliomas tend to arise in middle age, while metastatic tumors from other parts of the body are more common in the elderly.[29] Other frequent organic causes include medications, endocrine disorders, infections, and temporal lobe epilepsy.

Especially with the elderly, the interviewer should also consider dementia. Roughly 20 percent of patients with Alzheimer's disease demonstrate paranoid symptoms at some point. Paranoid delusions tend to occur later in the process with these patients, although suspiciousness may occur early on.[30]

The issue of paranoid symptoms raises a pertinent diagnostic point. Some elderly patients present with concrete paranoid delusions frequently accompanied by auditory hallucinations and some other features common in schizophrenia, almost as if these patients were presenting with a late-onset schizophrenia.

This particular syndrome raises some problems for the DSM-III-R, for these patients could technically be called schizophrenic (the DSM-III-R removed an upper age of onset limit of 45, which was present in the DSM-III for schizophrenia). But it is unclear whether these geriatric psychoses are genetically or phenomenologically the same as true schizophrenia. In the DSM-III-R, if the hallucinations are not prominent, one could probably use the diagnosis delusional disorder, other type. With prominent hallucinations, the diagnosis psychotic disorder not otherwise specified could probably be used reluctantly.

I say reluctantly because such presentations are neither uncommon nor atypical as the "grab-bag" diagnosis of psychotic disorder not otherwise specified suggests. One study revealed that at least 10 percent of patients who were admitted with psychotic features over the age of 60 presented as described above. It is here that European psychiatry may be able to offer some clarification. In Europe this type of presentation is frequently viewed as a separate diagnosis called paraphrenia.[31,32]

Paraphrenia typically presents in late life with well-organized paranoid delusions associated with hallucinations. In more severe illness the delusions may also become grandiose in nature. Before these overt psychotic symptoms appear, the patient may show prodromal symptoms for months or even years. These symptoms include suspiciousness, irritability, seclusiveness, and odd behavior. Unlike patients with schizophrenia these patients, even when grossly psychotic, do not usually show problems with peculiar affect or demonstrate a formal thought disorder. They also tend to respond reasonably well to antipsychotic medications.

An unusual associated finding is the fact that about 15 to 40 percent of these patients have some degree of hearing loss. It has been suggested that a hearing loss may predispose the patient to misinterpret the conversation of others in such a way as to create paranoid ideation. The clinician should be on the look out for this syndrome while interviewing the elderly. The diagnosis of paraphrenia may be included in future editions of the DSM.

For a moment let us review the diagnostic issues associated with Ms. Hastings. In this particular interview there was little time to explore for personality disorders, and the clinician would need to defer on this axis. She complained of peptic ulcer disease, chronic bronchitis, and the recent onset of a hacking cough associated with a long history of heavy smoking. With such a history of smoking the issue of lung cancer is certainly worth considering. Her diagnostic formulation would appear as follows:

Axis I: Delusional disorder (persecutory type)   297.10
         Rule out organic delusional syndrome   293.81
Axis II: Defer   799.90
Axis III: Peptic ulcer disease
         Chronic bronchitis
         Rule out lung carcinoma

On Axis III, as mentioned earlier, numerous entities should be ruled out. But for the sake of conciseness, it is probably more practical to only list those diagnoses for which the initial interview has raised some specific suspicions, as with the cigarette smoking history suggesting lung cancer in the case of Ms. Hastings.

Let us review the major issues that surfaced with the case of Ms. Hastings.

1. The diagnosis "delusional disorder" can be classified into six subtypes: persecutory, jealous, erotomanic, somatic, grandiose, and other type. (It should be noted, that at this time, it is not yet clear whether these subcategories will prove to have any association with etiology or treatment response.)

2. Outside of the delusional quality of their speech, people with paranoid disorders frequently appear and behave quite normally.

3. In any patient diagnosed as having a paranoid disorder one should rule out an organic cause of the paranoid symptoms.

4. Paranoid symptoms are not uncommon with people suffering from primary degenerative dementia (Alzheimer's disease).

5. Paraphrenia, although not currently recognized as a DSM-III-R diagnosis, may well represent a specific syndrome in elderly patients. It is characterized by a delusional system that is associated with hallucinations.

In the next case, we shall return to the basic definition of psychosis, for a thorough understanding of this term may have significant clinical importance as we shall see.

DISCUSSION OF MS. FAY

Ms. Fay was the twenty-three-year-old woman who had been seen two weeks earlier and given a diagnosis of generalized anxiety disorder. As she had appeared at her previous interview, she currently presents with an overwhelming sense of anxiety succinctly stated by Ms. Fay as, "I'm a nervous wreck." She flatly denies any overt signs of psychosis such as delusions or hallucinations. She does not demonstrate any marked evidence of a formal thought disorder such as a gross loosening of associations. She does not appear overtly psychotic, rather she seems consumed by her own anxiety.

It is this anxiety that warrants more careful exploration, for anxiety stands as one of the most frequent early signs in a developing psychosis. To further our understanding it may be useful to review what one might call the "life-cycle" of psychotic process.

In the first place, there exist certain overt signs of psychotic process, which, when present, are essentially conclusive evidence that the patient is psychotic. These hard signs of psychosis include the following: hallucinations, delusions, moderate to severe loosening of associations or other marked evidence of a formal thought disorder, gross disorganization, gross disorientation, and bizarre gesturing. In a strict diagnostic sense, unless these signs are present one does not call the patient psychotic by DSM-III-R standards. This conservative approach is probably good, for it eliminates the dangerous habit of loosely labeling people as psychotic. Such sloppy clinical work can lead to problems such as the inappropriate use of the diagnosis schizophrenia when the diagnosis schizotypal personality is more appropriate.

On the other hand, in a clinical sense, a patient can be quite psychotic without demonstrating these hard signs. The reason for this phenomenon can be found in the life cycle of a psychotic process. More specifically, most patients do not abruptly develop the hard signs of psychosis, as if the light switch of reason was suddenly snapped off. Instead patients generally move more slowly into the world of madness.

An excellent example of this concept can be provided by looking at one possible mode of development of a single psychotic symptom such as a delusion. The phenomenologist J. Lopez-Ibor has discussed this specific process in detail[33] (see Figure 6). In the following discussion we will follow his model with some minor adjustments.

In the beginning of a psychotic break the patient frequently develops what Lopez-Ibor calls a "delusional mood." During this phase the patient begins to feel that something is not quite right. There may be an intensification of perceptions such as sight and sound. In a sense, the world is almost clearer than before, for the environment appears more vivid. New details never before recognized take on new significance, for they may never have even been noticed before. There frequently exists an unsettling feeling that something ominous may be about to happen, although at other times life may seem refreshingly vibrant. The following excerpt captures this peculiar state of affairs:

> If I am to judge by my own experience, this "heightened state of reality" consists of a considerable number of related sensations, the net result of which is that the outer world makes a much more vivid and intense impression on me than usual. . . . The first thing I note is the peculiar appearance of the lights. . . . They are not exactly brighter, but deeper, more intense, perhaps a trifle more ruddy than usual. Certainly my sense of touch is heightened. . . . My hearing appears to be more sensitive, and I am able to take in without disturbance or distraction many different sound impressions at the same time.[34]

Eventually this process becomes more intense, developing a second phase, which can be called "delusional perception," a term clarified by the phenomenologist Kurt Schneider. With delusional perception, the perception itself is normal in a sensory sense, but the patient's interpretation of the perception is clearly distorted. The anxiety of the

LIFE CYCLE OF A DELUSION

delusional mood ⟶ delusional perception ⟶ concrete delusion

POSSIBLE INDICATORS OF PSYCHOTIC PROCESS

A) SOFT SIGNS

↓

Suggestive of Psychosis

↓

Can be caused by a variety
of non-psychotic processes

B) HARD SIGNS

↓

Conclusive for Psychosis

HARD AND SOFT SIGNS OF PSYCHOSIS

SOFTS SIGNS	HARD SIGNS
unusually intense affect	delusions
angry or agitated affect	hallucinations
glimpses of inappropriate affect	moderate or severe formal thought disorder
guardedness or suspiciousness	gross disorientation
vagueness	bizarre mannerisms and body language
evidence of a very mild formal thought disorder	
pre-occupation with an incident from distant past	
expectation of familiarity from interviewer	
inappropriate eye contact	
long latency before responding or thought blocking	

FIGURE 6. Life cycle of a psychotic process.

patient begins to snowball, as the patient becomes convinced that something is not right and that danger is present. In this phase, not only is the environment noticed in a more intense fashion, but the details of the environment are felt to be directly related to the patient. The world becomes at once both highly personalized and terrifying. Ideas of reference occur. In a sense, patients feel that people are talking about them, but do not yet know why.

> Not knowing that I was ill, I made no attempt to understand what was happening, but felt that there was some overwhelming significance in all this, produced either by God or Satan. . . . The walk of a stranger on the street could be a "sign" to me which I must interpret. Every face in the windows of a passing streetcar could be engraved on my mind, all of them concentrating on me and trying to pass me some sort of message.[35]

At this point the patient may already be showing marked changes in daily functioning, avoiding this person or that person, meticulously checking on people's behavior's, staying awake at night, and ruminating endlessly. In a very real sense of the word, these patients are already psychotic, for their perception of reality is markedly different than the reality of those around them. No hard signs of psychosis in a diagnostic sense have appeared yet, but they are just around the corner.

In the third phase, the phase of "delusional ideas," the slippery suspicions of the first two phases are transformed into concrete beliefs. Patients suddenly know what people are saying about them and why. The paranoid feelings become concrete delusions both more elaborate and entrenched. Here, indeed, the classic hard signs of psychosis flower. In a sense, as Clerambault stated, the psychosis is already old when the delusions have begun.

As mentioned earlier, psychotic process tends to fluctuate, and patients may move in and out of these various phases. For these reasons, the initial interviewer needs to pay keen attention to any evidence that the patient may be in one of the less obvious phases of psychosis. If such soft signs of covert psychosis are present, then the interviewer more carefully explores for the harder signs. These soft signs of psychosis are frequently overlooked by clinicians, as was the case with Ms. Fay during her first visit to the evaluation center. For this reason they shall be examined in more detail.

In the first place it is important to emphasize that the presence of the soft signs of psychosis does not imply that the patient is necessarily psychotic. Rather, their appearance suggests that psychotic process may be present and the clinician should thoroughly hunt for it. There exist many other nonpsychotic etiologies for the soft signs of psychosis, such as anxiety, an immature interpersonal style, or somewhat idiosyncratic interpersonal habits. For instance, a mild and infrequent loosening of associations, one of the soft signs, does not necessarily indicate that a patient is actively psychotic. Schizotypal personalities may routinely demonstrate this finding, in which case it represents an ingrained personality style, not evidence of psychosis. (see Figure 6).

There exist a variety of soft signs of psychosis, including the following: (1) mild or infrequent evidence of a formal thought disorder, such as a mild loosening of associations, infrequent bits of illogical thought, idiosyncratic speech, or mild to moderate tangential speech, (2) unusually intense affect, (3) angry or agitated affect, (4) infrequent glimpses of inappropriate affect, (5) guardedness or suspiciousness, (6) vagueness, (7) preoccupation with an incident from the distant past. (8) immediate discussion of personal details as if the interviewer already knew the patient well, (9) long latency before answering questions, (10) poor eye contact in a patient who does not appear depressed, and (11) inappropriate staring. The list could certainly be made longer, but the above signs serve as a good introduction. Note that both verbal and nonverbal clues may suggest underlying psychotic process (see Figure 6).

When a clinician notices some of the soft signs of psychosis, the clinician may want to expand the region of psychotic questioning in more detail, delicately probing for the hard signs of psychosis, such as evidence of delusions and hallucinations. The belief that psychotic patients will always spontaneously reveal their hallucinations and delusions is patently false. Frequently, one must ask for specific symptoms before they are proffered.

A few other points are worth mentioning. If the patient apears unusually affectively charged about a particular topic, it is often rewarding to gently guide the patient into a further discussion of this topic by appearing interested and asking clarifying questions. With this technique one structures very little. Instead, an attempt is made to unleash further affect, for as the patient becomes more and more involved, defenses may decrease, allowing more dramatic evidence of psychotic process to emerge. Eventually, as the patient senses a friendly ear, delusional material may be shared. It is not infrequent for interviewers to simply run-over these areas of intense affect, thus robbing themselves of a natural gate into the patient's psychotic world.

In a similar vein, when a patient uses an illogical or idiosyncratic phrase, it is often wise to ask for further elaboration. It is paramount that this request for clarification sound nonjudgmental and carry a tone of true interest. As the patient proceeds to explain the ideas behind the reasoning, it is not infrequent for further and more substantial evidence of psychotic process to emerge. The psychotic patient essentially guides the interviewer into regions of questioning more likely to unearth substantial evidence of psychosis.

At this point we can return to Ms. Fay, for an excerpt of her initial interview proves to be germane. In it we shall see some of the soft signs of psychosis, in particular the interviewer will follow up on an isolated piece of illogical thought.

> ***Clin.:*** Tell me a little bit more about what your anxiety has been like.
>
> ***Pt.:*** (giggles inappropriately) That's very hard to say . . . I get uptight and I just don't know what to do with myself. I suppose it all has to do with self-image and all that stuff.
>
> ***Clin.:*** How do you mean?
>
> ***Pt.:*** Sometimes when I'm alone I just get really frightened and . . . I don't know . . . well, I . . . I don't know if I'm coming or going. I guess I'm just too anxious to be a woman. I don't know what else to say. What else do you want me to talk about?
>
> ***Clin.:*** When you say that you are too anxious to be a woman, what exactly are you referring to?
>
> ***Pt.:*** I get panicky, you know all goose flesh all over. I never know exactly when it is going to happen but it always does.
>
> ***Clin.:*** But how does that tie in with your being a woman?
>
> ***Pt.:*** It just does. Women have to do certain things and I'm unclear what exactly they are. It was all so much simpler years ago when my mother was growing up. But today what with short skirts and rock videos, it is all more confusing and there is a lot more responsibility out there, so I'm just too anxious to be a woman and I'm also too anxious to be a man, so there you have it!

The phrase "I'm just too anxious to be a woman," is a curious one. The patient did not appear cognizant of this fact and made no spontaneous attempt to explain herself. At which point the clinician wisely asked for further clarification. Her subsequent explanation was also vague, although one can surmise to what she was probably alluding. Her subsequent reply was also somewhat illogical, giving even further suspicion that a psychotic process was at hand.

As the interview progressed she appeared to become more anxious, but she never displayed or related any hard signs of psychosis. Of course, during the interview she did display a variety of soft signs, including vagueness, guardedness, a few inappropriate giggles, some small bits of illogical thought, and the hint of a preoccupation with a distant past sexual event with her brother.

She described a variety of sustained symptoms of generalized anxiety, while denying any regularly occurring panic attacks. She also described periods of fleeting paranoia and magical thinking, but said she had always had such feelings " 'cause I grew up in a bad family." She denied any persistent symptoms of depression or mania. But she did describe episodes of angry outbursts and periods of being very moody. She was evasive when questioned about previous suicide gestures.

Ms. Fay represents an excellent example of a person who leaves the interviewer with the feeling that psychotic process is lurking beneath the clinical facade but cannot be clearly identified. Because of the presence of a large number of soft psychotic symptoms, the clinician would tend to arrange for both rapid and close follow-up care.

At the end of this interview her diagnostic conceptualization was as follows:

Axis I: Generalized anxiety disorder (provisional)   300.02
            Rule out psychotic disorder not otherwise specified
Axis II: Rule out schizotypal personality
            Rule out borderline personality disorder
Axis III: Defer

The diagnosis of psychotic disorder not otherwise specified (atypical psychosis) was employed because there were no strong indicators of an affective illness nor clear cut signs of schizophrenia or paranoid disorder, but the clinician was suspicious of some underlying psychotic process.

This suspicion proved to be well founded, for several weeks later Ms. Fay was admitted to the hospital with several striking paranoid delusions concerning her brother accompanied by many of the symptoms of mania. Apparently the clinician had caught her at a time when she was actively psychotic but had not yet developed the hard signs of psychosis. He had in essence seen her before the storm erupted, during the phase of delusional mood or delusional perception. Or she may have actually already had delusional ideas that she was not yet ready to share. Figure 7 summarizes the inter-relationships among the stages of the life cycle of a psychosis and the appearance of soft and hard signs of psychotic process. It also re-emphasizes the point that psychotic phenomena tend to fluctuate.

Later interviews with Ms. Fay and with her family revealed a history of intermittent affective instability with both manic and depressed features. Her psychotic symptoms appeared early on in the process. It was unclear exactly which appeared first, affective symptoms or psychotic symptoms. Consequently, her Axis I diagnosis was changed to schizoaffective disorder rule out bipolar disorder. Further observation and history would eventually determine whether she was experiencing a true bipolar disorder or not.

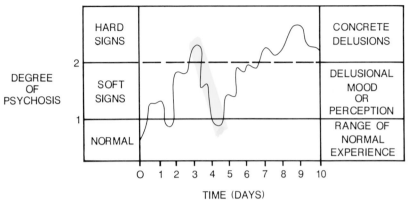

FIGURE 7. Evolution of a psychosis.

Fortunately, Ms. Fay eventually stabilized upon a combined treatment of Lithium and Haldol (haloperidol). Even during periods of stability, she continued to appear very manipulative. She also continued to have significant problems with anger and impulsive control. Her parents related these symptoms were lifelong in nature, lending further support to the idea that Ms. Fay might also have some severe characterological problems such as a borderline personality disorder.

Ms. Fay serves as an example of an intriguing study in the subtle signs of psychotic process and the need for the initial interviewer to constantly seek out the soft signs of psychosis. At times such a dedicated diligence, associated with prompt subsequent treatment, may help prevent from suffering the full-blown wrath of a psychotic illness.

Before leaving her case it is worth summarizing some of the major points it highlights.

1. A person may be psychotic in a clinical sense without demonstrating the hard signs of psychosis such as delusions or hallucinations.

2. The so-called soft sign of psychosis should always alert the clinician to the possibility of a smoldering psychotic process.

3. In the life cycle of a psychosis, hard signs of psychosis generally do not erupt without a prodromal phase of psychosis in which the patient's experience of reality is clearly abnormal but only the soft signs of psychosis are apparent.

4. Generally it is best to follow up on areas of intense affect for such areas may be outward manifestations of delusional material.

5. If the patient uses an illogical or idiosyncratic phrase, it is often useful to ask for clarification. In the process of clarifying, the patient may reveal further evidence of psychotic process.

6. A patient may have a severe psychotic illness on Axis I, such as schizophrenia, and still have a personality disorder on Axis II.

We can now leave the outpatient assessment clinic and return to the emergency room where Mr. Lawrence was hauled in by the police and a crisis worker, apparently suffering from an acute exacerbation of his chronic schizophrenia.

DISCUSSION OF MR. LAWRENCE

At first Mr. Lawrence presented in an agitated and violent manner. At one point he literally threatened to beat one of the nurses, and he subsequently tried to do so, eventually requiring restraints. There was a suspicion that somehow the nurse had been incorporated into a delusion, although the patient denied the typical delusions he had demonstrated in the past.

By the time I had arrived on the scene I was surprised to find that Mr. Lawrence was laying calmly on a cart and appeared quite cooperative. He denied any hard signs of psychosis and also denied any recent suicidal gestures, although he commented that he had been thinking of killing himself several days earlier. Eventually we were able to remove the restraints, at which point Mr. Lawrence took a peculiar turn in his clinical course.

He related that he needed to go to the bathroom. As he walked towards the toilet he appeared to stagger a bit. Once he reached his destination, he looked about as if plopped into an unfamilar space and asked, "What am I doing in here?" When told that he had wanted to go to the bathroom, he appeared puzzled and denied ever making such a request.

As the interview proceeded Mr. Lawrence began to appear drowsy, which he attributed to being up all night as well as drinking heavily. He could only repeat three or four digits forwards, whereas he had been able to repeat seven forwards earlier. He also began clutching at some invisible objects near his feet.

If at this point Mr. Lawrence is beginning to sound similar to our first patient, Mr. Williams, who presented with delirium tremens, it is because Mr. Lawrence is also suffering from a delirium, a delirium that would eventually threaten his life. The interview was promptly stopped at this point. An EKG revealed some subtle abnormalities. Roughly thirty minutes later Mr. Lawrence stopped breathing. Fortunately, his life was saved through the effective use of an artificial respirator.

In retrospect, the correct diagnosis was a tricyclic overdose leading to a paradoxical rage response. This rage was followed by a delirium. His case provides a springboard into a discussion of several important points. In the first place, it is important to note that it was initially assumed that Mr. Lawrence was merely experiencing an exacerbation of his paranoid schizophrenia, for he had frequently presented with violence in the past. And therein lies one of the more dangerous clinical traps when dealing with a patient who has been labeled with a chronic psychotic process. It is both easy and natural to assume that the old etiologic agent is at work without vigorously searching for a new one.

A useful point to remember concerns the idea that psychotic processes caused by a single etiology, such as schizophrenia, frequently present in a relatively similar fashion during each episode for a given individual. The soft signs, or early warning signs, are frequently similar from episode to episode, as are the subsequent hard signs. The psychotic process tends to leave an identifying fingerprint of sorts with each patient. Consequently, in any patient in which a new episode of psychosis appears distinctly different than in previous episodes, the clinician should become suspicous that something new has been added to the picture etiologically. In the case of Mr. Lawrence, he usually presented with delusions and hallucinations. In this case neither symptom was present. This is one area in which previous hospital charts can be useful, providing a history of the patient's past episodes.

The second major point has been stated earlier but certainly warrants repeating. Any patient presenting with a delirium requires immediate medical evaluation. This represents a clinical situation that frequently faces the crisis worker and for which the crisis worker must constantly be on the look out. It is critical for all initial evaluators to become adept at recognizing the clinical presentation of a delirium. With knowledge and common sense it is not necessarily difficult to recognize, yet this diagnosis is frequently missed, often by physicians themselves.

We can begin our exploration of the presentation of a delirium by reviewing the DSM-III-R criteria, which appear below:[36]

Delirium

A. Reduced ability to maintain attention to external stimuli (e.g., questions must be repeated because attention wanders) and to appropriately shift attention to new external stimuli (e.g., perseverates answer to previous question).

B. Disorganized thinking, as indicated by rambling, inrelevant, or incoherent speech.

C. At least two of the following:

(1) reduced level of consciousness, e.g., difficulty keeping awake during examination
(2) perceptual disturbances: misinterpretations, illusions, or hallucinations
(3) disturbance of sleep-wake cycle with insomnia or daytime sleepiness
(4) increased or decreased psychomotor activity
(5) disorientation to time, place, or person
(6) memory impairment, e.g., inability to learn new material or to remember past events, such as history of current episode of illness

D. Either (1) or (2):

(1) there is evidence from the history, physical examination, or laboratory tests, of a specific organic factor (or factors) judged to be etiologically related to the disturbance
(2) in the absence of such evidence, an etiologic organic factor can be presumed if the disturbance cannot be accounted for by any nonorganic mental disorder, e.g., Manic Episode accounting for agitation and sleep disturbance

It is important to note that not all delirious patients are disoriented.[37,38] Generally these patients develop disorientation, but at times, especially in the early stages of the process, they may be completely oriented. In this sense, deliriums can present in a variety of fashions, part of the reason they can be misdiagnosed.

The following guidelines provide a practical platform for clinical assessment. In the first place a delirium occurs when there exists a rather diffuse pathophysiological dysfunction in the brain. Such a diffuse dysfunction will frequently show itself by one of two ways, a fluctuating level of consciousness or a marked problem with attending to the environment. These two processes represent the keynotes that should alert the clinician to the possibility of a delirium. Indeed, if either of these processes appears in a patient demonstrating the soft or hard signs of psychosis, then one should strongly consider a delirium work-up.

It therefore becomes critical to evaluate these two points during the initial interview of any psychotic patient. Unfortunately, it is easy to overlook their significance if the patient is agitated, as was the case with Mr. Lawrence. Let us begin with the evaluation of the level of consciousness.

People with a delirium tend to present in one of three ways: (1)

hypoactive, (2) hyperactive, or (3) a mixed picture of the previous two states. In the hypoactive state, which represents the most common state, the patient may appear drowsy or literally be hard to arouse. This type of "quiet delirium" is common in geriatric patients. Their somnolent behavior is not bothering anyone, and consequently their condition may be overlooked. In the hyperactive state the patient is "wired." They appear unusually responsive to any stimulation from the enviroment and tend to appear driven. This is sometimes accompanied by marked agitation or aggression. We saw this presentation earlier with Mr. Williams, the man suffering from delirium tremens. Finally, patients may present with a mixture. One of the hallmarks of the delirious patient is the tendency for the level of consciousness to fluctuate. This fluctuation may be so extreme as to move the patient back and forth between hypoactive and hyperactive states.

If one is actively looking for changes in the level of consciousness, they are not hard to spot. But in a busy clinical situation the trick is to be aware of their importance. A problem arises in the fact that patients tend to move in and out of delirious states relatively quickly. An alert nurse may note a brief episode of delirium that will simply not be present during clinical rounds the following morning. A frequent physician error is to assume that if the patient looks good on rounds, then, "What's the fuss?" Unfortunately such a patient may be developing permanent brain damage during the periods of delirium. Consequently, this type of patient needs a medical work-up despite a good appearance during rounds.

In association with the tendency for the delirious patient to demonstrate a fluctuating level of consciousness, this phenomenon is usually paralleled by changes in the EEG.[39] In the hypoactive state, the EEG usually demonstrates a generalized diffuse slowing of the background activity. During the hyperactive state, fast activity is often seen. At times a normal EEG may be found.

With regard to determining whether or not the patient is having trouble attending to the environment, the task becomes more difficult. The difficulty lies in the fact that subtle problems with attention and concentration may not be apparent unless tested. At times the clinician may be able to determine that concentration is reasonably good, by noting the patient's ability to converse in a natural and intelligent fashion. At other times more formal testing is required, especially if the evaluator is truly suspicious of the presence of a delirium.

Four tests come to mind, which as a battery will generally pick up any significant problems with attending to the environment. These four tests are digit spans forwards and backwards, the vigilance test, constructions, and an examination of the patient's handwriting.

In the digit span test, one asks the patient to repeat a series of digits. The clinician begins with two digits and continues in successive steps to seven digits if the patient proceeds to answer correctly. It is important to say the digits in a steady rhythm. If said like a telephone number, the patient may find them artificially easy to remember. This test can then be done by giving a series of digits and asking the patient to repeat them backwards. With the digit span one should expect an average adult to be able to repeat about seven digits forwards and four to five backwards.

In the vigilance test the clinician recites a string of letters from the alphabet. The patient is asked to make a hand tap on the table every time the letter "A" is said. If the patient is experiencing problems attending to the environment both errors of omission and commission will tend to occur. A normal adult should make few if any errors. As the series continues some delirious patients will even forget what letter they are hunting for.

The patient may also be asked to make copies of constructions such as a cross or a cube. Once again the delirious patient may find such a task difficult. Finally, problems with writing (dysgraphia) are common and include spelling errors, clumsily drawn letters, reduplication of strokes in letters such as 'M" or "N," and problems with alignment and linguistics.[40]

These four tests represent an excellent screen for deficits in attending abilities, but one may have difficulty using them with a hostile patient. Not too many hostile patients are eager to demonstrate their artistic abilities or play word games. When these tests may be inappropriate, one can learn a great deal by carefully observing the patient. The delirious patient may demonstate attentional difficulties through an inability to follow commands, a problem remembering questions, a tendency to appear overly sensitive to noises and other outside stimuli, or simply an appearance of confusion, as was the case with Mr. Lawrence in the bathroom. The trick is in remembering to look for these processes on a routine basis when encountering a psychotic patient.

Thus far the focus has been on the two key characteristics of a delirium. It may be of value to review a few of the more common clinical characteristics.[41,42]

1. Hallucinations and/or illusions have been estimated to occur in 40 to 75 percent of delirious patients. Visual and auditory hallucinations are frequent, and the presence of visual hallucinations should always arouse suspicion of a delirious or organic state.

2. Rapidly changing delusions, especially of a paranoid nature, are common. These delusions tend to be of a much more fleeting and malleable nature than the delusions seen in schizophrena or one of the paranoid disorders.

3. Other problems with a formal thought disorder such as a loosening of associations or illogical thought may appear.

4. Short-term memory and orientation are frequently impaired.

5. Deliriums tend to fluctuate. In particular, patients tend to be more disoriented and delirious at night, a process that has been referred to as "sundowning."

6. Deliriums tend to emerge in a matter of hours or days, but this is not always the case. Insidious onsets can occur.

7. Although deliriums are generally believed to be related to organic etiologies, it is believed that stress and psychological mechanisms can lead to a delirious presentation in some instances.

8. Affect is typically abnormal, with a high incidence of emotions such as fear and anxiety.

9. A characteristic phenomenon is the tendency for the patient to misidentify the unfamiliar as familiar. For instance, a nurses aide may be identified as a brother or sister.

A variety of other odd behaviors have been reported during deliriums, ranging from wandering aimlessly about the hospital to drinking copiously from the toilet. A particularly peculiar process has been reported in which the patient continues habitual behaviors in totally inappropriate places. For instance, in an "occupational delirium," patients perform behaviors in the hospital that are normally only done at their place of work. The term "carphology" has been coined for the behavior of picking at one's bedclothes, another abnormal behavior sometimes seen in deliriums.

With regard to etiology the list is extensive. In Table 3 a practical list of common causes is presented. It is beyond the scope of this book to elaborate on the medical differential and on the appropriate laboratory and physical exam. The first and crucial step remains the uncovering of the delirium during the interview itself.

In a practical sense, interviewers must train themselves to rule out delirium any time a patient presents with a psychosis. Unless this active process of viewing delirium as a part of the differential becomes a clinical habit, one runs the risk of missing it. The patient is the one who pays for such an error, and the cost may be permanent brain damage or worse.

At this point let us summarize the DSM-III-R diagnosis on Mr. Lawrence.

Axis I: Delirium (secondary to antidepressant)   292.81
             Paranoid schizophrenia in remission   295.35
Axis II: None   V71.09
Axis III: Respiratory arrest secondary to overdose

Major points worth reviewing include the following:

TABLE 3. *Common Causes of Delirium*

Metabolic

1. Hypoxia, hypercarbia, anemia
2. Electrolyte imbalance, hyperosmolarity
3. Hyperglycemia or hypoglycemia
4. Abnormal levels of magnesium or calcium
5. End-stage liver or kidney disease
6. Vitamin B_1 deficiency (Wernicke's encephalopathy secondary to a thiamine deficiency)
7. Endocrine disorders (hyperthyroidism or hypothyroidism, hyperparathyroidism, and adrenal disorders)

Infections

1. Systemic (such as pneumonia, septicemia, malaria and typhoid)
2. Intracranial (such as meningitis, encephalitis)

Neurologic Disorders

1. Hypertensive crisis, stroke, subarachnoid hemorrhage, vasculitis
2. Seizures
3. Trauma

Drug Withdrawal

1. Alcohol hallucinosis, rum fits, DTs
2. Other withdrawal states (such as from barbituates, as well as acute intoxication with street drugs)

Intoxication

1. From agents such as digoxin, levodopa, anticholinergics, and street drugs

Postoperative sequelae

1. Especialy following cardiac surgery

---

1. Functional psychoses such as those seen with schizophrenia or bipolar disorder often present in a similar fashion from episode to episode.

2. If a patient's psychotic presentation seems different than is typical from previous episodes, then the clinician should strongly consider the possibility of a new etiologic agent.

3. The presence of a delirium always warrants an aggressive medical evaluation and can easily be missed in chronic patients.

4. The clinician should always consciously look for evidence of a fluctuating level of consciousness or a significant problem with attending to the enviroment in all psychotic patients, for these two characteristics are tip-offs that a delirium may be present.

At this point we shall look at a clinical case in which the outcome was unfortunately not as good as with Mr. Lawrence.

DISCUSSION OF KATE

Kate was the fourteen-year-old who had been depressed and was acting oddly. Her most bizarre behavior consisted of appearing at her parents' bedroom door topless. At several emergency rooms she had been diagnosed as hysterical and in need of outpatient psychiatric care.

In the interview it was easy to see why hysterical traits had been reported. She seemed preoccupied, as if pulled into an autistic cocoon. At one point she turned, and while looking me dead in the eye she dramatically said, "Tell me Doctor, what is reality?" She denied hallucinations, delusions, and other hard signs of psychosis. Her speech was halting and was interspersed with inappropriate giggles. At times she displayed thought blocking and seemed distracted. She was completely oriented, demonstrated an alert and stable consciousness, and when pressed, displayed no marked problems with attending to the enviroment, although her method of handling the conversation suggested that she might prove to have some problems in this area.

Her numerous soft signs suggested that a psychotic process was present, and she was hospitalized. Her physical exam was normal, and we were suspicious of drug abuse. Roughly one week following her admission, she lay dying in the intensive care unit. Her diagosis was viral encephalitis. Her admission bloodwork had revealed evidence of an infection, and a subsequet spinal tap revealed evidence of central nervous system involvement.

Diagnostically speaking, Kate did not present with a delirium. Not all organic causes of psychosis manifest as a delirium. While looking over the spectrum of organic etiologies of psychotic process outlined in Table 4,[43] it is important to remember that organic illness can present in a fashion suggestive of essentially any functional psychosis, such as schizophrenia or bipolar disorder. Frequently, delirium is not a part of the picture. This point once again emphasizes the need to "think organic" when evaluating a patient presenting with the onset of psychotic symptoms.

More importantly, in the emergency room, and even in the private office, one of the critical triage decisions involves ruling out a life-threatening cause of psychosis. The most common life-threatening illnesses that present with an acute psychosis include the following:[44]

1. Hypoglycemia
2. Hypertensive encephalopathy
3. Poor oxygenation (perhaps related to a heart attack, pulmonary embolus, anemia, or a hemorrhage)
4. Infections such as encephalitis or meningitis
5. Drugs, including medications, street drugs, withdrawal states, industrial toxins, and actual poisons.
6. Intracranial trauma (including hemorrhage, actual trauma related to head injury, and other causes of increased intracranial pressure.)
7. Wernicke's encephalopathy (not generally life threatening but should be viewed as a medical emergency, for if untreated, permanent brain damage can occur.)

TABLE 4. Organic Causes of Psychosis*

Space-occupying Lesions of the CNS
    Brain abscess (bacterial, fungal, tuberculosis, cysticercus)
    Metastatic carcinoma
    Primary cerebral tumors
    Subdural hematoma
Cerebral Hypoxia
    Anemia
    Lowered cardiac output
    Pulmonary insufficiency
    Toxic (e.g., carbon monoxide)
Neurologic Disorders
    Alzheimer's disease
    Distant effects of carcinoma
    Huntington's chorea
    Normal pressure hydrocephalus
    Temporal lobe epilepsy
    Wilson's disease
Vascular disorders
    Aneurysms
    Collagen vascular disease
    Hypertensive encephalopathy
    Intracranial hemorrhage
    Lacunar state
Infections
    Brain abscess
    Encephalitis and postencephalitic states
    Malaria
    Meningitis (bacterial, fungal, tuberculosis)
    Subacute bacterial endocarditis
    Syphilis
    Toxoplasmosis
    Typhoid
Metabolic and Endocrine Disorders
    Adrenal disease (Addison's and Cushing's disease)
    Calcium-related disorders
    Diabetes mellitus
    Electrolyte imbalance
    Hepatic failure
    Homocystinuria
    Hypoglycemia and hyperglycemia
    Pituitary insufficiency
    Porphyria
    Thyroid disease (thyrotoxicosis and myxedema)
    Uremia
Nutritional Deficiencies
    B_{12}
    Niacin (pellagra)
    Thiamine (Wernicke-Korsakoff syndrome)
Drugs, Medications, and Toxic Substances
    Alcohol (intoxication and withdrawal)
    Amphetamines
    Analgesics (e.g., pentazocine [Talwin], meperidine [Demerol])
    Anticholinergic agents
    Antiparkinson agents
    Barbiturates and other sedative-hypnotic agents (intoxication and withdrawal)
    Bromides and other heavy metals
    Carbon disulfide

TABLE 4. *Organic Causes of Psychosis* *(Continued)*

Cocaine
Corticosteroids
Cycloserine (Seromycin)
Digitalis (Crystodigin)
Disulfiram (Antabuse)
Hallucinogens
Isoniazid
L-Dopa (Larodopa and others)
Marijuana
Propranolol
Reserpine (Serpasil and others)

---

* Adapted from Bassuk, E. F., and Beck, A. W. (eds.): *Emergency Psychiatry.* New York, Plenum Press, 1984.

Other serious entities to keep in mind include hepatic failure, uremia, subacute bacterial endocarditis, and a chronic subdural hematoma. Fortunately this list does not represent a particularly extensive differential. If the clinician remembers to think of these entities, they are generally easy to rule out. But that is an important "if." In actuality, these entities are rare enough as causes of acute psychotic process that they are likely to be overlooked, unless clinicians train themselves to consistently consider them.

A brief, well-directed physical exam should uncover many of the life-threatening processes mentioned above. In fact, a patient presenting with the onset of a new psychotic symptoms should seldom, if ever, leave an emergency room without a screening physical exam.

This exam can be performed quickly and is geared towards uncovering evidence of a life-treatening dysfunction. To this end, it focuses upon the following five areas: (1) vital signs, (2) autonomic system dysfunction, (3) heart and lung dysfunction, (4) neurologic dysfunction and head trauma, and (5) abnormalties of the eyes.

Abnormal vital signs should be retaken. If they remain abnormal, an etiology for the dysfunction should be sought. Keep in mind that the pulse may be naturally elevated in an agitated patient, but agitation alone seldom causes pulses over 120 to 130.

Autonomic dysfunction is frequently present during a life-threatening illness. Agents such as the anticholinergic medications mentioned earlier frequently cause the patient to present with hyperthermia, blurred vision, dry skin, facial flushing, and delirium. The mnemonic "hot as a pepper, blind as a bat, dry as a bone, red as a beet, and mad as a Hatter" has been used to describe this toxic state.

A note of caution should be added, for the anticholinergic syndrome is often incomplete, or it may be hidden by other active agents such as opiates. For instance, Mr. Lawrence, who overdosed on Elavil, an antidepressant with many anticholinergic properties, presented with an increased pulse and a dry mouth, but his pupils were normal sized and reactive. His skin color was pale, not flushed, as would be expected in a classic anticholinergic syndrome.

This discussion also emphasizes the usefulness of looking at the patient's eyes. The clinician should look for abormal size or responsiveness of the pupils as well as asymmetry. Horizontal and vertical nystagmus should be sought. The eye grounds may reveal evidence of increased intracranial pressure.

Neurologically, one scans for evidence of focal weakness and changes in reflexes. Reflexes, including the suck reflex, snout reflex, palmo-mental reflex, and the Babinski sign, can be quickly screened. The clinician should check for signs of neck rigidity as well as for hemotympanum of the ears or other signs of a small skull fracture.

Finally the clinician should listen to the heart and lungs if an abnormality of the cardiovascular or respiratory system is suspected.

A screening physical as described above can quickly flush out a serious physical condition, sometimes even in the early stages. A common error in this regard is to admit extremely agitated patients directly to a seclusion room and subsequently fail to perform a follow-up physical exam when they have calmed down. Once the patient has calmed, the physician should attempt a screening exam no matter how late it is at night. If Mr. Lawrence had been sent to a seclusion room to calm down and a follow-up physical had not been performed, he could easily have died. At times when one is strongly suspicious of a serious illness, the patient may need to be physically restrained to allow for examination.

At this point we can return to Kate in an effort to summarize her DSM-III-R diagnosis. At the time of her admission, before any lab work had returned, her differential may have looked as follows:

Axis I: Psychotic process not otherwise specified (provisional) 298.90
Rule out (1) organic mental disorder (not otherwise specified) 292.81 related to an unspecified substance abuse, (2) organic mood disorder, depressed, 293.83, (3) major depression, single episode 296.20
Axis II: Defer   799.90
Axis III: Rule out organic causes of psychosis

Before leaving the topic of Kate's presentation, it may be of value to summarize some key points.

1. A delirium is not the only way in which a medical illness may manifest as a psychosis. Diseases such as encephalitis frequently mimic functional processes such as schizophrenia.

2. The clinician should routinely consider the various life-threatening illnesses when evaluating a patient who is psychotic.

3. A screening physical exam should be performed on any patient presenting with psychotic features.

4. The absence of all the typical signs of the anticholinergic syndrome does not rule out this syndrome, for it may present with only some of the physical signs.

Let us now move on to our final case presentation, for Miss Flagstone represents an anomaly among our other cases. She is not acutely psychotic.

DISCUSSION OF MS. FLAGSTONE

The reader will recall that Ms. Flagstone was the woman in her mid-thirties who presented with a dramatic flair and a long cigarette in hand. She related that several years earlier she had heard the voice of the angel Gabriel proclaim her with child. Upon further interviewing, the entire episode seemed to last roughly fifteen to thirty minutes. Moreover the voice of the angel was loud and distinct. At one point the voice actually conversed with the voice of God. Apparently, near the time of this episode she had been fired from a job and had also been feeling "slightly paranoid near my co-workers."

She also related that she undergoes periods in which she feels, "not quite myself, as if I wasn't quite real." These episodes last only for about ten minutes and occur during times of stress. She finds these episodes very disturbing. Further interviews would reveal that no true Axis I pathology existed with regard to Ms. Flagstone, yet how does one explain the voices and the episodes of depersonalization?

The answer lies in the fact that psychotic process is not limited to Axis I. A variety of personality disorders may present with "micropsychotic episodes." These episodes tend to last from minutes to hours. At times they may extend longer, but as soon as the episodes appear to be lasting a day or longer, one should immediately begin suspecting a process on Axis I. It is much more characteristic for these events to be short-lived, as demonstrated by Ms. Flagstone, who upon further interviewing seemed to fulfill the criteria for a histrionic personality disorder.

Micropsychotic episodes are characteristically precipitated by stress, or they may be unleashed by drug abuse. Processes such as fleeting paranoid ideation, depersonalization, and derealization are frequently experienced. If drug abuse or stress is frequent, then both the frequency and duration of the micropsychotic episodes may increase.

Diagnostically speaking, the following personality disorders may demonstrate micropsychotic episodes: paranoid personality, narcissistic personality, histrionic personality, schizotypal personality, and the borderline personality. These phenomena are frequent companions of the last two disorders mentioned.

This case also raises the important question as to whether this episode of voices should even be viewed as psychotic. Perhaps her religious beliefs suggest that this process is a normal one. At times subcultures may assert beliefs that other cultures do not accept. For instance, in North Carolina, where I trained in medicine, it was not unusual for people to believe in "rootwork." This was a magical belief similar to the idea that one has been cursed. In this subculture, a belief in rootwork did not necessarily indicate the presence of psychosis.

To help the clinician decide whether a belief is delusional, two avenues suggest themselves. One method is to explore vigorously to what degree the reported episode is typical for the culture in mind. It is advisable to talk with friends or family. At times the clinician will discover that people holding the same belief system feel that the patient in question is "beyond this belief system." By way of example, one of my patients suffering from chronic paranoid schizophrenia routinely attends an Evangelical church in which her father is the minister. Despite the intensity of the Evangelical practices, such as speaking in tongues, both the patient and her father can tell when her religiosity is becoming abnormal.

The second avenue for clarification is born from an understanding of the life cycle of a psychotic process as discussed earlier. As had been noted, patients are frequently engulfed by psychotic process long before the hard signs of psychosis, such as delusions and hallucinations, manifest concretely. When talking with the patient, the interviewer may elicit information suggesting that soft psychotic signs were not a part of the process. If such processes as delusional mood and delusional perception are absent as was suggested by the lack of soft signs, it gives further weight to the idea that the process is cultural, not psychotic. Looked at in context of the Evangelical movement, "speaking in tongues" is a special but normal aspect of an Evangelical religious life. In contrast, if the patient were psychotic then speaking in tongues may have become a nagging preoccupation, which develops an ominous significance for the patient long after the patient leaves the church.

With regard to Ms. Flagstone, her voices and depersonalization episodes probably warrant the label of micropsychotic episodes. They are always brought on by stress, and further interviewing revealed that they tend to be preceded by mood states suggestive of the soft signs of psychosis. It should be born in mind though that micropsychotic episodes, unlike their counterparts on Axis I, can occur fairly abruptly.

After the first interview, the differential on Ms. Flagstone looked something like the following:

Axis I: Defer-probably none 799.90
(because of her tangential speech and mood shifts an entity such as cyclothymic disorder or dysthymia could be kept in mind.)

Axis II: Histrionic personality disorder (provisional) 301.50
Rule out personality disorder not otherwise specified (mixed with histrionic, schizotypal, and borderline traits)

Axis III: Rule-out temporal lobe epilepsy

The Axis III diagnosis may surprise the reader, and rightfully so, for I have not yet included some pertinent information. Ms. Flagstone reports that she has become extremely interested in a variety of philosophical and religious issues. She has filled nearly twenty journals with her thoughts, none of which are psychotic in nature. She also reports brief episodes of feeling very uncomfortable in her abdomen, a sensation that seems to move upwards into her throat area. All of these phenomena could be components of temporal lobe epilepsy, including her periods of depersonalization and her mood shifts.

Temporal lobe epilepsy is the "masquerader par excellence." It can mimic essentially any psychiatric disturbance and is particularly good at presenting as a psychotic disturbance. A query should be made for temporal lobe epilepsy in any patient presenting with psychotic symptoms.

Psychotic symptoms may emerge during the seizure itself or between seizures (the period known as the interictal phase). The seizure activity sometimes begins with a phase known as the aura, in which patients may experience a variety of odd sensations, including fear and anxiety. Patients may feel that they are experiencing a given situation for a second time (known as déjà vu), or they may have the opposite feeling that nothing is familiar (known as jamais vu). Strange and pungent odors may also be a predominant symptom. Peculiar abdominal feelings are very frequent. In some instances, these feelings are the only symptoms, and the patient is said to have "abdominal seizures."

As the seizure develops patients lose consciousness and usually display various automatisms such as picking at themselves, wandering about, and displaying bizarre mannerisms or odd behaviors. To uncover such processes, a useful question remains, "Have you ever found yourself somewhere and you didn't know how you got there?" Two other pertinent questions are, "Have you ever had periods of losing consciousness?" and "Have your friends or family ever told you that they have seen you doing very odd things that you don't remember?"

Curiously, personality changes and/or psychotic-like activity may appear between seizures.[45] Ms. Flagstone reported some of the more common interictal phenomena: preoccupation with religious or moral issues, a tendency to write copiously, decreased sexual drive, intense mystical experiences, a deepening intensification of emotions, and what has been called interpersonal viscosity. This latter term refers to a tendency to want to keep talking and being near people.

It is certainly not always possible to explore all these issues during the initial interview because of time constraints. But in later sessions these questions should be rigorously pursued. It is an unfortunate error to label someone as having schizophrenia when the actual problem is temporal lobe epilepsy. Such a person would be robbed of the chance to benefit from a course of antiseizure medications.

At this juncture we are rapidly drawing to a close on our case discussions. It seems appropriate to summarize some of the points brought forward by the case of Ms. Flagstone.

1. Some personality disorders may present with psychotic symptoms, so-called micropsychotic episodes.

2. These micropsychotic episodes tend to extend from minutes to hours and are often triggered by stress or drugs. Paranoia, depersonalization, and derealization are common.

3. Temporal lobe epilepsy may present with psychotic symptoms, both during seizures or between seizures.

4. Consequently, questions should be asked concerning both the symptoms commonly seen during a seizure as well as the interictal personality change.

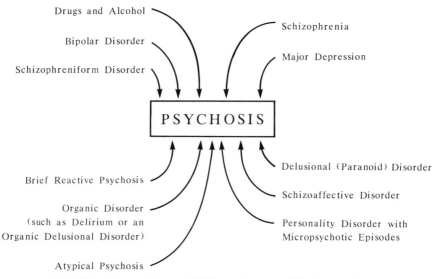

FIGURE 8. Diagnostic possibilities when considering psychosis.

We have now concluded our survey of diagnoses that may present with psychotic symptoms. Figure 8 illustrates the rich diversity of etiologic agents that may present as a psychosis. As mentioned earlier, the word "psychosis" is not a diagnosis. The presence of psychotic symptoms forces the clinician to delineate the possible etiologic agent or diagnosis, as seen in Figure 8.

In order to interview effectively we must possess a sound and flexible knowledge base concerning diagnosis. The first part of this chapter has attempted to provide just such a base. We now can turn to the equally important issue of understanding what it is like to experience a psychotic process. From such an understanding, both our interviewing skills and our abilities to empathize will undoubtedly mature. Moreover, few topics remain more fascinating or puzzling.

SECTION II: THE UNDERSTANDING OF PSYCHOSIS

In this unnerved — in this pitiable condition — I feel that the period will sooner or later arrive when I must abandon life and reason together, in some struggle with the grim phantasm, Fear.

Edgar Allan Poe, The Fall of the House of Usher

Poe aptly describes the fear and anxiety that so frequently walk hand-in-hand with the process known as psychosis. In this section we will attempt to move system by system, as we did in the previous chapter on depression, in an effort to better comprehend the intense fear associated with "going mad."

Fields of Interaction

I: THE PHYSIOLOGICAL SYSTEM

One of the major physiological moorings of our daily lives is the routine appearance of the phenomenon known as sleep. If one's sleep patterns are disturbed, one quickly begins to feel "not quite oneself." It appears as no surprise then that a sleep disturbance often appears early in the psychotic process.

As psychotic process begins to gain momentum, patients often experience severe problems falling asleep. In some instances the patient will eventually undergo a day/night reversal, in which sleep occurs during the daylight hours and the night becomes a bed of agitation. Patients may also experience other sleep disturbances, such as early morning awakening, especially if the psychosis is part of a major depression.

This difficulty with falling asleep stands as a sensitive sign of impending psychosis, frequently appearing during periods of delusional mood or delusional perception. Patients sometimes deny this sleep disturbance. Consequently, it is useful to ask family members about the patient's sleep, for they have frequently been awake themselves, coping with the growing restlessness of their relative.

Psychotic process tends to disrupt the normal control of activity levels, resulting in patient behavior ranging from agitated catatonia, in which the patient cannot stop moving, to stuporous catatonia, in which the patient shows little movement at all. It is to this peculiar state of stuporous catatonia that we shall turn our attention briefly.

At one time catatonia was generally believed to be primarily associated with schizophrenia. More recently, it has been viewed as a symptom complex that is not only seen in schizophenia but also in affective disorders, hysterical dissociation, and in a variety of medical illnesses.[46]

Stuporous catatonia is often associated with mutism, lack of movement, negativism (as shown by a tendency to not comply with any requests), and ambitendency. This latter trait reveals itself as a hesitancy to complete behaviors, demonstrated by actions such as extending one's hand to shake and then removing it. All of these behaviors have been referred to as the "negative symptoms of catatonia." Stuporous catatonia is also associated with the so-called positive symptoms, such as the holding of bizarre postures, the senseless repetition of the clinician's words, and waxy flexibility. This latter phenomenon manifests itself as a bizarre willingness to hold one's body in any position to which it is moved.

The initial interviewer is faced with the question of how to approach a catatonic patient. It is not clear exactly what such patients are experiencing, and most likely the experience varies from patient to patient. Apparently some patients seem well aware of what is going on around them while others may be lost in peculiar feelings of timelessness and autism.

In the previous chapter various verbal techniques for dealing with the catatonic patient were discussed. A logical question arises as to whether one should attempt a nonverbal technique such as touching the patient. Generally speaking I believe that in an initial interview the answer is no, primarily because one simply does not know what these patients are experiencing. If delusional or actively hallucinating, the patient may perceive the clinician as attacking. Moreover, some of these patients can move almost immediately from stillness into hyperactive states.

I am reminded of one such patient who I inadvisedly touched. She was laying on the floor in an unresponsive state. We were concerned about the possibility of an overdose. When she did not respond to loud questions, I shook her shoulders. To my shock she immediately grabbed me and attempted to bite me. Apparently, drugs were not the issue.

On the other hand, in certain unusual instances the clinician may decide that it would be useful to touch the catatonic patient. If such a decision is reached, then some simple principles should be followed. In the first place someone else should be in the room, and safety officers should be aware that the patient may be unpredictable. The patient should be told in a calm and reassuring voice exactly who the clinician is and what the clinician is about to do. Patients should also be told why they are being touched and that if at any point they want to be left alone they should simply say so. The clinician should be prepared to quickly take evasive action.

I am reminded of a woman in her mid-thirties, suffering from schizophrenia. During the interview she sat with her head wrenched straight back while wincing with pain. For about ten minutes she refused to answer any questions. Her neck continued to hyperextend, as her face further contorted in pain. A second clinician stepped in at this point and said the following, "Ms. Jackson, I am one of the physicians here. I can see that you are in some kind of pain. I am concerned that you may be having a type of drug side effect (dystonic response to her neuroleptic) and I would like to see if I can help relieve your pain. In a moment you will feel me touching the back of your head. I will be trying to see if I can get your neck to move more freely. If you want me to stop, just tell me." The clinician proceeded to do just as he said, while continuously informing the patient as to his next move. In about a minute, the patient's neck straightened, allowing the interview to continue, although she proceeded to speak in a disorganized fashion. Her neck spasm was hysterical, not medication related.

Leaving the area of catatonia, one is confronted with another possible somatic concern of the patient suffering from psychotic process. Namely, these patients frequently have literal problems with determining the limits of their bodies and in a parallel sense the limits of their sense of self, their "realness" so to speak.

It has been suggested that patients experiencing psychotic process often regress to an infantile state in which the body is viewed as part self and part object.[47] At such points the person may experience intense feelings of depersonalization and/or derealization. This type of experience was vividly described by one patient as follows:

I look at my arms and they aren't mine. They move without my direction. Somebody else moves them. All my limbs and my thoughts are attached to strings and these strings are pulled by others. I know not who. I have no control. I don't live in me. The outside and I are all the same.[48]

When intense, these feelings of depersonalization may be associated with a terrifying sense of impending annihilation. Perhaps this is the almost otherworldly fear that Roderick Usher felt was his destiny in Poe's story. It is important to realize the intensity of these fears for they provide insight into the sometime violent and drastic measures of psychotic patients.

The above quotation also leads into an extension of the concept of poor ego boundaries. One can view psychotic patients as possessing a "porous ego." The world seems to invade their skins in a distinctly unpleasant fashion. They experience a variety of sensations, which seem to enter from the outside world while becoming one with them. It is this unidirectional invasion of of their integrity that is partially responsible for their fear and anxiety.[49]

Kurt Schneider included these types of invasion experiences in his list of first rank symptoms of schizophrenia. He mistakenly thought that the presence of any of these symptoms guaranteed the presence of schizophrenia. This did not prove to be the case (although they are frequent in schizophrenia), but his symptoms are an excellent inventory of common psychotic phenomena whatever the etiology, and questions concerning them should be part of any interviewer's repertoire.

Schneider described eleven symptoms, of which seven are characterized by this odd feeling of invasion by the outside world. These seven symptoms are somatic passivity exeriences, thought withdrawal, thought insertion, made feelings, made impulses, made volitional acts, and delusional perception. The remaining four Schneiderian symptoms are audible thoughts, voices arguing, voices commenting upon one's actions, and thought broadcasting. These four symptoms will be described later.

With somatic passivity experiences the patient is the reluctant recipient of bodily sensations, such as suddenly feeling that his intestines are wriggling about inside his abdomen against his will. It is easy to see how such a peculiar sensation could subsequently plant the seed of delusional material, such as a paranoid fear that someone is purposely twisting the patient's insides.

Unfortunately, the patient's porous ego may also leak outwards. The result may be fears that aggressive fantasies will be heard by others in the room, or even worse, that in a magical sense, these violent ideas may automatically become reality. A common feeling is that the patient's thoughts are being broadcast, one of the four remaining Schneiderian symptoms, as poignantly described below:

My difficulty is an outgo of my silent thought. It goes as it comes. I may think whatever I please, but whatever I do think goes as it comes. I suppose the constant irritation and annoyance they have kept up around me has affected the tension of nerve, so that unlike others who have the same phenomenal power, it goes as rapidly as my mind thinks. I have but to think a thought and it reaches other minds in sound without an effort on my part, and is sounded for a distance, I suppose, of two or three miles.[50]

One can quickly sense the inherent strangeness of a world encountered with a porous ego. One can more easily intuit why these patients frequently seem preoccupied or lost in thought. It requires tremendous attention to try to sort out the meanings of so odd and intrusive a world. The clinician must also bear in mind that these patients are frequently attempting to determine which of their sensations are real and which are false. To the degree that they possess a "distance" from their psychosis, they will realize that much is unreal. As the psychosis deepens, this distance is lost, and the inexplicable becomes a reality that needs no explanations.

Thus far the focus has been upon the somatic sensations and physiological ramifications of psychotic process. But with the advent of neuroleptic medications, which have remarkably enhanced our ability to decrease psychotic process, a new set of problems has unfortunately appeared. Patients may develop significant side effects. Earlier the side effect was discussed in which the patient's affect becomes blunted secondary to an antipsychotic-induced Parkinson's syndrome. This blunting could be mistaken for the blunted affect so characteristic of schizophrenia.

A second side effect, akathisia, can also confuse the initial interviewer, for it can be mistaken as evidence of psychotic agitation. Akathisia represents a symptom in which patients feel that a part or all of their body needs to move. It is a deep-seated feeling of restlessness. Generally it will show itself as the physical sign of moving about in an agitated fashion, sometimes with a prance-like step. It is important to remember that akathisia is a subjective symptom and not a physical sign. In this sense the patient may not always appear agitated but may still be feeling extremely restless. By way of illustration, if in addition to akathisia the patient has also developed the stiff-like Parkinson's syndrome described above, the patient may move very little despite an intense drive to move. Needless to say this type of paradoxical situation creates an extremely discordant sensation for the patient.

It is easy to mistake akathisia for psychotic agitation; consequently the interviewer must be alert for it. In a severe form akathisia represents a new and bizarre sensation that a patient, already having problems with psychotic process, certainly could do without. Some authors have reported incidents in which they felt akathisia either worsened a psychotic state or at times predisposed the patient to inflict self-damage.

In the following direct transcription a young professional will describe his experiences with akathisia. At the time of the transcript he was no longer psychotic. When the medication had been utilized, he had been suffering from a frightening delusional system. He had also been told about akathisia and its transitory nature, but his psychotic process appears to have disrupted this information. I have never heard akathisia or its interplay with psychotic process so eloquently described:

Pt.:   I was very aware of a different kind of feeling from what I usually have. It felt as if it was most immediately recognizable in the morning, in that I felt that I just couldn't go through with my normal morning routine, like taking a shower and shaving and everything I do to get ready for work. It felt more like I couldn't do it because I couldn't stand to wait that long, to go through those things which were such routine motion.

Clin.:   Like, what are some of things that were routine?

Pt.:   Well, like standing under the shower. It just seemed impossible to stand under the shower for any much longer and once I got done with the shower it seemed impossible to stand there and dry myself.

Clin.:   Ok. What do you mean when you say it wasn't possible. What was it that you felt would happen if you did stay there?

Pt.:   That I would break out of my skin or something like that. But, uh, that I would be so upset and und unsettled that I would just be totally destroyed I think. It's just very unsettling.

Clin.:   Now, did the experience change over time? In other words, were there parts of the day where you would feel worse than other parts?

Pt.:   It was pretty much general all day. When I got to work, I have a sit-down job. I do remember that it was hard to stay put. It was really hard to sit. I do a lot of reading in my job and it was very hard to concentrate on the things I have to read, and as a consequence it made me feel ineffectual in my work. I just felt totally wiped out at work. I felt like I really couldn't keep working if I were to keep having this feeling.

Clin.:   You mentioned the ineffectual feeling. Did you start to feel upset about being ineffectual?

Pt.:   Oh, sure. Yeah, I felt that I was going to be a failure, really, if I were to keep feeling this way. I thought it would become evident right away to all the people around me that I was really screwing this up and that I really couldn't do my job anymore. And, in fact, I even got a little panicky about that.

Clin.:   Describe that to me.

Pt.:   Yeah, I just felt like being between a rock and a hard place because the feeling was that I had to sit there and keep doing my work because I was at work. On the other hand, my body felt like I just couldn't keep doing that anymore, and, uh, it was like you were in a crisis every second is what it was really like. Between wanting to stay there and do your job and being unable to do so.

Clin.:   Did you have any fears that somehow or other that this state would not go away? You know, that this was going to continue?

Pt.:   Definitely. I had the fear that the drug had set off something in my system whereby, even if I stopped the drug, that I was going to continue to have this feeling. What was definitely very much a part of the feeling was the fact that how could I go through the rest of my life feeling this way? That was very much a part of it.

Clin.:   Now, what types of things did this sort of lead you to think then, that you couldn't do your work and that this state might not change?

Pt.:   Uhm, I felt depressed about it, and, uh, it led me to feel scared and afraid that something was going to happen.

Clin.:   Do you think that you got more frightened or nervous than you had been before? In other words, did the unpleasant sensation increase your own anxiety just because you were having it?

Pt.:   Oh, yes. Definitely. I was very anxious being around other people, that they might perceive that I was in this agitated state.

Clin.:   Did you have any feelings that you should try to hurt yourself or that you might hurt yourself? . . . because of the . . .

Pt.:   Yes, it did seem, it did occur to me that it would be easier not to live than to live this way. That probably seems really heavy, but that did occur to me. I did, I had a resurgence of suicidal thoughts during those feelings.

Clin.:   What kinds of things were you thinking at the time?

Pt.:   Uh, usually blowing my head off. Really, I was thinking about that and just ending it all because it just, I think every drug I ever took, I always had the fear that it would do something, that it would never go away again.

One aspect that can help the interviewer attempt to sort out akathisia from psychotic agitation is the fact that akathisia represents a true bodily sensation. Patients will generally describe a need to move, an actual restlessness within the limbs. This is not generally the case when the agitation is caused by psychotic process. If the patient lacks other psychotic symptoms that could be triggering intense anxiety, then it is also more likely that akathisia is the main problem. But at times the only way to distinguish akathisia from psychotic agitation is to attempt to treat one or the other process. Fortunately with the patient described above the akathisia was greatly relieved by lowering the dose of the neuroleptic.

II: THE PSYCHOLOGICAL SYSTEM

Auditory hallucinations remain one of the trademarks of psychotic process. To the lay person, the presence of "voices" is practically synonymous with madness. In actuality auditory hallucinations represent one of the true hard signs of psychosis.

But the determination of whether a patient is having hallucinations is not as easy as one might think, for the clinician must, for the most part, depend upon the patient's self-report. Errors in validity appear more frequently when one must depend upon patient opinion as opposed to the elucidation of behavioral incidents. To clarify this dilemma, it may be best to start with a definition of an auditory hallucination.

For quite some time, clinicians tended to clump reports of auditory hallucinations into two categories: pseudohallucinations and true hallucinations. This distinction may well have found its most fertile roots in the writings of Karl Jaspers, who we have discussed before in Chapter 5. Jaspers seemed to believe that there was no continuum between hearing one's thoughts and hearing true hallucinations. Patients either had hallucinations, or they did not. With true hallucinations he felt that two elements were always present. First, the hallucination was substantial in the sense that it seemed real and had many of the perceptual qualities of a real perception. Second, the hallucination seemed to occupy space. With an auditory hallucination this suggests that the voice came from a given area outside the head.

But Jaspers may not have been correct, as Fish and others have pointed out, and modern clinical experience has borne out.[51-53] There does appear to be a continuum, and I have talked with many schizophrenic patients who describe their voices as "being in my head." In some instances, as the psychotic process progresses, these voices move out into space and truly seem more real at that point. In other cases, the voices always seem to be originating from outside the patient's head. But the bottom line remains that auditory hallucinations can be experienced in both ways. And the DSM-III-R accepts both voices from inside and outside the head as representing hallucinatory phenomena.

In an even more classic sense, the concept of the apparent localizability of a hallucination is probably best viewed with regard to whether a voice is heard within the mind (which has no location) or outside the mind (where a location can be assigned). In a pure pseudohallucination, the voice is only within the mind. In a pure hallucination the voice can be physically located, and this location may even be reported as being inside the patient's head as with "A radio transmitter is broadcasting from inside my head, where my neighbor implanted it." The internal terrain of the body can actually represent a geographic space and a source of hallucinatory phenomena in this regard.

It is also interesting to explore what is meant by the word "real," for patients may tell the clinician that the voices are quite real but do not sound exactly like normal voices. It is not uncommon for psychotic patients to be able to identify their hallucinations as abnormal voices. Sometimes they may even possess names for them.

If a clinician is attempting to decide whether or not a patient is faking hallucinations, these points become important. A patient who is malingering may tend to describe the voices as sounding just like normal voices, which remains possible in psychosis but not typical. The malingerer may also describe the voices as happening all of a sudden, unaware that hard psychotic symptoms usually have subtle prodromal phases such as delusional mood and delusional perception. Moreover, the voices found in processes such as schizophrenia are frequently hostile in nature and often hurl unusually obscene insults at the patient.

Because of the importance of auditory hallucinations, three of Schneider's eleven first rank symptoms concern voices. One of these symptoms consists of the patient experiencing audible thoughts, in which the patient's thoughts are repeated aloud. Or the patient may hear an undecipherable voice whose content becomes clear a few seconds after hearing it. The other two symptoms consist of arguing voices and voices commenting on the patient's activities.

The following excerpt vividly presents the eerie world created by such phenomena.

Seated on a steamer chair on the boardwalk of Coney Island, I heard the voice for the first time. It was as positive and persistent as any voice I had ever heard. It said slowly, "Jayson, you are worthless. You've never been useful, and you've never been any good." I shook my head unbelievingly, trying to drive out the sound of the words, and as if I had heard nothing, continued to talk with my neighbor. Suddenly, clearer, deeper, and even louder than before, the deep voice came at me again, right in my ear this time, and getting me tight and shivery inside. "Larry Jayson, I told you before you weren't any good. Why are you sitting here making believe you're as good as any one else when you're not? Whom are you fooling? You're no good," the voice said slowly in the same deep tones. "You've never been any good or use on earth.

There is the ocean. You might as well drown yourself. Just walk in and keep walking." As soon as the voice was through, I knew, by its cold command, I had to obey it.[54]

In the last analysis, there exists no better method of learning about hallucinations than the experience of asking questions about auditory hallucinations to numerous people, ranging from psychotic to normal. Only in this manner will the clinician develop a sound sense of the range of normal and abnormal responses. The following types of questions can both convey to patients that the interviewer is genuinely interested in their experiences, as well as helping the clinician learn about hallucinations themselves:

    a. When you are feeling very distressed, do your thoughts ever get so intense that they sound almost like a voice? (If answered "yes," consider the following.)
    b. Tell me what the voices sound like to you.
    c. What do they say to you?
    d. Do they sometimes taunt you or say mean things about you?
    e. Are they male or female voices?
    f. Do you have names for them?
    g. Do they seem to be inside your head or do they come from outside your head?
    h. Are they loud or soft?
    i. When you first heard the voices, what did you think they were?
    j. What feelings do you have as you hear the voices?

The wording of the first question allows the topic to be broached in a fairly nonaffrontive fashion, for the interviewer is tying the phenomena directly into the patient's pain. The clinician asks if the patient's thoughts sound *like* a voice, a phrasing that offers a backdoor to the reluctant patient who fears being viewed as crazy. In a typical first assessment, the interviewer may not have time to ask all of these questions, but as time permits the clinician can pick and choose, constantly learning more about the phenomenology of hearing voices.

Besides abnormalities of perception, the psychotic patient's thought process itself is often disrupted by the psychotic process. Thoughts may become speeded up and racing in nature, as is also seen in mania. It becomes difficult to concentrate as evidenced by the following patient description:

I just can't concentrate on anything. There's too much going on in my head and I can't sort it out. My thoughts wander around in circles without getting anywhere. I try to read even a paragraph in a book but it takes me ages because each bit I read starts me thinking in ten different directions at once.[55]

This excerpt also hints at another disquieting characteristic sometimes seen. Psychotic thinking has an internally "contagious" quality to it, in the sense that it triggers a multitude of associations, sometimes close in nature and at other times distant and disjointed. This abnormality in thought process will frequently show itself with a loosening of associations in the patient's speech. This trend of creative but dystonic associations, which are not in the patient's control, is nicely captured in the following excerpt:

My trouble is that I've got too many thoughts. You might think about something — let's say that ashtray — and just think, oh yes, that's for putting my cigarette in, but I would think of it and then I would think of a dozen different things connected with it at the same time.[56]

At other times thought processes may become, perhaps because of the previously mentioned abnormalities, somewhat disrupted. Patients may stop in midsentence and be unable to return to their original topic. This process is known as thought blocking. It represents a strongly suggestive soft sign of psychosis. It is useful to quietly ask patients what has happened at these moments. Sometimes the patient has been derailed by an auditory hallucination. If the clinician suspects this process, the clinician can ask if this was the case.

It is important to know if a patient is actively hearing voices during the interview, for the patient may feel that the clinician is producing the messages. Generally, it is not good for rapport to be perceived as calling the patient a drunken slob or threatening to chop off the patient's fingers and other appendages. This active state of hallucinosis represents the type of situation in which violence can erupt.

It has already become apparent that the patient's thought processes are frequently affected during a psychosis, although this is not always the case. One common problem is the presence of truly illogical thought. One of the more frequent breakdowns in formal logic is the appearance of what Rosenbaum has called predicative thinking. This means that the person views things as similar or identical because they are connected by the same predicate (verb). The following example shows this process at work:

Major premise: Jesus Christ was persecuted.
Minor premise: I am persecuted.
Conclusion: Therefore, I am Jesus Christ.[57]

Other distinct problems with logic, as well as the emergence of magical thought, as seen in young children, frequently accompany psychotic process. But it is not necessarily a black or white phenomenon. Many patients will demonstrate varying degrees of normal logic.

This knowledge that the psychotic patient may be losing an ability to think logically is of immediate practical use when approaching patients who are both psychotic and agitated. It is probably a mistake to immediately assume, before talking with the patient, that the patient either can or cannot be talked down. Instead the interviewer should gently attempt to engage the patient in conversation. While doing this, the clinician can decide to what degree the patient's logic is intact. If it is reasonably intact, the interviewer may try to talk with the patient and perhaps alleviate some of the patient's anger. If, with this technique, the patient begins to escalate or if the patient's logic is severely impaired, it is probably best to quickly back off from the patient and proceed with appropriate safety procedures.

To further attempt to reason with such a patient does not make much sense, for the patient is not processing the clinician's words in a normal fashion. Further interaction may push the patient towards violence. The key lies in carefully assessing the impact of one's interaction and proceeding appropriately.

A similar situation arises if the clinician discovers that the patient has incorporated the clinician into a delusional system. This brings to mind a patient with whom I observed the interview as a supervisor. She was ragged appearing and sat in her chair spitting her words into a hostile world. As soon as I sat down she yelled out, "You're the one who called me a prostitute the other day. You're the one who has been spying on me!" I had never seen her before and even if I had, I doubt I would have spoken to her as she was suggesting.

No matter what I said in my defense she immediately grew angrier, and so I quickly shut up. Such a retreat is not only the better part of valor, but also represents a sound clinical maneuver, for this patient was not hearing a word I was saying. It becomes easier to understand her hostile position, if the clinician realizes that she truly believed that I had belittled her publicly. Clinicians cannot quickly detach themselves from such a delusional web.

In most patients the initial interviewer has much more access to the process of blending. The question then becomes one of how does one broach topics like paranoia without offending the patient. Paranoid ideation is often easily entered by keying off the content of the patient's conversation, utilizing natural, implied, or referred gates as follows:

> **Pt.:** I don't know what to do with myself. I just, I just feel the whole thing is a mess. Probably, I don't know, probably the baby is even aware of our arguments. When we were first married, everything was so much better. But when the mill shut down a third time and he lost his job for good, well it all became history.
>
> **Clin.:** It sounds like an ugly situation at home. Has the tension ever gotten so bad that he has struck you?

> ***Pt.:*** Thank god no. I'd leave him, honestly I would.
>
> ***Clin.:*** Do you think that in any way he is trying to hurt you, perhaps even trying to get your friends against you?
>
> ***Pt.:*** Oh he's tried to hurt me in the sense of making me feel guilt, but he knows better than to mess with me or my friends.

In this fashion, the clinician has smoothly made a foray into the paranoid region. The patient's comments do not suggest paranoid ideation. There is probably no need to explore further. By now most paranoid patients would probably have nibbled at the "bait." The clinician has scouted for paranoid ideation without the patient having any idea that such an exploration of psychotic material has occurred.

This point leads to the more general issue of broaching other psychotic topics in a nonthreatening fashion. For most interviewers this type of questioning is most difficult when interviewing a patient in whom the clinician doubts the presence of psychotic process. Some authors have suggested that interviewers should never ask questions about voices and other psychotic phenomena unless they strongly suspect the presence of these phenomena. To do so, they argue, will disengage the patient.

But I have my doubts about such a blanket admonition, and in practice I generally ask all patients about psychotic process at some point in the initial interview. I believe this represents a sound practice for three reasons. (1) A patient whose psychotic process is fluctuating or whose psychotic process is part of a character disorder may look remarkably intact during any given interview. For instance, to not ask about ideas of reference or episodes of depersonalization invites the cover-up of diagnoses such as a schizotypal personality. (2) I have seldom, if ever, seen such questioning result in any lasting problems with engagement in a nonpsychotic patient. I have seen patients balk at it, but with skillful engagement techniques, the blending is quickly restored. Moreover, most patients do not seem offended at all. (3) And when patients do balk at such questioning, their emotional overreactions provide an open window into their defenses and psychodynamics. This psychodynamic window is one of the best reasons to routinely ask such questions, as seen in the following:

> ***Pt.:*** Let's get it straight, things have been tough all over for everybody involved and I've been damn upset.
>
> ***Clin.:*** When you are really feeling upset, have your thoughts ever gotten so intense and bothersome that they sound almost like a voice?
>
> ***Pt.:*** Oh great, here come the crazy questions. (Said angrily)

> Well I got news for you. I'm not crazy and I've been asked
> all those questions before. (The patient reaches over and
> squeezes her boyfriend's hand, smiling at him while sub-
> sequently tossing a little sneer to the clinician.)

This hostile display is not a typical response to this question. Indeed, it suggested to the interviewer that the patient might have some type of personality disorder, as evidenced by her sense of entitlement and manipulative actions. Such a response may suggest the expansion of diagnostic categories not considered earlier. In this case, further interviewing revealed a full-blown borderline personality disorder.

Once entering the psychotic region it is not necessary to beat it into the ground. Quickly, the clinician will achieve some idea as to whether the region is worth expanding further. If hints of psychotic process emerge, then a full expansion may be warranted. If no hints emerge, the topic may be left quickly after only a few probing questions. Part of the art lies in learning how to smoothly enter these psychotic regions.

Some questions that may be used effectively as gates into psychotic material are shown below.

a. Have you had experiences that seemed odd or frightening to you?

b. Earlier we talked about your nightmares. Have you ever had similar types of frightening images bothering you during the day?

c. You had been talking about some of your talents. Have you ever felt that you had some unusual abilities such as ESP?

d. You mentioned earlier that one of your favorite activities is watching T.V. Have you even been frightened by the T.V.? (depending on what the patient says one might pursue this with a question such as follows) Did it ever seem like the people on T.V. were watching you or that they literally were aware of private aspects of your life?

e. You had mentioned earlier that your sister had apparently been hearing voices. Have you ever had similar experiences?

Another excellent method of entering psychotic material is through the discussion of religious issues as shown below:

Pt.: I have always been a fairly religious person. My father was a devout Lutheran. Religion runs in our family.

Clin.: On a moment by moment basis, how much is God a part of your life?

Pt.: (long pause) He is my life and my breath, so be it.

Clin.: It sounds like He is a very important part of your life.

> Sometimes people who are close to God feel that He has a special mission or role for them to play. Do you feel that you may be lucky enough that God has such a role for you?
>
> ***Pt.:*** Yes, I do. I am to bring peace to all nations. And I shall bring a calmness to all that I touch.

Clearly it would be worth exploring the psychotic region more thoroughly with this patient. But the important issue from our viewpoint is the naturalness of the gate provided by religious discussion. Even as the topic was first entered, the intensity of the patient's feelings probably suggested to the clinician that something was up.

In this sense it may be of value to examine the impact of the psychotic patient on those with whom they talk, in short, the dyadic system.

III: THE DYADIC SYSTEM

It is not infrequent for psychotic patients to become socially withdrawn. In particular, when the psychosis is secondary to schizophrenia, episodes of social withdrawal are extremely frequent.[58] This social withdrawal could be related to the tendency for the patient to enter a more autistic world. In an effort to sort out the tremendous number of peculiar sensations and thoughts, the person suffering from a psychotic process may find it necessary to withdraw. Social contact becomes painfully disruptive. In other patients in which aggressive drives may be building to a pitch, people may be avoided because of a fear of loss of control.

But there is another aspect to this entire issue, which brings us directly to the dyadic system itself. Frequently, these patients' behaviors are socially inappropriate. As we had seen in the chapter on nonverbal behavior, psychotic patients generally show some disturbance in the normal nonverbal rules for coversation. This may range from sitting or standing inappropriately close to the clinician to displaying markedly abnormal affects. Because of the tremendous need of these patients to attend to the troubled thoughts in their own minds, their ability to empathize is frequently strikingly diminished.

Clinicians should also be aware of their own feelings of confusion that may develop as they interview psychotic patients. This confusion in the clinician may be caused by psychotic processes in the patient, such as a subtle loosening of associations. If the clinician can recognize the subjective feeling of confusion, then a more thorough pursuit of psychotic process and content may be suggested. The confusion in the clinician mirrors the confusion or disorganization of the patient.

A word of caution seems in order here. Clinicians lucky enough to be gifted with an intuitive sense of empathy can fall into a trap. The patient may be displaying subtle signs of disorganized thought, but the clinician ignores them because he or she understands "what the patient is thinking." And indeed the clinician might. But the patient is still psychotic. In hunting for evidence of formal thought disorder the question is not whether we understand the patient, but whether a normal person would be confused or not. At the other extreme, sometimes a well-trained clinician will recognize a formal thought disorder before it would even be evident to a layperson.

All of the above disturbances in dyadic communication may lead to an uncomfortable sensation in a clinician. The sensation has been described as not being able "to feel" with the patient, in short, an inability to experience an empathic bond with the patient. This peculiar sensation has been called the "precox feeling."[59] It is felt to be particularly suggestive of schizophrenia. Used in the appropriate sense, as an intuitive guide suggesting the need to carefully explore for the criteria of schizophrenia, the precox feeling is a useful tool. It should never be used as a criterion of schizophrenia or as a justification for labeling someone as having schizophenia.

People with psychotic process can also create feelings of frustration in the initial interviewer. This may result when the patient's lack of insight pushes the patient to reject various avenues of help such as medicaton or hospitalization. It can be particularly frustrating to work with a paranoid patient who clearly needs help but feels strongly "nothing is wrong with me."

In these instances, it is important to accept the naturalness of one's frustration while avoiding a demonstration of this frustration to the patient. These countertransference problems tend to surface as extensive and sometimes heated attempts to convince the patient of his or her illness. Such attempts are probably far more counterproductive than productive. It is often best to calmly discuss one's views and then acknowledge openly that the patient and oneself seem to have a difference of opinion. The patient should know that if the patient feels a desire to talk again or experiences a change of opinion, that the clinician is always available for another appointment.

Frustration may also evolve when the interviewer feels that the patient is somehow in control of the psychotic process, "flipping it on" when it is advantageous to do so. At some level this manipulation may acutally occur at both the conscious and unconscious plane. I remember a man of about thirty years old who would begin talking in a disorganized and delusion-littered fashion. But as he felt more comfortable with me, his thinking would become more organized. If I then probed even in a subtle fashion into his personal life, he would quickly become disorganized and mumble about "the cheesedogs that were going to drop a nuclear warhead on Pittsburgh." Oddly enough I do not think he was particularly conscious of this process.

One can better conceptualize such behavior if one assumes that at some level, to the degree that the patient has both insight and motivation, the patient may be able to partially rein in psychotic process. This self-modulation must require a considerable amount of effort and concentration. Perhaps at times, and depending upon the interpersonal situation, the patient might find it simply easier to just let things go as they may. At such points the psychotic process may emerge in a more pressing fashion as seen above. To the degree that we understand this process our frustration levels may decrease.

Frustration may also arise with patients suffering from schizophrenia who are persistently negative during the interview. As Michels suggests, the interviewer may gently point out that automatically saying "No" to everything is as much a relinquishment of control as saying "Yes" to all the clinician's requests.[60] Jointly agreeing upon a topic to discuss may also open up avenues for better engagement.

Thus far the emphasis has been on the patient's effect on the clinician. With psychotic patients, it is also important to realize that clinicians may need to monitor their own impact on the patient. In earlier chapters we have already discussed in detail some of the changes in style that may help facilitate blending with paranoid patients, such as decreasing the use of complex empathic statements. It is also important to realize that because of disturbances in logic and reality testing, normally well-received statements by a clinician may be hostilely received. Michels points out, for instance, that with one of his patients the word "leg" had taken on a highly sexualized meaning.[61] Consequently, when the clinician would use the word, it was received as a sexual topic, probably carrying a variety of unwanted overtones.

Sometimes when psychotic patients are cooperative but frightened, it goes a long way to simply reassure them that they are in a safe enviroment. Especially if such patients are disorganized as well as frightened, it is useful to tell them what is happening, ask them to bring up any questions they may have, and structure the interview for them. If the patient is forced to handle an unstructured interview, filled with open-ended questions, gentle commands, and pregnant pauses, the interview itself may become traumatizing. Gentle structuring will sometimes actually result in a more organized production of speech as the psychotic defenses recede.

Along similar lines, in some instances an empathic interviewer may so decrease the anxiety level of a subtly psychotic patient that the observable psychotic process temporarily disappears or recedes significantly. Ironically, the clinician's style will have distorted the clinical picture, amply reminding us that as the interview proceeds we become a part of the dyadic system, whether we intend to or not. In a similar fashion, an involvement with the psychotic process itself awaits the friends and family members of the patient. Unfortunately, unlike clinicians, they are not generally trained to handle such bizarre interactions.

IV: THE FAMILY SYSTEM AND OTHER GROUP SYSTEMS

Psychosis, despite its propensity for autistic withdrawal, is a family matter. No person in the immediate vicinity of the patient will be able to remain uninvolved for long. Few processes can so ravage a family and its underlying structure. This is particularly true when the process is chronic in nature, such as with schizophrenia or a bipolar disorder. For these reasons, family members will become an important source of information as well as a targeted group for therapeutic intervention.

Most family members are sorely ill equipped with the knowledge that could help them understand and cope with the bizarre behaviors of their loved ones. One can imagine what it is like for family members to become the object of the penetrating hatred that may erupt when one is perceived as part of a patient's delusional system. In some instances family members are physically assaulted, and in rare instances, killed by the very people they have loved most. Obviously, both family and friends must cope with powerfully ambivalent feelings, including embarrassment, guilt, fear, compassion, helplessness, bitterness, love, and the desire to abandon the patient.

I remember working with one family whose plight illustrates some of the many processes at work in the family system. The family was of Creole background. The patient was an attractive woman in her midthirties who sat with a defiant jut to her jaw. Upon her head she wore a faded scarf that lent a sad elegance to her. She had become progressively depressed, and her mind was swarming with religious delusions. She had had to stop work and had been living with her mother and a brother, both of whom were taking care of her children. These family members had not wanted her to seek professional help, for they felt that whe would get over it with God's help.

But she had recently spent several days with another brother who had angrily insisted that help be sought. Already the psychosis was beginning to dig its claws into the structural foundations of the family. It is commonplace for family tensions to crystallize around issues such as, "What to do with Jim or Sandy."

While waiting in the emergency room, the patient, who we shall call Ms. Jenkins, stood up and began to perform a ritualistic chant. It was sad indeed to watch the mother and brother hide their embarrassment as they struggled to get her back in her seat. Later, this same mother and brother would undercut our efforts to hospitalize Ms. Jenkins. Her mother wearily looked at us saying, "I don't think there is much really wrong with her. I don't think she needs to be in a hospital. She'll pull out of it on her own. But thank you for your help." Her thanks were sincerely given.

The next day the Jenkins family was back. Ms. Jenkins had been acting bizarrely throughout the night. In the waiting room the mother sat with her arm around her daughter, her eyes red from the painful recognition that her daughter was no longer the same person she had raised.

In this regard, it appears useful to remember that at some level family members will be mourning the loss of "the person they knew." As with any mourning process, various stages such as denial, anger, mourning, depression, and acceptance will intermingle and be entered at different times. The Jenkins family highlights a common problem facing the initial interviewer, the presence of a powerful system of denial among family members. By understanding the mourning of family members, it may help decrease the angry countertransference feelings arising from their rejection of the clinician's help.

From the above discussion, it can be seen that in few cases does the initial interview with a psychotic patient end with the patient. At some early point, the family warrants an assessment as well as a chance for later counseling. Keep in mind that some family members may become seriously depressed and perhaps even suicidal. Psychosis is indeed a family affair.

The tensions of the family may at some level precipitate or aggravate the psychotic process itself. Research such as the EPICS (Environmental/Personal Indicators in the Course of Schizophrenia) Project has shown that families in which members are overly involved or antagonistic to the patient may hinder recovery even when the patient complies with medication use. Family counseling seemed to significantly decrease relapse rates. This emphasizes the importance of assessing the family and beginning an alliance with them. Frequently, the initial interviewer is the first person to meet the family and consequently represents a key person in the attempts to build the much needed alliance described above.

Not only is the family affected, but other important social networks may begin to collapse around the patient. Jobs may be lost and friendships tattered. It is difficult to remain friends with a person who has developed a severe psychotic process. Frequently, both friends and family members may be dealing with feelings of guilt. A simple phrase said early during an interview may be comforting such as, "I just finished talking with your friend, who seems very disturbed. I bet you've gone through a lot recently. It was nice of you to come with him today." As with the patient, engagement issues remain critical during the opening phases of collateral interviews.

With depressed patients we had talked about the importance of understanding the patient's subculture. This is equally true with psychotic patients. Here, though, we encounter a new and somewhat disturbing twist, for patients with chronic psychotic processes such as schizophrenia frequently become a new subculture. As these patients lose their friends, spend long stays in hospitals, and wear out their welcome with relatives, they end up spending progressively more time with each other.

In essence these patients form a social caste of sorts. Even as clinicians, most of us, when speaking honestly, would admit to doubts about hiring these patients or choosing them as new friends. These people frequently become outcasts from the mainstream of the society. It is important for the initial interviewer to understand these dynamics, for they may appear as a veiled hostility from the patient. And sometimes this animosity is not so veiled.

Each subculture composed of chronic patients may affect the views of the patient towards treatment itself. It is useful for the clinician to learn about these biases. For example, the local patients may develop prejudicial views on certain medications. If all the friends of the patient hate the drug Thorazine(chlorpromazine hydrochloride), it does not make a lot of sense to send the patient out on Thorazine, when a different neuroleptic may be just as effective, but not blackballed by the subculture.

V: THE FRAMEWORK FOR MEANING

In the arms of a psychosis the problem is not so much a world that is meaningless but rather a world that is too meaningful. As the patient copes with a suffocating mixture of bizarre and unscreened sensory experiences, the world is gradually transformed into a desert filled with burning bushes. The patient finds little rest from the intensity of the delusional world, and this intensity creates the driven quality so characteristic of psychotic process.

One of the saddest aspects of psychotic process remains the irony that it can make a patient so religiously preoccupied that religion is no longer a practical support system. Instead of providing a calm guidance, relgious issues become disturbing. This type of overzealous religious ideation is frequently seen with schizophrenia.

In this regard, the clinician should not be afraid to hear about the patient's religious beliefs. These areas can provide avenues for entrance into psychotic process, as mentioned earlier, and more importantly, may help us to understand the patient's world view. By listening attentively and nonjudgmentally, the blending process may also be facilitated. If for some reason this type of discussion seems to be agitating the patient, then the clinician can skillfully guide the conversation to other topics.

Psychotic religious preoccupation may represent an intensified effort to replace previous areas that had provided a sense of meaning to the patient. For instance, the patient's family ties may have become critically weakened, thus depriving the patient of a powerful framework for meaning. In some unfortunate instances, patients may actually come to view themselves as burdens upon their families. In such situations, one can easily see why a grandiose religious delusion may serve as a source of much needed solace. It could represent a very real resurrection of sorts, a resurrection of the patient's self-esteem.

This process brings to light a curious aspect of the psychotic patient's search for a framework for meaning. With some patients the psychotic delusions literally become the focal points of their lives. When these delusions disappear, so can the meaning behind life.

In this regard I worked briefly with a young man suffering from schizophrenia, who believed he could broadcast his thoughts. As he phrased it, "I'm the best there is. Nobody can send their thoughts faster or further than I." As he came out of his psychosis, his delusion began to fade. One day as we talked by his bedside he turned to me saying, "I've come to realize that I can't really send my thoughts out like I told you I could. And you know what I also just realized, I realized that I'm just not a very special kind of person." At which point, he began to cry. I have since discovered that several years later he shot himself to death.

I raise these issues, because the initial interviewer will undoubtedly be working with patients in various stages of belief and disbelief of their delusions. It is useful to attempt to understand the significance of these beliefs to the patient at the time of their presentation.

Even if the patient's psychosis is being caused by primarily biological dysfunction, the fact remains that the content of the delusions are directly related to the patient's psychological constitution, including the patient's upbringing, memories, values, and beliefs. In that sense, one may find important clues to underlying fears and issues in these seemingly illogical fantasies.

In closing, the reader will recall that we began this chapter with the writings of Gerard De Nerval, who would eventually take his own life. Who knows what the voices were saying to him or in what personal hell he found himself. What we do have are his words. As we reread them, perhaps from the understanding gained from this chapter, we will hear them with a new respect for both their brilliance and their sadness:

I seemed to myself a hero living under the very eyes of the gods; everything in nature assumed new aspects, and secret voices came to me from the plants, the trees, animals, the meanest insects, to warn and to encourage me. The words of my companions had mysterious messages, the sense of which I alone understood.

References

1. Hammacher, A. M.: *Phantoms of the Imagination.* New York, Harry N. Abrams, Publisher, Inc., 1981, pp. 136–138.
2. Symons, Arthur: Essay on Gerard de Nerval. In *The Symbolist Movement in Literature.* New York , E.P. Dutton and Co., 1985, pp. 14–17.
3. American Psychiatric Association: Diagnostic and Statistical Manual of Mental Disorders. Third edition, revised. Washington D.C., APA, 1987, pp. 194–195.
4. Fish, F.: *Clinical Psychopathology.* Bristol, Britain, John Wright and Sons Ltd., 1967, pp. 19–26.
5. Roberts, J. K.: *Differential Diagnosis in Neuropsychiatry.* New York, John Wiley and Sons, 1984, p. 263.
6. Asaad, G., and Shapiro, B.: Hallucinations: Theoretical and clinical overview. *American Journal of Psychiatry* 143:1088–1097, 1986.
7. West, L. J.: A clinical and theoretical overview of hallucinatory pheomena. In *Hallucinations: Behavior, Experience, and Theory,* edited by R. K. Siegel and L. J. West. New York, John Wiley and Sons, 1975, p. 308.
8. Lehman, H. E., and Canero, R.: Schizophrenia: Clinical features. In *Comprehensive Textbook of Psychiatry IV,* edited by H. I. Kaplan and B. J. Sadock. Fourth edition. Baltimore, Williams and Wilkins, 1985, p. 683.
9. West, L. J., 1975, p. 308.
10. Roberts, J. K., 1984, p. 262.
11. Sellers, E. M., and Kalant, H.: Alcohol intoxication and withdrawal. *The New England Journal of Medicine* 294:757–760, 1976.
12. Sellers, E. M., 1976, p. 758.
13. Hackett, T. P.: Alcoholism: Acute and chronic. In *Massachusetts General Hospital Handbook of General Hospital Psychiatry,* edited by T. P. Hackett and N. H. Cassem, St. Louis, The C. V. Mosby Company, 1978, p. 19.
14. Hackett, T. P., 1978, p. 20.
15. Goldfrank, L. R., Lewin, N. A., and Osborn, H.: Dusted (PCP). *Hospital Physician,* May 1982, pp. 62–67.
16. Lydiard, R. B., and Gelenberg, A. J.: Treating substance abuse, Part I. *Drug Therapy,* April 1982, pp. 57–66.
17. Goldfrank, L. R., 1982, p. 65.
18. Goodman, L. S., and Gilman, A.: *The Pharmacological Basis of Therapeutics.* New York, Macmillan Publishing Co., Inc., 1975, pp. 514–532.
19. Guze, S. B.: Schizoaffective disorders, In *Comprehensive Textbook of Psychiatry IV,* edited by H. I. Kaplan and B. J. Sadock. Fourth edition. Baltimore, Williams and Wilkins, 1985, p. 657.
20. Lehman, H. E., 1985, p. 690.
21. Haier, R. J.: The diagnosis of schizophrenia: A review of recent development. *Schizophrenia Bulletin* 6(3):417–427,1980.
22. Guze, S. G., 1985, p. 757.
23. DSM-III-R, 1987, pp. 208–209.
24. Tsuang, Ming T.: Schizoaffective disorder. *Archives of General Psychiatry* 36:633–634, 1979.
25. Guze, S. B., 1985, pp. 756–759.
26. DSM-III-R, 1987, p. 202.
27. Walker, J. I., and Brodie, H. K.: Paranoid disorders. In *Comprehensive Textbook of Psychiatry,* edited by H. I. Kaplan and B. J. Sadock. Fourth edition. Baltimore, Williams and Wilkins, 747-755, 1985.

28. Walker, J. I., 1985, p. 75.
29. Bannister, Sir Roger: *Brain's Clinical Neurology.* New York, Oxford University Press, 1978, p. 197.
30. Walker, J. I., 1985, p. 751.
31. Raskind, M.: Paranoid syndromes in the elderly. In *Treatment of Psychopathology in the Aging,* edited by C. Eisdorfer and W. E. Fann. New York, Springer Publishing Company, 1982, pp. 184–191.
32. Bridge, T. P., and Wyatt, R. J.: Paraphrenia: Paranoid states of late life: European research. *American Geriatrics Society* 28(5):193–200, 1980.
33. Lopez-Ibor, J.: Delusional perception and delusional mood: A phenomenological and existential analysis. In *Phenomenology and Psychiatry,* edited by A. J. J. Koning and F. A. Jenner. New York, Grune and Stratton, 1982.
34. Bowers, M. B.: *Retreat from Sanity: The Structure of Emerging Psychosis.* Baltimore, Penguin Books, 1974.
35. McDonald, N.: Living with Schizophrenia. *Canadian Medical Association Journal* 82:218–221, 1960.
36. DSM-III-R, 1987, p. 103
37. Roberts, J. K.: *Differential Diagnosis in Neuropsychiatry.* New York, John Wiley and Sons, 1984, p. 158.
38. Murray, G. B.: Confusion, delirium, and dementia. In *Massachusetts General Hospital Handbook of General Psychiatry,* edited by T. P. Hackett and N. H. Cassem. St. Louis, C. V. Mosby Company, 1978, p. 98.
39. Roberts, J. K., 1984, p. 164.
40. Murray, G. B., 1978, p. 96.
41. Murray, G. B., 1978, p. 93–116
42. Roberts, J. K., 1984, pp. 161–164.
43. Barsky, A.: Acute psychoses. In *Emergency Psychiatry: Concepts, Methods, and Practices,* edited by E. F. Bassuk and A. W. Beck. New York, Plenum Press, 195–218, 1984.
44. Barsky, A., 1984, pp. 195–218.
45. Bear, D., Freeman, R., Schiff, B. A., and Greenberg, M.: Interictal behavorial changes in patients with temporal lobe epilepsy. In *APA Annual Review,* vol. 14, edited by R.E. Hales and A.J. Frances. Washington, D.C., APA, 1985, pp. 190–210.
46. Roberts, J. K. A., 1984, p. 239.
47. Hedges, L. E.: *Listening Perspectives in Psychotherapy.* New York, Jason Aronson, 1983, pp. 239–243.
48. Mendel, W. M.: A phenomenological theory of schizophrenia. In *Schizophrenia as a Lifestyle,* edited by A. Burton, J. J. Lopez-Ibor, and W. M. Mendel. New York, Springer Publishers, 1974, pp. 106–155.
49. Lopez-Ibor, J., 1982, pp. 135–152.
50. Landis, C., and Mettler, F. A.: *Varieties of Psychopathological Experience.* New York, Holt, Rinehart and Winston, 1964.
51. Fish, F., 1967, p. 16.
52. Asaad, G., 1986, p. 1091.
53. West, F. J., 1975, p. 307.
54. Landis, C., and Mettler, F. A., 1964.
55. McGhie, A., and Chapman, J.: Disorders of attention and perception in early schizophrenia. *British Journal of Medical Psychology* 34:103–117, 1961.
56. McGhie, A., and Chapman J., 1961, pp.103–117.
57. Rosenbaum, P.: *The Meaning of Madness.* New York, Science House, 1970, pp. 73–99.
58. Lehman, H. E., and Cancro, R.: Schizophrenia: Clinical features. In *Comprehensive Textbook of Psychiatry IV,* edited by H. Kaplan and B. Sadock. Baltimore, Williams and Wilkins, 680–713, 1985.
59. Lehman, H. E., and Cancro, R., 1985, p. 704.
60. MacKinnon, R., and Michels, R. P.: *The Psychiatric Interview in Clinical Practice.* Philadelphia, W. B. Saunders Co., 1971, p. 236.
61. MacKinnon, R., and Michels, R., 1971, p. 235.
62. Hogarty, G. E., Anderson, C., Reiss, D., Kornblith, S., Greenwald, D., Javna, C. and Madonia, M. Family education, social skills training, and maintenance chemotherapy in the aftercare treatment of schizophrenia. *Archives of General Psychiatry* 43:633–642, 1986.

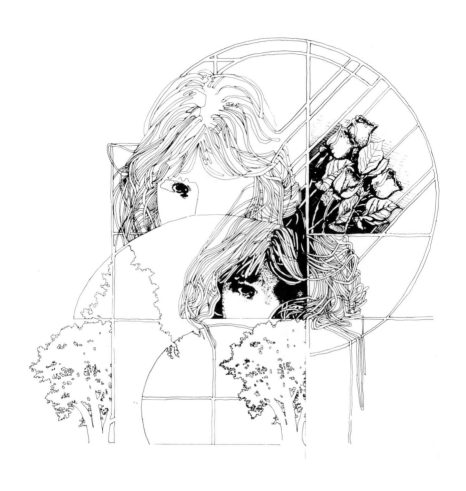

7

Personality Disorders: Reflections of the Social History

> The passionate hand is fleshy, resisting, hard, sometimes dry, always strong. The fingers are thick and rather short. . . . The passionate character is believing, powerful, active, inspired. It proceeds by a feeling for things and produced by a natural abundance. Capacity for work. Keen, enthusiastic, absorbed worker.
>
> *Anonymous, The Encyclopedia of Occult Sciences*

As the above quotation illustrates, for ages humans have enthusiastically attempted to classify each other. Such behavior seems to represent a trademark of the species, for better or worse. In previous centuries chirologists attempted to determine the currents of personality in the physical characteristics of the hand. Today, such viewpoints have been appropriately relegated to the niche of the historically curious, an intellectual antique of sorts.

But personality theory remains as intriguing today as it did for the chirologists of the eighteenth century. In a sense, tremendous advances have been made in understanding both the normal and abnormal aspects of personality development. On the other hand, much remains to be learned. To be successful in the art of personality assessment, it is important to understand the limitations of current conceptualizations. It is also of value to arrive at an understanding of some of the controversies surrounding the various personality disorders, for probably more controversy is associated with this collection of disorders than with Axis I disorders. If these complicating factors are not understood by the clinician, they can seriously hamper the clinician's ability to utilize these diagnostic categories effectively in a fashion that may guide the clinician towards better methods of care.

Coupled with the fact that there are eleven specific personality disorders in the DSM-III-R, the above points suggest a slightly differ-

341

ent approach than has been taken in the previous two chapters. Rather than attempt the exhaustive task of representing each diagnosis by a separate case presentation, smaller case illustrations will be liberally used to delineate diagnostic principles that may be generalizable to any personality disorder. The emphasis will remain on practical clinical points, utilizing both case histories and clinical dialogues. The task will consist of interweaving the controversies and subtleties surrounding these diagnoses into an understanding of the people beneath these labels.

To achieve this complex goal, the chapter will be divided into two sections. In Section I, Clinical Principles Concerning Character Psychopathology, the needed theoretical background is examined in detail, including basic definitions, a survey of the diagnoses, and discussions of various controversial issues regarding personality disorders. In Section II, The Approach to the Interview, the effective utilization of this background in clinically problematic areas is directly addressed in a comprehensive fashion. Without further introduction, let us begin an exploration of an area of psychopathology that some would say represents the most enigmatic field of study that clinicians encounter on a daily basis.

SECTION I: CLINICAL PRINCIPLES CONCERNING CHARACTER PSYCHOPATHOLOGY

In Search of a Definition

To begin the discussion it is useful to look at an actual clinical presentation. We will refer to the patient as Mr. Fellows and begin by examining his history, which will then be complemented by a recreation of a brief bit of dialogue from the initial interview.

Mr. Fellows was referred for outpatient psychotherapy. He had originally been seen in the emergency room with a subsequent referral for possible group therapy. After attending two group sessions he left because "the therapist spent too much time listening to all those screwball people. And he was also an inexperienced therapist, that's for sure. I just didn't like him."

Mr. Fellows presented in a dirty plaid shirt and an unkempt army jacket. He was short in stature with a balding head from which his black hair emerged. His hair had clearly met a comb, but the meeting had not been for long. He quickly conveyed a feeling that he did not really want to be in the room. His handshake had been overly firm and then suddenly weak, as if purposely avoiding prolonged contact. He had worn a jaunty cap, which was a little worse for wear and had now found itself in his lap, a plaything for his fidgeting hands.

With regard to his history he had come from a tough neighborhood, and he had seldom felt at home there. "I didn't belong there, I'm a sensitive guy, and I felt things those other kids could never feel. But I beat it." He related having a very high IQ, and he indeed appeared quite knowledgeable and well read. But he had always encountered intermittent problems in school. He had frequently been involved in arguments with teachers and tended to be a loner. He had had no problems with the law and seemed strongly opposed to violence and criminal activity. Drugs were viewed as bad things, yet he hesitantly admitted to drinking problems in the past.

He had never liked his father, who viewed him as a complete failure and had beaten him in the past. Over the years he had lost contact with most of his family and was generally not welcome in their homes. He viewed himself as talented, especially with regards to writing. Indeed, he had been working on a novel for years. He also boasted of his tendency to protect others from violence and carried a small canister of tear gas repellant with him.

Despite his abhorrence of violence, he reported a life-long history of "finding the nearest argument." Apparently he often tended to dominate conversations because "in all honesty I'm smarter than most of the people I meet." In short he had developed the rather nifty habit of alienating people almost upon first contact. He was true to his style during our first session. The following dialogue occurred during the early phases of the body of the interview:

> **Pt.:** That last therapist was a real loser. And I really don't see much sense in group therapy anyway. In fact if I really look at this realistically, I don't really need any help at this time.
>
> **Clin.:** With that idea in mind what were some of your reasons for coming in for an evaluation today? Apparently you had been referred for outpatient psychotherapy.
>
> **Pt.:** In the first place I don't really like psychotherapists. I don't think you guys really know what you're doing any way. I mean I had seen a therapist off and on for six or seven years, he was O.K. but he charged more than he was worth. What you need to do for me today is to write a note saying that for medical reasons I need to live in a new halfway house. The one I'm at is situated in too dangerous a neighborhood. And that's all I need or want from you.

Mr. Fellows was clearly not meant for public relations work. At least he quickly got to his point. In the next session, when he was reminded that further evaluation was needed before I would consider his request, he became actively hostile commenting, "You don't give a damn do you, Doctor! For all you care, I could be mugged tomorrow, and it would be no sweat off your back. I hope someday you're being murdered and when you call the police, they say further inquiry will be necessary before we respond to your call!"

With regard to diagnosis, Mr. Fellows was eventually given the primary diagnosis of a narcissistic personality disorder. He also displayed antisocial, borderline, and paranoid traits. Indeed a rule-out secondary diagnosis was a mixed personality disorder consisting of those three traits. On Axis I he continued to demonstrate alcohol abuse intermittently, although he had not been drinking for several months.

Subsequent therapy revealed that throughout his life Mr. Fellows had suffered from an intense feeling of vulnerability. The question, "Am I really worth loving?" was a rather constant companion, a shadow, from which he could not step away, no matter how hard he tried to inflate his self-esteem. He developed a series of defenses to protect himself from his pain, including a sense of entitlement, a tendency to put others down, fantasies and preoccupations with grandiosity, and a coolness in interpersonal contacts. This coolness could serve to protect him from the danger of imminent rejection, a rejection that had first surfaced in the form of abuse from his father.

And now we are beginning to perceive the subtle workings of a personality disorder. In these conditions, the individual develops a series of defenses that can temporarily and in certain circumstances protect them from significant pain. Unfortunately these same defenses become rigid and small in number. The patient is left with a defensive structure that is inflexible and frequently ineffective in decreasing pain in the long run. Mr. Fellow's cool indifference and his tendency to put others down may indeed protect him from the potential pain of losing a loving figure, but it ironically will prevent him from ever developing such a relationship in the first place. But Mr. Fellows does not know how to function otherwise. There lies the tragedy of the situation. The intensity of the loneliness and self-loathing can be enormous.

This point is important for the clinician, for it serves to reframe the obnoxious and irritating behaviors of the various personality disorders in the light of a response to their pain and anxiety. Such a realization can help to decrease angry countertransference feelings, while serving to increase a sense of compassion. For instance, the same Mr. Fellows, who was so patently rude and demanding in these initial sessions, would later cry during the termination phase of his psychotherapy.

The story of Mr. Fellows also highlights another, sometimes easily missed, point. The key to understanding adult psychopathology lies in an understanding of childhood and adolescent development. An adult psychiatrist cannot work in an intellectual vacuum, as if adult patients spontaneously appeared at age eighteen. Many critical therapeutic interactions parallel parent-child behaviors and feelings. Indeed these patients can quickly arouse parental responses in the clinician even during the initial interview. If unaware of these responses, initial interviewers can inadvertently disrupt blending.

With these ideas in mind let us look at the definition of a character disorder as viewed in the DSM-III-R:

> The manifestations of Personality Disorders are often recognizable by adolescence or earlier and continue throughout most of adult life, though they often become less obvious in middle or old age.
>
> The diagnostic criteria for the Personality Disorders refer to behaviors or traits that are characteristic of the person's recent (past year) and long-term functioning since early adulthood. The constellation of behaviors or traits causes either significant impairment in social or occupational functioning or subjective distress.[1]

Several key points are beginning to emerge. In the first place, a personality disorder (or character disorder as it is sometimes described) is a historical diagnosis. The critical criteria for making the diagnosis lie in the patient's history not in the patient's behavior in the interview itself. The patient's immediate behavior in the interview often provides important clues to underlying psychopathology, but the criteria for establishing the diagnosis lie in historical evidence. In a sense, a personality disorder leaves historical tracks.

The nature of these tracks varies significantly, but one of two elements will be present. Either the patient's rigid defenses result in behaviors, which are disturbing to other people, or to feelings, which are unsettling to the patient. By way of illustration a person with an antisocial personality may steal the life savings of an employer who trusted the patient implicitly. The patient may have no regrets about such actions, but clearly the patient's behavior will have had a disastrous effect on the employer. Such behaviors are called ego-syntonic, for they do not disturb the patient. At the other extreme, a person with an avoidant personality may shun almost all social contact, while living in a self-imposed interpersonal tomb. This behavior may not really harm anyone else per se but results in significant personal distress. These types of behaviors are referred to as ego-dystonic, for they directly create subjective pain in the patient.

Many patients show a combination of ego-dystonic and ego-syntonic symptoms. But in patients who display primarily ego-syntonic behaviors, an important point surfaces. These patients frequently are not strongly invested in receiving help, for their behaviors are not disturbing to them. Family members, lawyers, or administrators may have pushed such patients into therapy; consequently these patients may be unusually difficult to engage in therapy. For the interviewer, functioning as a consultant, the presence of primarily ego-syntonic behaviors may suggest the recommendation that an experienced staff member be assigned to the case as opposed to a trainee.

But whether ego-syntonic or ego-dystonic, the behavioral manifestations of a personality disorder tend to result in specific types of interpersonal patterns, including parental relations, sibling relations, dating relations, employment patterns, and friendship patterns. In this fashion, the historical tracks of a disordered personality are usually found in the soft ground known as the social history.

The social history is not merely a sterile recording of "what job was held when" but represents an extremely sensitive mirror in which the reflections of a personality disorder may first appear to the alert clinician. Stated even more boldly, a totally normal social history is not compatible with a personality disorder. Somewhere along the line the pathological personality traits will disrupt interpersonal relationships. Later in this chapter various methods of effectively gathering the social history in this light will be described.

In uncovering personality disturbances the clinician must actively search for consistent patterns of behavior, demonstrated from adolescence onwards, without major disruption of these patterns. In this regard, Mr. Fellows serves as an apt illustration. His defensive patterns appeared early in his life. His social history was littered with weak relationships, a poor job history, an unending string of arguments, and a maladaptive grandiosity. These behaviors were consistent over time, undeniably crystallized by the time of late adolescence.

A natural next question focuses upon the etiology of such unchanging patterns of behavior. Theoreticians could spend — and have spent — a large amount of time discussing the numerous conflicting theories regarding etiology. But a recapitulation of their work would not be time well spent in a text of this type. Instead a simplified and unifying approach will be described, which can help guide the interviewer towards a more sophisticated understanding of the person seeking the clinician's help.

The shaping of a personality structure can be viewed as a matrix of sorts, consisting of three interdependent factors: (1) physiological factors, (2) psychological factors, and (3) environmental/interpersonal factors. Together, these fluctuating influences will eventually determine the anxieties and need states that will result in the development of specific unconscious defense mechanisms and conscious coping strategies of the organism.

In the physiological realm, Thomas and Chess have emphasized the point that small infants display characteristic temperaments, which can persist into later stages of life.[2] These variables include intensity of reaction, activity level, attention span, threshold of response to stimulation, mood, and distractability. Both genetics and intrauterine factors could influence the development of such traits. One can easily see how such factors could play a significant part in the determination of personality structure.

For example, if a child was born with a propensity to be easily distracted, the child may have significant problems with learning and also with obeying rules. The child might literally have problems attending to a parent's commands. And here we see the matrix effect. For this physiologic component will both affect and be affected by the other two realms mentioned earlier. The child's seemingly intentional disobedience and poor school performance may disturb the child's parents. Frustration and anger may result, even in high-functioning parents, who may tend to show displeasure and subtle rejection of the child. Perhaps a sibling will become "the apple of Daddy's eye."

Considerably more problems will arise if the child has been born into a family already steeped in psychopathology. An alcoholic parent may beat the child, probably only resulting in a child who is further unable to concentrate and learn secondary to fear and agitation. The cycles begin to feed and regenerate each other. Marital disharmony may intensify as arguments ensue regarding the management of the bad behavior of the child. On the other hand, a child with a relatively normal attention span may be born into such a chaotic household. Soon the child may become chronically anxious, and in this sense environmental influences may actually trigger physiological changes.

In any case, the child will begin to develop psychological defenses in order to function at a reasonable level of anxiety. The theoretical child, described above, could easily become more reclusive and timid. Or the child may develop a conception of itself as inferior and unwanted. The result may be the development of distancing tactics that protect the child from rejection or the development of grandiose thinking. These tactics function to buffer the child from its feelings of worthlessness. Perhaps these were the types of factors that jointly combined to create Mr. Fellows, the theoretical child in the flesh.

No easy explanations exist. It is relatively meaningless to bicker over which element of the matrix was most instrumental, for with each individual this mixture will vary. Moreover, in most instances, the resulting personality is a reasonably healthy one. This chapter concerns itself with those instances in which an inflexible set of defenses emerge.

In the DSM-III-R, an attempt is made to characterize behavior, not to explain it. In this modest fashion the DSM-III-R may help provide more reliability in the labeling process, thus allowing research to eventually provide more clues as to etiology and hopefully improved treatment techniques. In this vein, the criteria for determining personality diagnoses in the DSM-III-R are not etiologic in nature. The DSM-III-R acknowledges the fact that any of the factors listed above may play a part in the development of character psychopathology.

To serve as an illustration, let us look at the criteria used in the diagnosis of a narcissistic personality disorder, the diagnosis used with Mr. Fellows.

Narcissistic Personality Disorder[3]

A pervasive pattern of grandiosity (in fantasy or behavior), lack of empathy, and hypersensitivity to the evaluation of others, beginning by early adulthood and present in a variety of contexts, as indicated by at least five of the following:

(1) reacts to criticism with feelings of rage, shame, or humiliation (even if not expressed)

(2) is interpersonally exploitative: takes advantage of others to achieve his or her own ends

(3) has a grandiose sense of self-importance, e.g., exaggerates achievements and talents, expects to be noticed as "special" without appropriate achievement

(4) believes that his or her problems are unique and may be understood only by other special people

(5) is preoccupied with fantasies of unlimited success, power, brilliance, beauty, or ideal love

(6) has a sense of entitlement: unreasonable expectation of especially favorable treatment, e.g., assumes that he or she does not have to wait in line when others must do so

(7) requires constant attention and admiration, e.g., keeps fishing for compliments

(8) lack of empathy: inability to recognize and experience how others feel, e.g., annoyance and surprise when a friend who is seriously ill cancels a date

(9) is preoccupied with feelings of envy

These criteria are fairly representative of the criteria used in the DSM-III-R for the delineation of personality disorders. The criteria range from those traits of a more subjective nature, such as fantasies of unlimited success, which the clinician would depend upon patient self-report to determine, to more objective criteria such as rage in response to criticism, which are more behavioral in nature and could be reported by friends or family. Of special interest is what is not here. Specifically, the DSM-III-R purposely avoids criteria that would be tied to a specific etiologic theory.

For example, one does not find criteria such as "the patient has not adaptively integrated his grandiose imago with his idealizing imago." This particular criterion would represent one of several psychoanalytic models, in this instance the work of Heinz Kohut. It can be seen that the inclusion of such etiologic criteria could lead to many problems, including clinician bias away from diagnoses because of a disagreement on theoretical grounds, clinician ignorance of the meaning of specific terminology, and the need for clinicians to "read into" the facts in order to recognize a diagnostic criteria. All of these factors could lead to disturbingly poor inter-rater reliability, a flaw that essentially prohibits productive research. In this attempt to produce more reliable criteria, the DSM-III and its revision represent an important advance.

As with most advances, there are some accompanying limitations, and the DSM-III-R system is no exception. As clinicians it is important to remember that these diagnostic labels do not necessarily shed significant illumination on the person behind the label. This is the penalty one pays for not basing the diagnoses on dynamic formulations. It also emphasizes the fact that these diagnostic labels serve a valuable function only when the clinician understands their development and limitations. They do provide a foundation for predicting treatment selection and a powerful method of learning from the writings of previous clinicians who are using the same criteria. But they do not explain the person sitting in front of us. The DSM-III-R has never purported that diagnoses should be used as explanations. Instead they serve as useful maps, suggesting possible avenues of exploration, as the clinician attempts to understand the reasons that this particular patient has developed these particular behaviors.

In order to use these diagnoses intelligently, another ramification of their development deserves attention. Some of these diagnoses, such as the antisocial personality, are based upon extensive empirical research and historical validity. Other categories, such as the narcissistic personality, have little empirical research behind them. Indeed, some authors feel that this lack of empiricism may result in the inclusion of diagnoses that will not survive the "test of time"; in short, they may lack validity.[4]

But let us see how all this controversy can affect the clinician directly. The narcissistic personality serves as a good example. A significant problem consists of the fact that in attempting to read about a specific diagnosis, various authors may be describing strikingly different types of people, while applying the same diagnosis. For example, the criteria for the narcissistic personality tend to follow the conceptualizations of Theodore Millon. The emphasis is upon a person who tends to exude a sense of overconfidence and superiority. As long as the patient's abilities parallel the existing expectations, these people may be reasonably happy and certainly may function at a high level of achievement. The personality structure is supposed to develop from a parenting pattern of overattention and favoritism. This is the classic "spoiled child," who can be so frustratingly pompous and demanding as an adult.

In contrast to this relatively well-functioning individual, albeit a rigidly structured personality, the DSM-III-R criteria could also be met by a person with a remarkably different history and psychological structure. Kohut and his colleagues have elegantly described this type of personality. These people also appear grandiose and demanding, but these defenses are the result of poor self-esteem. The world is seen as hostile and threatening, a place teeming with rejection and competition. Their poorly evolved sense of self results in marked periods of depressed mood, even in relatively benign environments. Anger and resentment are daily personality accessories. Mr. Fellows is an excellent example of such a person. These people are strikingly more disturbed than narcissists described by Millon, and yet both types of people could conceivably fulfill the criteria of the DSM-III-R for a narcissistic personality. This overlap suggests a diagnostic category whose criteria are too broad to ensure appropriate discrimination.

We have reached a point in which our search for a definition has begun to wind down. An attempt has been made to demonstrate that to intelligently utilize the diagnoses subsumed under the category of personality disorders one must understand the development and limitations of the system. The case of Mr. Fellows has served to illustrate some of the complexities inherent in the system. In retrospect one could say that just as a species must evolve, each individual personality must also undergo a gradual evolution. This development can be affected by the elegant interplay of various factors, including physiology, environment, and psychology. When such evolution is disrupted, maladaptive behavior patterns emerge, which have been described as personality disorders. To understand the pain of these patients, the clinician must move beyond the label into a study of the patient's personal development. In this idiosyncratic history, the interviewer will find the constellation of factors that have spawned the aberrant behavior, essentially trapping the individual in a prison defined by the unyielding walls of his or her own personality structure. At this point it may be of value to take a closer look at these puzzling disorders as they actually present to the clinician.

Survey of DSM-III-R Personality Disorders

One cannot begin a discussion of these disorders without touching upon the unifying concept of Axis II itself. In DSM-I and DSM-II a multiaxial approach was not taken. This unidimensional scheme of conceptualization ran the risk of leading unwary clinicians into simplistic formulations. One of the great advances of the DSM-III was the introduction of a diagnostic formulation that essentially forced clinicians to view the patient as an integrated whole not just a "case study." On these five axes the clinician was to explore not only evidence of hard-core psychiatric illnesses such as schizophrenia, but would also consider the patient's personality structure, the physiological factors, the immediate stressors, and the abilities of the patient to function adaptively.

Axis II was created in an effort to emphasize the importance of assessing the patient's character structure in all instances. In certain individuals, it was felt that disorders of personality could be primarily responsible for psychiatric dysfunction, without an accompanying Axis I diagnosis. Even in the presence of Axis I psychopathology, such as a bipolar disorder or an anxiety disorder, it was felt that the underlying character structure could significantly affect the manner in which the Axis I disorder would manifest itself. For instance, the development of a bipolar disorder, at age twenty-five in a person with an underlying borderline personality, may present a strikingly more complicated picture than a bipolar disorder in an otherwise high-functioning individual. Questions also began to arise as to whether certain personality disorders might predispose individuals to develop specific Axis I diagnoses.

Brief mention should be made of the fact that Axis II also serves as the region in which the clinician notes specific delays in the cognitive functioning of the patient. These so-called developmental delays include entities such as the developmental reading disorder, the developmental language disorder and more serious problems such as autism and mental retardation. Once again the inclusion of these disorders on a separate axis was intended to push clinicians to view the patient in the context of a developmental history as opposed to a "case to whom one simply feeds medications." In this sense the DSM-III heralded a significant and important attitudinal change in clinical conceptualization. Most clinicians conceptualized patients within a sophisticated developmental context, but the DSM-III has now made this type of conceptualization a standard for all clinicians.

DSM-III also advocated an extremely flexible system of nomenclature, which has been further developed in the DSM-III-R. If the patient fulfilled the criteria for more than one personality disorder, then each disorder should be listed separately. A separate category was created for those individuals who did not fulfill the criteria for any specific disorder but demonstrated a personality disorder that seemed to be created from bits and pieces of different disorders. These patients are to be listed as a personality disorder not otherwise specified (mixed personality disorder) with the specific traits listed. It should be noted that this diagnosis is only for patients who do not fulfill the criteria of any of the already described personality disorders. A common mistake would be exemplified by taking a patient who fulfills the criteria for both an antisocial personality and a histrionic personality and labeling him as a mixed personality. Instead, such a patient should have both diagnoses listed separately, as mentioned above.

The DSM-III-R demonstrates ultimate flexibility by also allowing the clinician to essentially use diagnostic labels not even delineated in the DSM-III-R itself. For example a clinician may find a utility in the diagnosis of an inadequate personality, which is not listed in the DSM-III-R. The clinician could utilize this diagnosis by writing personality disorder not otherwise specified (inadequate personality). Theoretically one could even coin new personality disorders under this heading. In this regard several potentially new personality disorders, the self-defeating personality and the sadistic personality, have been included in the appendix of the DSM-III-R.

But perhaps the most telling advance in flexibility generated by the DSM-III and its revision is the concept of personality traits, which should also be listed on Axis II. By a personality trait, the DSM-III is recognizing that all people develop healthy coping mechanisms similar to those seen in the personality disorders. These healthy mechanisms are flexible and diverse. For instance one could not become a sound physician if one did not possess a healthy dose of compulsive traits. Otherwise, nasty things like sponges are left in patient's abdomens during surgery. The enduring qualities of a powerful marriage are related to the abilities of both spouses to display healthy dependent and trusting characteristics, as well as being appropriately narcissistic to convey expectations and needs to the partner. Each individual's personality may be highlighted by one or more of these traits. The DSM-III-R suggests that these healthy characteristics should be noted. For further clarification, let us look as the distinction between trait and disorder as worded in the DSM-IIIR:

> Personality traits are enduring patterns of perceiving, relating to, and thinking about the environment and oneself, and

are exhibited in a wide range of important social and personal contexts. It is only when personality traits are inflexible and maladaptive and cause either significant functional impairment or subjective distress that they constitutue Personality Disorders.[5]

The concept of emphasizing personality traits introduces the idea that the clinician should also be searching for evidence of mental health as well as mental illness. In a similar attempt to provide a more realistic picture of the patient, the DSM-III-R also suggests the listing of defense mechanisms (such as denial, isolation, and repression) on Axis II. All in all, it can be seen that the development of Axis II, despite some of its problematic issues, represents many important innovations in clinical emphasis, which many would say were long overdue.

With the above ideas in mind, we can begin our survey of the diagnostic entities themselves. It is crucial that the clinician become thoroughly familiar with the actual criteria, for the diagnoses are made by a careful expansion of these diagnostic regions. On the other hand, the criteria are somewhat sterile sounding in nature. One of the first steps in gaining a proficiency is the development of a general sense of what the core characteristics of each disorder actually look like. The clinician must gain a sense of these disorders not as checklists but as living individuals. In the following survey an effort will be made to provide some flesh to the individual disorders, while pointing out some of the distinguishing characteristics between similar disorders. The reader should supplement the descriptions below by a parallel reading of the actual DSM-III-R criteria.

To aid in the familiarization process, the 11 specific personality disorders recognized by the DSM-III-R will be clustered into three broad groups. These groups contain disorders that have some similar core characteristics with regard to how the patient experiences life. If during the course of the initial interview, the clinician recognizes these more pervasive world views, then an immediate cluster of diagnostic regions for more extensive expansion suggests themselves. Each clinician can determine his or her own ways of organizing the personality disorders. The following system merely represents a method that I have found practical. In any sense, the three broad categorizations are as follows: (1) anxiety prone disorders, (2) poorly empathic disorders, and (3) psychotic prone disorders (referring to a more frequent tendency to develop micropsychotic episodes as described in the previous chapter). It should be noted that the DSM-III-R clumps the diagnoses in a slightly different fashion using broad categories related to oddness of behavior, dramatic behavior, and anxious or fearful behavior.

ANXIETY PRONE DISORDERS

This cluster includes the following four disorders: compulsive personality, passive-aggressive personality, dependent personality, and the avoidant personality. All four of these disorders share the common thread of an existence riddled with tension and anxiety. They differ in how this anxiety manifests itself and with which methods it is controlled. This is not to say that other personality disorders do not become anxious, for they can. Instead it merely suggests that anxiety is often a keynote feature of these four disorders. These patients are also prone to intermittent bouts of depression, which may occur when their needs are not met or their defenses are not adequate.

The Obsessive Compulsive Personality

The obsessive-compulsive personality sees life from the inside of a pressure cooker. It is a pressure cooker constructed from the patient's own set of perfectionistic goals and demands. In short, these patients are hard on themselves. Driven by an internal sense that any failure is an ultimate failure, they help to form the army of workaholics, who both love and resent their work. In a sad sense, these people frequently function under a covert belief system that they must prove themselves worthy of being loved. Thus there is no time for fun, and they often appear too serious for their own good, while presenting a somewhat cool and distant exterior. Deep inside there seems to be a fear that they are about to lose control. Consequently life becomes a series of contests, that are won through discipline and endless lists and work schedules. Patients with an obsessive compulsive personality truly show their colors when they produce an innately paradoxical "schedule for play." Even free time is a commodity to be well-spent. Moreover, major decisions rapidly become major hurdles, for the patient becomes terrified of the chance of making a wrong decision. Life is viewed as a long corridor of one-way doors, few of which lead to "success." It is a costly lifestyle, filled with stress. It is a way of life in which tears may not be shown but are felt nevertheless.

The Passive-Aggressive Personality

Like the compulsive personality, the passive-aggressive personality plays hide-and-seek with a hostile world. But the goal is not to prevent the loss of control, for control has already been lost. To these patients life appears to be inconsistent. There is no guarantee that anyone will ever really care, and rejection and punishment become expected nightmares. And like a person suffering from nightmares, they metaphorically do not know whether to enter sleep or not. Consequently they sometimes give of themselves in relationships and at other times hold back. Their tremendous anxiety often finds its roots in this perplexing sense of ambivalence.

To protect themselves from failure and reprimand, they become half-hearted and negativistic. They too see the rainbow but are quick to point out that the pot of gold is probably empty. If a new plan is suggested, they produce a surprisingly astute list of reasons why it will fail. This negativism can disrupt their coworkers and, ironically, bring on the world of rejection, which they knew was always there. Because they fear open rejection, while harboring an intense bitterness, they attack by passive means. They have perfected the art of dawdling, lateness, intentional ineffectiveness, and carrying out the new rule so rigidly that it is bound to fail. They live on a tightrope of never feeling that they are a welcome visitor. They literally do not know what exactly to do to win love, and the result is a world lived through the eyes of someone bitterly resigned to sitting on the bench. Tragically, their dour attitude will probably assure that on the bench is where they will stay.

The Dependent Personality

As with the previous two disorders, the dependent personality views the world as a place pregnant with disaster. But the resulting anxiety is handled in a different fashion. The compulsive throttles the anxiety by fiercely attempting to control all possible situations. The passive-aggressive mutes the anxiety by saying, "I never expected much from this lousy show anyway." In contrast the dependent personality runs from the anxiety, straight into the arms of some unsuspecting surrogate parent. Life is spent hunting for this savior. White knights are not the inhabitants of fairy tales; they are the invited dinner guest. These patients are exquisitely rejection sensitive, but they are willing to risk humiliation if the reward is eventual safety. Consequently they are often warm and giving, bordering precariously on the cusp of obsequiousness. They are more than willing to bend to the needs of others; indeed they thrive on receiving the chance to prove their irreplaceable devotion. Because they view themselves as weak and ineffectual, they do not want to make decisions. Moreover their intensely low sense of self-esteem traps them into a fear that they could not make it on their own. These are people who cannot leave the wife-beater, and whose unfortunate answer to insecurity is the safety of slavery.

The Avoidant Personality

Affection and love are two conditions that people with an avoidant personality hope for desperately. Unfortunately these goals remain mere dreams, for these patients suffer from such low self-esteem, that they dare not risk making an attempt at friendship. If ever there were people who followed the credo "Any club that would accept me, I wouldn't want to belong to," it is this group of patients. Like dependent personalities, they feel inadequate, but their low self-esteem seems laced with a more brutal self-ridicule. These people literally do not generally trust themselves and essentially become socially phobic. Unlike the dependent personality, they frequently appear aloof and cool, so as to protect themselves from the rejection they feel is a future certainty. They also tend to alienate other people with self-denigrating comments such as, "You probably don't want me along, but can I come to the movies too?" Such testing comments beg for a statement of acceptance from their targets, who may quickly tire of providing reassurance. Their timid demeanor may provoke ridicule from bullies and those predisposed to cruelty. Moreover they do not search for the "white knight" of the dependent personality, for they would not even dare to address such a figure if found. It is a lonely existence. These are the patients who live in cities for years without making an effort to secure a friendship unless they feel absolutely certain that rejection will not occur. Every night is lost in the white flickering of television characters, who have no method of inflicting pain and who will reliably show up for the next date.

POORLY EMPATHIC DISORDERS

These personality disorders share a peculiar inability to empathize in the same sense, or with the same regularity, as most people. Their personal history may be littered with a trail of people who have felt betrayed and manipulated. On the other hand, the lack of empathy may be a reflection of a true lack of interest in human contact, as seen with the schizoid personality. In any case, during the initial interview, one may catch glimmers of a world in which the feelings of other people are of little worth to the patient. The manner in which this self-centered approach manifests may vary strikingly among the following four disorders comprising this group: the schizoid personality, the antisocial personality, the histrionic personality, and the narcissistic personality.

The Schizoid Personality

The schizoid personality represents the classic picture of the quiet loner. If one were to picture an animal analogue, some type of mollusk comes to mind, slow moving, limited ability to reach out, yet more than capable of living a shell-like existence, content to function as an isolated unit. There is a blandness to the world of these patients, both in their internal and external worlds. They tend to form few relationships and prefer the role of a wallflower. Emotions run neither high nor deep. Tenderness tends to be neither felt nor sought. They exhibit a relatively bland indifference to what others may think of them. Their lack of affective color may suggest the cool stamp of one looking down from the pedestal of superiority. This is seldom the case. In actuality, their "colorless" quality represents a muted palette. These people tend to lack both the need and the social skills to actively engage other people.

On the surface, they may sound somewhat like an avoidant personality. But the avoidant personality is a hotbed of anxious emotions stirred by a perpetual duel with predicted humiliation. The avoidant personality actively flees people, whereas the schizoid personality effortlessly glides through people with a minimum of contact. There is no fear of rejection, for there is no desire for acceptance.

Some mention should be made of another diagnosis with which the schizoid disorder is sometimes confused, but which, in reality, shares little resemblance, except with regard to the spelling of their names. The schizotypal personality, like the schizoid personality, may also have few friends and appear somewhat aloof and distant. But these patients are generally but not always rejection sensitive, much more like an avoidant personality. Moreover their world is seldom bland. To the contrary it is extremely active, rich with bizarre and idiosyncratic emotions and conceptualizations, a bit like a dream on feet. Moreover the schizotypal personality seems to be somehow related to schizophrenia and may later develop this Axis I diagnosis. To the contrary there appears to be no relation between the schizoid personality and schizophrenia. Indeed the schizoid personality is not generally prone to the micropsychotic episodes seen with certain other personality disorders.

The Antisocial Personality

The antisocial personality is a chameleon. At times they may appear somewhat withdrawn like the schizoid, but more frequently they appear actively involved with others. With certain people they may appear belligerent and nasty. On a different night or with a different person, they may present as the epitome of charm. The reason for the deftness in style lies primarily in the fact that these patients are participating in a continual game in which other individuals exist as pieces to be manipulated and utilized as deemed fit. As a result, antisocial personalities are frequently at odds with the law and noted for lying, cheating, drug fencing, job hopping, and paternity suits. Sex is a one-night affair, and the word "responsibility" is not listed in their dictionary. At their worst, these patients may be cruel, sadistic, and violent. It has been suggested that they seldom feel anxiety and certainly infrequently feel the anxiety born from guilt. Indeed, they live a life in which a superego seems to have never set foot in their psyche. In a surprising sense, these people frequently see their problems as arising from flaws in other people, as opposed to their own inadequacies.

Obnoxious as these patients may sound, Vaillant makes the humanizing point, that, in reality, they probably do or at least did feel pain.[6] Indeed, their amoral behaviors and world view probably are at least in part a reflection of defenses developed to deflect relatively intense pain. For instance, the apparent callousness of their relationships may in some cases represent a defense, protecting the patient from a fear of being engulfed by intense dependency needs. Ironically, people with an antisocial personality may very well be as entrapped as their victims, their distancing defenses taking them so far from human emotion that they may appear as monsters. But in the last analysis, they are all too human.

The Histrionic Personality

There are probably few personalities as pleasant as a happy histrionic personality disorder and few as miserable as an unhappy one. On this adult see-saw, these patients attempt to live life as a child, hoping to find a perch on Daddy's knee. The world is seen through the eyes of an Impressionist painter, popping an occasional hallucinogen. They do not look at details and seldom remember them. The past is a blur of impressionistic images. Whereas the compulsive personality collects the world in neat categories and cages, the histrionic gleefully unlocks all the doors. They feel little responsibility and demonstrate an unnerving sense of devil-may-care. With a forced eviction lying only days ahead, the histrionic may be focusing attention on courting a date met on last Friday night's dance floor. Somehow or another a new apartment is supposed to materialize.

There is no doubt that life is exciting for them, for they view themselves as if their life were part of a movie. They tend to demand center stage, and if lucky enough to be good-looking and/or talented, they may well end up center stage. Their life is a long string of over-reactions, tantrums, and lost loves. Beneath the dramatics is a painfully fragile self-esteem that is easily crushed. Behind the glamour, intense feeling of inferiority and neediness hide. They are powerfully dependent upon the applause of others for their own sense of self-worth. Keenly sensitive to rejection, they are constantly searching for reassurance and praise. People are manipulated to achieve these needs, and the histrionic personality can little afford to empathize with the needs of those who may lie in his or her way. Suicidal gestures are not uncommon, but may be followed several days later by a bright smile, if "Mr. or Mrs. Right" has entered the picture. This ability to change moods rapidly, depending upon environmental circumstances, is a hallmark feature. Like a child throwing a tantrum, one needs only to distract the histrionic in order to make things better. Somehow, there is tragedy in all this glamour. Adults were not made to live as children.

The Narcissistic Personality Disorder

As mentioned earlier, this category seems to house two rather distinctive types, which, for want of a better title, can be referred to as the stable and unstable variants. In the stable variant, the patient's narcissism appears to be well rooted. These patients actually view themselves as superior and frequently enjoy their own company. In contrast to this picture, with the unstable variant, the narcissism appears more as a defensive front, a pseudonarcissism of a sort. With these patients the grandiosity is more of a charade, hiding an intensely frightened ego.

Let us look at the stable narcissistic personality first. To these patients, other people exist as objects, whose reason to be is to comfort the patient. Other people are objects made to serve the "self" of the patient. This tendency, seen in both stable and unstable narcissistic personality disorders, has been referred to as conceptualizing the world through "self-objects." The narcissist finds it difficult to view others as having needs. The world revolves around one god and the god is "I." Like a small child, the narcissist's views of others may rapidly change from idealizing to denigrating. Mother is great if she buys the toy airplane and is a hated object if she denies the purchase. Stable narcissists are often the product of a spoiled upbringing, in which sharing was not common. Consequently they never develop the ability to think of other's needs. It simply does not cross their minds. Naturally, few narcissists are born with nearly the talents and skills they feel they have. Daddy's little girl may merely be another average kid to the rest of the world. To deflect this painful realization, these patients may pre-occupy themselves with grandiose fantasies. It has been said that neurotics build castles in the air, while psychotics live in them. Narcissists try to rent them. In many respects stable narcissists, especially if talented, may be reasonably happy, although they may be difficult to get along with. Problems arise if, for whatever reason, adulation and subservience do not come their way. In such instances they may pout, stomp about, or become depressed.

In contrast, the unstable narcissistic personality tends to live in a much more hostile world. The sense of ego is actually poorly developed and life is a constant threat. There lurks an incipient feeling of annihilation and a piercing feeling that they are truly worthless. This is defended against by the production of a grandiose style, not unlike that seen in the histrionic personality. But the stakes are high, and these patients are easily wounded. Their defense may consist of a vicious rage, and they can turn on a friend in moments. Few people are trusted, and bitterness becomes a way of life. They are constantly fleeing humiliation, while gloating over the embarrassment of others. If dinner is not on the table on time, then one may find it angrily thrown on the floor. Tantrums and rages become second nature. They expect to be at the head of the line, and when this does not happen, a scene is to be expected. They are almost impossible to please and are prone to severe depressive episodes, as their needs are not met. Their personality structure is quite primitive, and they are prone to micropsychotic episodes. Unstable narcissists are often not successful in life, for their behaviors prevent advancement, while their mood swings make consistent work difficult. In other instances, they may demonstrate reasonably good impulse control in public or on the job, demonstrating their more primitive qualities in specific relationships such as with their therapist. Unlike the stable narcissist, the unstable narcissist is frequently sad and angry. Every day is a battlefield. They pretend to be Napoleon, but deep in their hearts they know they are a sham. Worse yet, they fear that others recognize the sham as well.

THE PSYCHOTIC PRONE PERSONALITY DISORDERS

This collection of disorders includes the borderline personality, the schizotypal personality, and the paranoid personality. If one looks at the patient's sense of self in these disorders, as indicated by their ego structure and spontaneous coping defenses, one finds that these people appear to be seriously delayed developmentally. Their defensive structure is reminiscent of the defenses used by tiny children, including magical thinking, preoccupation with internal fantasy worlds, and tendencies to act impulsively or out of rage. When pressured, they may experience micropsychotic episodes, as these defenses sweep them into a false reality. For this reason they are being clustered as "psychotic prone." They could just as easily be referred to as the primitive personality disorders referring to the developmental immaturity of their ego structure. In this regard the histrionic personality and the unstable narcissistic personality, of the last section, at times may also function as primitive personalities. Let us begin our survey of these disorders with a special attention to the intense pain that coats their reality with a distinctive sense of impending chaos.

The Borderline Personality Disorder

The borderline personality experiences life as if there was no sense of inner self. If one could feel inanimate, like a piece of clothing hanging forlornly in a closet, then one can begin to appreciate the hollowness that haunts these people. Like the clothing, they feel empty unless filled by the presence of others. And like the clothing, they depend upon others to give meaning to life. Consequently, they intensely dislike being alone, for it can lead to sensations of impending annihilation and destruction. As a friend leaves the apartment, they may literally feel empty, as if a part of themselves was now absent. Their need for others is so great that they cannot understand how anyone who really cares about them could leave them alone. Thus their dependency quickly becomes a hostile one, as they resent the pain that others inflict upon them. When they feel slighted, they can rapidly escalate into rages, throwing glasses, breaking furniture, and screaming profanities. In this sense they are unpredictable, for they are so exquisitely sensitive to being hurt, that friends and lovers quickly tire of apologizing, eventually growing angry themselves. A high level of interpersonal stress is the standard price required to befriend these patients.

Without the presence of others, these patients frequently view life as colorless and boring. Consequently, coupled with their intense feelings of weakness and self-loathing, they may ceaselessly seek stimulation using drugs, sex, and eating to satisfy their feelings of emptiness. Their impulsive behaviors unfortunately may bring them into contact with superficial people, who promptly proceed to abuse them, thus fulfilling their worst fears. Fear of abandonment becomes a nagging companion, stoked by the fact that their unpredictable behavior and manipulative attitude frequently result in actual rejection.

Suicidal thought arises almost with a predictability. It may be coupled with a peculiar tendency to enjoy self-mutilation. These patients are notorious for delicately cutting at their wrists, burning themselves with cigarette butts and matches, and overdosing. When cutting themselves, they frequently report no pain. The self-mutilation seems to serve as a release for intense feelings of rage. Such bizarre gestures are often preceded by an argument or broken date. These periods of analgesia, while cutting themselves, probably represent fleeting periods of psychotic depersonalization. Other common micropsychotic processes include derealization and paranoia. In the last analysis these patients face a harsh world over which they feel they have little control. The picture is further darkened by the sense that they themselves are also out of control. They represent the stuff of which soap operas are made. They are "the glass people," delicate to touch, easily broken, and dangerous when shattered.

The Schizotypal Personality

Like the borderline personality, the schizotypal personality seems to lack a core. They too are stalked by a rather unsettling sensation that they are somehow empty. This blandness becomes an invitation to an inpouring of vivid fantasy and psychotic-like process. The world becomes peopled with clairvoyant messages, ghostlike presences, magical hunches, and secretive glances. Like a child withdrawn into a world peopled with pretend playmates, the schizotypal personality silently retreats from life. Unlike the schizoid personality described earlier the schizotypal personality is frequently rejection sensitive. They want contact but do not know how to make it. There is a desperate quality here, in which the eccentric professor finds more solace in his books than with others of his species. One of my adolescent patients would spend endless days running with stray dogs in the woods near his house. Apparently they were kinder companions than the children at his school. Moreover, he was "the king" of his dogs, whereas he was merely "the dog boy" at his school. Thus these fantasy wanderings may provide a firmer sense of self-esteem to these patients. Because of their withdrawal into their private worlds, these patients may develop idiosyncratic ways of thinking and using words, tending to become metaphorical and vague. Unfortunately these traits result in further problems with socialization. When stressed, the schizotypal personality may decompensate into micropsychotic episodes, including delusions and hallucinations. In a sense, they live life from "the inside of the bottle," peering at others as if watching a different species, worried that someone may poke a finger or two into their private worlds.

The Paranoid Personality

The world of the paranoid personality is blanketed by a thick covering of restless worrying. Probably more than any other disorder discussed so far, these patients see the world as a hostile environment. These patients have never evolved the ability to trust other people. As a consequence they are suspicious and guarded by nature. They scour their interactions with others for the subtlest hints of deception, often ignoring the bigger picture as they fixate on a slip of the tongue or an errant look. Their paranoid ideation, except during micropsychotic episodes, is not delusional in quality, but nevertheless, they seem driven by it. It is as if they feed on their own concerns. One is left with the feeling that without their fears, they would feel awkward and without purpose.

Their defensive guardedness has generally arisen to protect them from a deep-rooted sense of inferiority. Moreover, they fear that their weaknesses will leave them vulnerable to attack. In response they become haughty, finding it extremely difficult to admit mistakes. All new faces represent potential enemies, not potential friends. Everything needs to be checked out. By way of illustration, during an initial interview one of my patients suddenly produced a notebook in which he began vigorously scribbling down our dialogue. He related that, "I'm just keeping a record so that people on the outside know what's going on in here." It is a lonely existence. It is also one in which delusional thinking can erupt, for the paranoid patient's isolation prevents the patient from receiving corrective opinions from others. These brief delusional micropsychotic breaks are often accompanied by tremendous feelings of rage and indignation. These patients are also predisposed to more severe disorders on Axis I such as a paranoid disorder. In the final analysis they are exquisitely unhappy. In a true sense they lead tortured lives, for everywhere that they look they see men with black hoods. Ironically, it is their own projection that provides the hoods.

We have now completed our survey of the various personality disorders. The above descriptions are meant to convey a general feeling for the manner in which these disorders may present. An attempt has also been made to convey, in a phenomenological sense, some of the ways in which these patients experience life. Only with this type of compassionate feeling for the patient can the clinician become skilled at detecting the possibility of a personality disturbance during the initial interview. It remains important to realize that the above descriptions are, in actuality, caricatures of a sort, useful as they may be. In reality patients present with nuances and variations that a short description cannot hope to convey. Only by listening carefully to many patients while attempting to actively empathize can the clinician gain a clearer understanding of the individuality of the person seated across from them.

Having completed our survey, it may be of use to examine some of the problems associated with the diagnostic system in actual practice.

Common Problems Associated with Determining an Axis II Diagnosis

A variety of problematic issues arise when attempting to utilize the concepts described thus far. These problems cluster into two main areas: (1) problems with diagnostic reliability and validity and (2) problems created by the interviewers themselves.

Looking at the first area, one difficulty that strikes the eye is the fact that many of the personality disorders seem to share characteristics with each other. All the disorders that we have collected under the heading of psychotic prone personalities also tend to experience anxiety on a frequent basis. In this sense they share this quality with the disorders described as the anxiety-prone disorders. On a more specific level, a significant degree of people with a borderline personality will also fit the criteria of a histrionic personality. The more overlap found in a diagnostic system, the more likely that the system will have trouble distinguishing between entities. At some level this is a problem of sorts for the DSM-III-R, which manifests as a propensity for patients to carry multiple diagnoses on this axis. It is hoped that in the future this overlap will be decreased, but some overlap is a natural outcome of the complexity of personality structure. One would expect to see considerable overlap in this area for, in actuality, these diagnostic categories are merely labels into which reality is sometimes uncomfortably forced to fit.

A second and perhaps more disturbing problem is the issue of cultural bias in the DSM-III-R. For instance, some of the criteria listed with the antisocial personality may appear abnormal to the white middle class but not be unusual or deviant in a different culture. Occupational history is a good example of this problem. Some individuals simply enjoy switching jobs relatively frequently, and their culture may accept this behavior as reasonably normal.

Even more interesting is the fact that the criteria listed in the DSM-III-R such as criminal behavior, frequent fighting, drunken driving, and the use of aliases seem to describe a personality type that is commonly known as a criminal. And these are the characteristics of an antisocial personality as seen in the lower socioeconomic classes. But are there no sociopaths among the educated elite?

The problem is that the DSM-III-R will not pick them up readily. The white collar sociopath frequently shows criteria not listed in the DSM-III-R, including tax evasion, sexual harassment of employees, stealth in business dealings, broken committments, backbiting, slander, and long-standing extramarital affairs. The psychodynamics of this person may be little different from the pimp on Eighth Avenue, but the DSM-III-R might not even acknowledge such a person as having a specific personality disorder.

This criticism leads to a related problem. Some of the criteria used in the diagnostic descriptions tend to be vague or depend upon subjective interpretation by the interviewer. For example, in the diagnosis of a histrionic personality we find the following types of items listed:

1. expresses emotion with inappropriate exaggeration
2. has a style of speech that is excessively impressionistic and lacking in detail
3. is overly concerned with physical attractiveness
4. is inappropriately sexually seductive in appearance or behavior[7]

Although these characteristics appear simple enough, one wonders how flirtatious one has to be in order to fulfill criterion 4. And what exactly does an exaggerated expression of emotions look like in order to be viewed as pathologic? Obviously each clinician is left to decide these issues somewhat idiosyncratically. One of the real dangers arises when clinicians are unaware of their own personality traits both pathologic and not pathologic. In these instances the clinician may accept clearly pathologic behavior in the patient as not bad enough to fulfill a specific criterion. For example a clinician may possess a hefty dose of dramatic and reactive behavior. This clinician may subsequently view the patient's dramatic behavior as "quite all right, I might do the same thing myself if feeling pressured." Such blind spots can significantly affect the inter-rater reliability of the Axis II diagnoses.

This discussion leads into the second category of diagnostic problems, those problems related not so much to weaknesses in the diagnostic system but to clinician misconceptions. The first common problem to be avoided is the tendency to make personality diagnoses too rapidly, without actually determining whether the patient truly fulfills the criteria or not. This problem manifests itself frequently, when clinicians diagnose in an impressionistic fashion, saying things such as, "That patient is clearly a borderline, she was so manipulative during that interview." The behavior of the patient in the interview and the clinician's intuitive feeling for the patient's pathology are extremely useful tools. But they are tools whose usefulness rests in guiding the clinician towards diagnostic regions that merit further detailed exploration, perhaps even in future interviews if time does not allow appropriate immediate exploration. The major point remains the fact that personality disorders are historical diagnoses and the patient's behavior in the interview provides suggestive, not conclusive, evidence.

This point is far from academic in nature. It is extremely important clinically. So far we have emphasized the overlap among various Axis II diagnoses. In actuality, superficial overlap may exist between diagnoses on Axis I and II when one considers the immediate behavior of the patient in the interview itself. A patient may present in a dramatic fashion with a seductive blouse and brightly colored pants. The patient may talk with a mild pressure to her speech, demonstrating a knack for telling a colorful tale. The same patient may act coyly and be caught by the clinician in several trivial lies.

An inexperienced clinician may immediately label this patient as a histrionic personality, but this diagnosis is being made on the recent and immediate behavior of the patient. In actuality, the patient may be in the early stages of a first break manic episode. A careful interview might have uncovered that this extroverted behavior is quite atypical for this patient historically. In addition the patient may have a long history of depressive episodes as well as a positive family history for bipolar disorders. With regard to treatment this patient may benefit significantly with a trial of lithium. Unfortunately the impressionistic diagnostician may not "get the point" until the patient turns the corner into a blatant manic crisis. A dramatic patient presentation could also be seen with other Axis I diagnoses, including an atypical bipolar disorder, a cyclothymic disorder, and amphetamine abuse or some other drug-related disorder. An even more ominous problem would exist if this abnormal behavior was secondary to an organic agent such as a brain tumor.

The impressionistic diagnostician can also run into problems around the issues of countertransference and labeling theory. Stated simply, the various diagnoses on Axis II often carry a connotation to them, frequently pejorative in nature. If a clinician takes a rapid dislike to an abusive patient, then the patient may rapidly become "just another god damned sociopath." One would like to think that one is "above that process," but few if any clinicians are. In this sense it is important for clinicians to explore what these diagnoses mean to them on a personal and emotional level. It also serves as a reminder that these diagnoses should not be made casually, for they can greatly affect the future course of therapy for the patient. I have certainly seen patients refused by a clinic because "he's a borderline and we don't treat borderlines."

It also serves to warn us not to fall into the trap of using these diagnoses as stereotypes. In a positive sense they can provide valuable information that allows the clinician to learn from the writings of others and to eventually lead to a better understanding of the patient. But they do not delineate the specific characteristics or prognosis of any patient. It may be true that people with an antisocial personality tend to do poorly in therapy, but it does not necessarily mean that the patient sitting in front of the clinician will do poorly. Within each of these personality disorders there exists a wide range of characteristics and responses.

The above cautionary points are important in guiding the clinician towards a wise use of these diagnostic entities. But if these cautionary points are taken to their extreme interpretation, they become damaging in themselves. In this sense clinicians can become essentially phobic towards the idea of making a personality diagnoses in a single hour. One might hear the clinician state, "I never make a personality diagnosis in an hour, it takes much longer to know a person and make sure they present in the same way over several sessions." Ironically this misinterpretation of the concept of a personality disorder hinges on the exact same error in thinking seen with the impressionistic interviewer. Specifically, the clinician is stating that the diagnosis is being made primarily upon how the patient presents. But we have just seen that a hypomanic patient could present for months in a style totally consistent with a histrionic personality.

The pertinent point remains that personality disorders are not made primarily upon the basis of the patient's presentation. They are historical diagnoses. The issue is not whether the patient presents for seven sessions with histrionic behaviors but whether the patient has displayed histrionic behavior consistently for years dating back to adolescence.

In this light the limiting factors in making the diagnoses in the initial session are twofold: (1) Does the clinician have enough time to explore the past history of the patient appropriately and (2) Is the patient providing reasonably valid information. If the above two criteria are met, then one can safely make a personality diagnosis in an hour. The truth of the matter appears to be that some diagnoses are more easily made in an hour and some may be difficult to make in an hour. Those that are easier tend to have behaviorally oriented criteria that do not depend much upon the subjective opinions of the clinician. For instance, the antisocial personality, the borderline personality, and the schizotypal personality depend heavily upon fairly concrete criteria. As a case in point, either the patient has or has not been suspended from school. Either the patient has demonstrated self-mutilating behaviors outside of periods of Axis I pathology or no such behaviors have occurred. These behaviorally oriented diagnoses can fairly frequently be made in a single hour, as long as the patient is telling the truth.

On the other hand, those disorders in which the criteria are highly subjective may be quite difficult to make in an hour, for the clinician must cover a wide variety of historical circumstances in order to determine whether or not the patient typically demonstrates the behaviors in question. This category of disorders, which are difficult to diagnose in an hour, includes entities such as the histrionic personality and the narcissistic personality.

In actual practice a talented clinician who actively pursues clues to personality dysfunction and who persistently hunts for diagnostic criteria will usually have a good idea as to whether a personality disorder is present or not. With the more behavioral diagnoses this may result in an actual diagnosis or perhaps a provisional diagnosis or at least a set of rule-out diagnoses. In the more elusive diagnoses the clinician should at least have a feeling for possible rule-out diagnoses and, at times, even the elusive diagnoses may be made in an initial assessment. Interviews with family members and other collaborative sources are particularly valuable in clarifying personality diagnoses when the picture is not clear.

The interviewer who appears overly cautious risks a variety of consequences. In the first place the attitude itself tends to make these interviewers sloppy in approaching these diagnoses for, "if you can't make the diagnosis, then why try?" In a sense they become self-fulfilling prophets. Because they do not practice delineating the skills needed to make these diagnoses efficiently, they indeed cannot make them efficiently in one or two interviews. But even more important is the fact that it may be a dis-service to the patient to not spot these diagnoses until it's too late.

This is particularly true in the case of the consultant or the intake interviewer, who may be asked to suggest treatment approaches or may actually triage the patient. If the patient is determined to either fulfill or nearly fulfill the criteria of a borderline personality, the head of an outpatient psychotherapy clinic would be ill-advised to refer this patient to one of the inexperienced clinicians or worse yet to a clinician demonstrating serious psychopathology. In short, it is of value to recognize these diagnoses early. As another example, a psychotherapist may significantly change such parameters as the frequency of sessions, depending upon the presence or absence of a primitive personality disorder. It might be detrimental to accept for therapy such a patient if the clinician intended to move from the area in the next six months.

We have ended our discussion of the numerous factors that can effect the clinician's ability to utilize Axis II diagnoses effectively. It is hoped that the survey of the disorders also provided a beginning sense of the enormous pain that sometimes envelops these patients and the people who care about them. In the next section we shall get down to the actual art of interviewing these patients, who represent a complicated challenge even for the experienced clinician.

SECTION II: THE APPROACH TO THE INTERVIEW

Sometimes she [Emily Dickinson] would only talk to acquaintances from behind a closed door. She fled from approaching visitors and refused to appear when friends or guests came to see her. She surprised one visitor, who was permitted to see her, by allowing him to choose between a glass of wine or a rose from the garden. Whenever possible, she avoided conversation, preferring to communicate with people in writing.

A. M. Hammacher, Phantoms of the Imagination

A) Eliciting Sensitive Material

When one speaks of the approach to the interview, one is in some sense speaking of the clinician's approach to life as well. More precisely, a clinician, who is prone to passing moral judgments will probably have great difficulty in both interviewing and subsequently working with people who have developed the character structures that we label as pathologic. A gentle compassion is needed in order to convey the unconditional positive regard of Carl Rogers discussed in Chapter 1.

This point is of importance because many of the traits that the clinician must explore in order to detect the presence of character pathology are traits that may arouse considerable guilt in the patient. If the clinician conveys a judgmental attitude, this guilt will generally be intensified, frequently to the point that the patient will feel uncomfortable, undergoing not a therapeutic exchange but a public humiliation. A clinician's parental glance may punish as effectively as a scarlet letter.

Besides unsettling the patient, such behaviors by the clinician serve to sabotage the interview itself, for the more that the patient's self system is activated, the more likely that information will be distorted or withheld. Indeed the skill of a clinician to uncover character pathology seems to greatly parallel the ability to ask questions regarding sensitive material in an unassuming and natural fashion. The sensitive material may range from inner feelings of despair, which are not necessarily viewed in a negative light by society but that are viewed as intimate feelings by the patient, to activities such as drunkenness, promiscuity, and criminal activity, which are clearly frowned upon by the society. It is not that the clinician condones such activities, but rather that the clinician views them as aspects of the human condition, reflections of human pain. The clinician listens in an effort to understand the patient, not in an effort to chastise the behaviors chosen by the patient.

In this regard a variety of techniques exist that can help the clinician to approach sensitive material without conveying that the clinician is "digging for bad material." Some of these techniques are also specifically geared to decrease the likelihood of deception, thus increasing the likelihood of a valid data base. When utilized effectively, these techniques can result in the elicitation of sensitive material that one might think would never be revealed in an initial assessment. And indeed it would not be revealed had not the patient been provided a safe environment for sharing.

Let us look at one technique, "shame reversal," which operates upon a clever premise. The problem with many sensitive questions lies in the fact that if the patient answers positively they are in essence admitting a failure. The natural result is a feeling of shame, which can clearly act as a deterrent to open expression on the part of the patient. For example if the clinician asks, "Do you have a drinking problem?"

many patients will answer negatively, unless they have already reached a degree of insight that has led them to acknowledge their alcohol abuse. But in the following example we will see a different approach:

> **Pt.:** I guess some of my best times are with my friends. I really would rather be with my male friends than with my wife and some of her losers. Talk about boring, they invented the word.
>
> **Clin.:** Are these the same guys who are your drinking buddies?
>
> **Pt.:** Yep. They're the ones.
>
> **Clin.:** Well where do you guys like to go for a brew?
>
> **Pt.:** All over the place (patient chuckles). We'll tie one on anyplace anytime.
>
> **Clin.:** Well it sounds like you enjoy your drinking and your friends. You know, some people have problems holding their liquor. How about you, can you hold your liquor pretty well or do you have problems holding it down?
>
> **Pt.:** Oh, I don't have any problems holding my liquor. I'm not the best mind you, but I can hold my own.
>
> **Clin.:** Can you hold down a pint or a fifth in a single night?
>
> **Pt.:** Sure, no problem.
>
> **Clin.:** How often in a given week do you put down a pint or more, in all seriousness.
>
> **Pt.:** In all seriousness . . . I'd say two or three nights a week. Well, make that two nights. It's usually only on weekend nights that I really go after it.

In this example the clinician has phrased the question in such a way that if patients answer affirmatively, then they are actually stroking their egos as opposed to admitting a flaw. In fact to admit that "I have problems holding my liquor," represents the answer more likely to produce shame, hence the name shame reversal. This exchange is both more comfortable for the patient while also much more likely to yield valid data than a standard question such as, "Are you an alcoholic?" Of course one must also make sure that the patient is not purely bragging. This can usually be accomplished by subsequently delineating the actual drinking history via specific questions aimed at eliciting behavioral incidents, as this interviewer was just beginning to do.

This technique is so valuable that we ought to see it in a different context. In this instance the clinician is suspicious that the patient has had problems with angry exchanges on the job and has probably been fired several times. But the patient appears somewhat cagey around this topic. Consequently the clinician utilizes the technique of shame reversal to create a safer environment for the patient.

Clin.:	What have your jobs been like?
Pt.:	Oh, nothing special, I've always gotten along O.K.
Clin.:	Ever have any problems on the job?
Pt.:	Nah, none worth mentioning.
Clin.:	How about with bosses, have you had any bosses who really seemed like they needed to be "big shots," you know, the kind that just like to get on somebody's case?
Pt.:	Now that I've been asked, more than I care to think about.
Clin.:	What do you do, do you tend to take the abuse or are you the kind of guy who likes to let the boss know where you stand?
Pt.:	Oh, I let them know where I stand alright, nobody is going to just push me around.
Clin.:	Well, what might you do if the boss seemed out of line?
Pt.:	I'd tell him to get off my back, that's what I'd do.
Clin.:	How do they usually react?
Pt.:	Most of them back off.
Clin.:	Any of them ever get mad and fire you?
Pt.:	A couple have, but I didn't want to work for them anyway.
Clin.:	How many times have you been fired, would you say five times, ten times?
Pt.:	Hmm . . . maybe around five times, somewhere around there.

The actual phrase that represents the shame reversal was, "What do you do, do you tend to take the abuse or are you the kind of guy who likes to let the boss know where you stand?" Once again the technique takes away the judgmental shame associated with a positive answer. Imagine the difference in response that might have followed a line of questioning that began with, "Are you unreliable at work or have you ever been fired?"

An important point to remember with regard to the technique of shame reversal is that the clinician must be careful not to side with the patient or condone the described behavior. Such overidentification gives a false impression to the patient and also conveys an inaccurate moral judgment. Instead, the clinician attempts to suspend judgment, while voicing the question in such a manner that the patient may respond from the perspective of how the patient sees it. Thus although the sociopath frequently sees other people as the trouble makers, the clinician neither agrees or disagrees with this stance. Moreover the phrasing of the question allows the sociopath to express the world as it is seen through the patient's own eyes.

This clinician also demonstrated another technique, "symptom amplification." In this technique the clinician acknowledges the fact that patients, especially around topics such as drinking and drug abuse, tend to minimize the amount that they are taking. Assuming that this process may be true, the clinician allows the patient to minimize but sets the suggested limit so high that even though the patient minimizes, it is still apparent that substance abuse and/or tolerance is present. In the above example the clinician asked if the patient had been fired around ten times. Now as the patient minimizes downwards to five, the clinician still receives valid information that being fired is hardly a foreign experience for this patient.

Another useful process consists of asking specific questions as opposed to generic questions, if the evaluator is truly suspicious of drug usage by a patient. Instead of asking, "Have you ever used any street drugs?" the clinician asks a series of questions concerning specific drugs. It is generally more difficult to shade the truth in response to a specific question as opposed to a generality. In the following example, the clinician will use symptom amplification as well as a series of drug-specific questions.

Clin.:	What types of street drugs have you used in the past?
Pt.:	Oh . . . I like to smoke a joint or two, get a mild buzz on now and then.
Clin.:	Do you smoke roughly a couple of joints per day, a little less, a little more?
Pt.:	I guess you could say about two or three joints per day.
Clin.:	How about coke?
Pt.:	No no, not really, it's too expensive.
Clin.:	How about if someone gives it to you?
Pt.:	(patient smiles) Hey, I'm no fool. Sure, I'll run in the snow if it's falling.
Clin.:	Would you say about a couple times a week?
Pt.:	Nah, maybe three, four times a month.
Clin.:	How about when you were younger, has there ever been a time when you used more coke?
Pt.:	Oh sure, when I was in the first couple of years of college, I was probably snorting a couple of lines a day?
Clin.:	What about speed?
Pt.:	Now that's a drug that I can take or leave.
Clin.:	What's it like for you?
Pt.:	I just don't like it that much. I don't like coming down off it, crashing is no fun.
Clin.:	Even though you don't like it very much, how many times have you used it in the last month?

> ***Pt.:*** The last month, let's see, hmm, maybe two or three times.
> ***Clin.:*** Was there ever a time in the past where you speeded for days at a time?
> ***Pt.:*** Sure, when I was in college I might speed for two, three weeks at a time. Hey, I was a Hunter S. Thompson. I was on the road to Vegas (patient chuckles), sort of wish I was there now.

The clinician's persistence is paying off. It is not infrequent for patients initially to deny or downplay the use of a drug. But if asked specifically about past use, a patient may then admit to heavier usage. Thus it is often a good idea with a drug history to probe both for the recent past and the distant past.

So far we have been discussing the elicitation of material that many patients would view as potentially incriminating. There are other areas that both patients and clinicians have difficulty talking about openly, such as sexuality. With these types of questions it is critical that the clinician's paralanguage and body language appear exactly as they do when asking less sensitive questions. In other words the clinician avoids telegraphing that a sensitive area has been broached. In this regard, it is frequently of value for clinicians to practice these questions either in front of a mirror or during role playing until they can be asked smoothly and with a natural intonation.

It is also useful with these types of questions to eliminate the patient's fears that he or she is the only one who has ever experienced these activities or problems. Examples of sensitive methods of approaching delicate informational areas follow:

a. It is not unusual for men at some point in their lives to have experienced problems with maintaining an erection. Have you had this type of experience in the past year or so?

b. It can be pretty difficult to control a temper sometimes. Have you ever done anything that you really regretted when you flew off the handle such as striking your wife or your child?

c. Sometimes a parent can be really pushed to their limit, and they're so upset they just feel like hitting their kid if they cry just one more time. Have you ever felt like that yourself?

d. Women vary a great deal on how frequently, if ever, they have an orgasm. What percentage of the time do you think you have an orgasm, 5 percent, 20 percent, 80 percent, almost never?

The last question illustrates another useful point emphasized by Pomeroy, Flax, and Wheeler.[9] When seeking a specific frequency of an activity, the clinician should attempt to avoid leading questions that may be interpreted as indicating what answer the clinician is expecting. Thus one would avoid saying, "Do you have orgasms about 80 percent of the time?" Instead, as shown above, the clinician provides a broad range of frequencies, thus providing no indication that a particular number is either normal or abnormal.

A less specific question may also lead to invalid information, as compared to a question which provides a range. For instance the question, "What percentage of the time do you experience an orgasm?" leaves patients alone with their projections of what they think the clinician is looking for. The provision of a range by the clinician eliminates any projected idea that a specific answer is expected.

All of the questions listed above attempt to help the patient to relate difficult material, without feeling shame. Once a patient can admit a problem such as child abuse, the patient may be able to get some help. As long as such abuse is kept a secret, little can usually be done. A sensitive interviewer can help a patient make this first step.

Some patients will feel guilt about activities for which there is not necessarily a reason to feel guilt such as homosexuality. Once again the clinician attempts to raise the topic in such a way that the patient does not feel awkward. For example, one useful method of approaching homosexuality is via the developmental history as follows, "As adolescents mature they frequently experiment with different life styles and sexual preferences. When you were an adolescent, did you ever experiment with homosexual contact, perhaps to see what it was like?" One can continue the questioning into adulthood simply by asking, "In the long run some people prefer homosexual sex to heterosexual sex or vice versa. Do you have any preference at this point in your life?"

Another useful maneuver, as suggested by Pomeroy, Flax, and Wheeler, is to ask questions in such a way that the clinician gently assumes that the patient may have experienced the behavior in question. For instance incest may be approached sensitively as follows, "Different families and cultures have different views on who it is appropriate to have sex with; who is the closest relative, if any, that you have had a sexual contact with?" The technique of "gentle assumption" as illustrated by this question, may make it more difficult to flatly deny an activity if indeed it has occurred. As was seen with the previous questions, this example also attempts to decrease the guilt that may accompany a positive reply. Victims of incest may be acutely experiencing shame on many different levels, including guilt over their own role in the incest or guilt that they should not "tell on Daddy." The phrasing of the above question neither condemns nor approves of incest, thus allowing the patient to feel that a moral judgment is not about to be pronounced.

We have reviewed a variety of techniques, such as shame reversal and symptom amplification, that may help a patient to feel more comfortable while relating sensitive material. At this time a more extended example of a clinical dialogue will demonstrate the utility of such techniques in clinical practice. In this example the patient was a lanky male around the age of twenty-seven. He had come to the evaluation center on his own initiative because, "I just think things are going poorly at Trellway House (fictional name for a local drug rehabilitation center)." Although the patient complained of feeling depressed, he gave the impression that all of his problems were the result of the weaknesses of others. He was dressed in jeans and a faded plaid shirt. Apparently he was in the process of growing in a goatee that was tugged at intermittently. We will pick up the conversation well into the body of the interview, at a point at which the clinician decided to expand the antisocial personality region.

> **Clin.:** Tell me a little more about what is bothering you the most back at Trellway House.
>
> **Pt.:** To begin with man you got to understand that I been living at Trellway for a couple of years now. And it used to be that we were really trying to get off the drugs and if you didn't pull your own way, hell, they'd let you have it, really have it. But not now, now they let them get away with too much, hell, I've seen guys regularly toking up on the back porch.
>
> **Clin.:** It sounds like you don't really like some of the new people who moved in. Have you tried to talk to any of them about the changes that are happening?
>
> **Pt.:** Hell, I talk to them man and they don't listen. These guys don't give a damn.
>
> **Clin.:** Do some of them try to hassle you?
>
> **Pt.:** Yeah sure, but that's all part of the game.
>
> **Clin.:** Have any of them tried to push you around?
>
> **Pt.:** Yeah, a couple of them but I set them straight.
>
> **Clin.:** How do you mean?
>
> **Pt.:** I kicked their asses.
>
> **Clin.:** Well, you look like you're in pretty good shape, I imagine you can take care of yourself pretty well. What about in the past, what types of fights have you been in?
>
> **Pt.:** Oh, I been in a few now and then. People know not to mess with me. I grew up in a tough neighborhood and you had to know how to fight to survive.
>
> **Clin.:** When you were fairly young let's say between the ages of say fifteen and twenty-five, how many fights do you think you were in, twenty, thirty?

Pt.: I'm bad but not that bad . . . oh, let's see, maybe about fifteen, who knows, it could have been as high as twenty.

Clin.: Did you ever get hurt?

Pt.: Nah, not really, but I did a number on a few of those guys.

Clin.: Did you ever put anyone in the hospital?

Pt.: Yeah, there was one dude that I cut up pretty good, but he really deserved it, trust me.

Clin.: Earlier you told me that you drank a fair amount in the past but have completely stopped now, which you deserve a lot of credit for. Back when you were drinking, did you sometimes feel on edge almost like you needed a good fight, so you went looking for one, perhaps the alcohol making it a little more difficult to control your anger?

Pt.: Sometimes, yeah sometimes . . . especially if I was pretty strung out I would be just plain nasty, and I started my fair share of fights. But usually I was just protecting myself or the guy really had it coming to him.

Clin.: It certainly sounds like you know how to handle yourself in a fight. Did you used to run in a gang or how did you learn how to defend yourself so well?

Pt.: Like I said, where I grew up you had to learn how to fight, and I did hang out with a gang for a couple of years.

Clin.: Oh, what were they called?

Pt.: The Blades. And we were a tough group, but not crazy, no way crazy, not like . . . like some gangs.

Clin.: Did you ever get back at people by slashing tires, smashing windows, any kind of vandalism?

Pt.: Yeah, but I grew out of that phase. It looks pretty stupid now.

Clin.: Did you ever get suspended from school because you were out with the gang?

Pt.: Oh yeah, I was suspended maybe three, four times.

Clin.: What for?

Pt.: Fighting, cutting classes, the usual stuff.

Clin.: How do you look back at this stuff now?

Pt.: Well, I think a lot of it was pretty stupid, but it's what I needed to do. There were a lot of stupid people in that school and the principal came on way too strong.

Clin.: How did all the hassles at school affect your grades?

Pt.: I did all right, grades weren't a big hassle.

Clin.: What types of grades did you get?

Pt.: Mostly B's and C's. You see, I did some growing up back then and I eventually left the gang. I even did pretty good in history.

Clin.: Oh, what kinds of grades did you get there?

Pt.:   Mostly B's and I even pulled a couple of A's.

Clin.:   Sounds like you did real well there. What did you like about history?

Pt.:   Uh, I liked learning about the past and I got into things like the Korean War and the Civil War. It's interesting, and the way I figure it you got to learn from the past, even from your own past, like my father he never learned from his mistakes, and that's why he is and always will be a jerk. But I learn from my mistakes.

Clin.:   You mean sort of like how you turned your drug habit around?

Pt.:   Exactly. I don't mess with nothing now, and I don't intend to in the future.

Clin.:   You really did do well in history, did you ever have some difficulty with some courses?

Pt.:   Sure, didn't everybody?

Clin.:   Did you ever flunk a course?

Pt.:   Yeah, I flunked algebra and I also flunked social studies, but that teacher was a farce. I'd like to catch up with her now.

Clin.:   Did you ever have to repeat a year?

Pt.:   No, but I had to go to summer school twice (chuckles). What a joke, I skipped out on that more than I skipped out during the regular school year.

Clin.:   Jim, you mentioned earlier that your father had given you a rough time and that he would beat you if he felt you were pulling a fast one. Did you find that in order to protect yourself, you had to lie to him, keep him in the dark if you know what I mean.

Pt.:   Yeah he was easy to fool. I could lie to him all over the place. I once told him that I was staying at school during remedial period for help in math, but that they had begun remedial periods an hour earlier than they used to. The old man bit on that one.

Clin.:   What about now, do you feel like if you have to you are pretty clever at deceit or are you a lousy liar?

Pt.:   (chuckles) I can lie if I have to.

Clin.:   In what kinds of situations would you lie if you had to?

Pt.:   Well I'll tell you one thing, I ain't telling the old lady if I'm having an affair (patient chuckles) I ain't that dumb.

Clin.:   You had been telling me about your childhood and it sounds like both of your parents were unpredictable and tough to be around at times. Did you ever run away to get away from it all?

Pt.:   Yeah.

Clin.: How many times?

Pt.: Around three times, but I always came back in a day or two. I don't know why but I did.

Clin.: To get back at them, did you ever do things like set fires?

Pt.: No.

Clin.: Did you ever try get revenge by sort of punishing them, perhaps by hurting one of their pets?

Pt.: No, but I did like to tease cats for awhile, a couple of us were doing that.

Clin.: What would you do?

Pt.: We'd stick a cat in a can and then kick it or sometimes we sprinkled the cat's tail with lighter fluid and then lit it.

Clin.: How do you view those behaviors now when you look back.

Pt.: That was weird and I don't think I'd do any of that now. I've learned that there's no use hurting things in this life man, and I'm really pretty much of a pacifist. I'm not out to push anybody around.

In this excerpt the clinician is eliciting a powerful history, filled with evidence of sociopathy, and yet the patient appears to feel comfortable. Part of this comfort may be related to the sociopath's tendency to not feel guilt, but a considerable part seems to be related to the clinician's skill at handling sensitive material. It certainly warrants taking a closer look in an effort to see the smooth intermingling of the various techniques utilized by the clinician.

In the first place the clinician is not taken in by the patient's superficial appearance of "being a good guy just minding my own business." In this light, people presenting with an antisocial personality frequently see themselves as the victims of circumstance, highlighted by a tendency to point their finger at a variety of nearby villains. In this interview the patient presents himself as a rehabilitated drug addict who is incensed that the rehabilitation program is not as strong as it ought to be. He may actually have many of these feelings, but there is more to the picture than he spontaneously presents, such as the fact that he has been in fights with several of his fellow residents. The deftness with which this clinician manages to uncover the underlying material results in many ways from his ability to take advantage of the patient's trait described above, namely of seeing others as the cause of his problems.

For example the clinician chooses to enter the potentially loaded topic of fighting by asking, "Do some of them try to hassle you?" referring to the patient's fellow residents who are supposedly abusing the system. In this fashion the topic of fighting has been brought up in a manner in which the patient will openly discuss his participation in fights, for no accusation has been made that he is starting them. And this is probably exactly the fashion in which this patient views most of his fights.

Once the patient is talking freely about fights, the clinician takes the opportunity to focus the interview towards a historical perspective by asking, "When you were fairly young let's say between the ages of say fifteen and twenty-five, how many fights do you think you were in, twenty, thirty?" It is important to focus the patient on specific periods of his life as opposed to just asking generally about the past. With a more specific focusing the clinician will gather much more data efficiently. Moreover, this question also illustrates the effective use of symptom amplification.

The clinician needs to discover whether the patient is indeed someone who is involved in fights primarily because of a violent neighborhood or whether the patient is frequently the instigator. This is not done by prematurely asking questions such as, "Do you pick a lot of fights?" Instead the clinician has waited until fighting itself has become a topic that has been discussed in detail and with ease. At this point the clinician moves towards uncovering the patient's role in these fights. If the patient denies any provocative role the clinician does not know whether to believe the patient or not. On the other hand, if the patient openly admits to self-incriminating behavior, then the validity of the information is probably reasonably high. Towards this end the clinician's phrasing has associated the tendency to pick fights with the use of alcohol, thus providing the patient something else to blame, in this case the bottle, for his own tendency to lose control.

A similar technique is used when entering the issue of grades. The clinician asks, "How did all the hassles at school affect your grades?" as opposed to asking something such as, "Did you have any problems with grades at school?" Once again the clinician has allowed the patient to blame the hassles at school as the culprits as opposed to poor study habits. At this point we see the implementation of an important principle in effectively expanding a personality disorder region.

The clinician has been gently but persistently focusing the interview into the content region of sociopathy. But when the patient brings up a bright spot in his academic career, the clinician flexibly takes time to talk about this bright spot and to stroke the patient for his accomplishment with the question, "Sounds like you did real well there. What did you like about history?" This ability to skillfully pepper the expansion of the content region with facilitory excursions and empathic interludes is pivotal to the development of the powerful blending needed to pursue sensitive material.

After allowing the patient to describe his interests in history and providing some positive feedback, the clinician reapproaches the topic of poor grades. This transition is made upon the tails of the positive reinforcement with, "You really did do well in history, did you ever have some difficulty with some courses?" The clinician eventually asks specifically about any failing grades. This quiet persistence frequently pays off with material that would otherwise be hidden or downplayed. Indeed this patient had previously stated that, "I did all right, grades weren't a big hassle." If the clinician had accepted this self-evaluation by the patient, then the truth that this patient had failed several courses and been required to attend summer school twice would never surfaced. This is a reminder of the need to hunt for behavioral incidents when the emphasis is upon validity.

Eventually the interviewer utilizes a referred gate to bring the discussion back to the patient's childhood in an effort to search for evidence of early sociopathic traits. The referred gate was as follows, "Jim, you mentioned earlier that your father had given you a rough time and that he would beat you if he felt you were pulling a fast one. Did you find that in order to protect yourself, you had to lie to him, keep him in the dark if you know what I mean." With this transition, the clinician has also managed to inquire about deceit in a fashion that is not antagonistic, once again offering a possible rationalization for the activity to the patient.

With his follow-up query, the clinician effectively utilizes the technique of shame reversal, "What about now, do you feel like if you have to you are pretty clever at deceit or are you a lousy liar?" With these techniques the clinician has actually reached a point in which the patient is openly admitting negative traits without any significant lowering of the blending process. This situation is providing a more valid data base for the clinician, while also making the interview far less threatening for the patient. It is more likely that this patient would return to this interviewer than to one who probed for sociopathic material in a rigid and checklist fashion, as if interrogating the patient.

This example also illustrates a major point. Although this represents a rather lengthy excerpt, the actual time involved in the interview is probably no more than around fifteen minutes. In this relatively short span the clinician is already close to having enough information to make not just a tentative diagnosis of sociopathy but an actual diagnosis of an antisocial personality disorder. This diagnosis could probably be shored up in another five to ten minutes. In this regard a personality disorder is being uncovered in roughly twenty to twenty-five minutes of interviewing time, emphasizing that lengthy interviews or multiple interviews are not always needed in order to make these diagnoses.

We have completed a review some of the techniques that may be useful in delineating a specific personality disorder. What remains is to examine the methods through which the clinician first gather hints as to which personality disorders may be present in the patient. We will also examine the reasoning that helps the clinician to choose the specific disorders to expand in detail, for the clinician can only hope to fully expand a few personality disorders or perhaps only one in a given hour.

B) Passively Scouting for Clues to Personality Dysfunction

Throughout the interview the clinician has the opportunity to reflect upon both the patient's words and actions. In this sense, without actively searching for clues to personality dysfunction, the astute clinician frequently picks up on a variety of hints as to which disorders may be worth pursuing in more detail. In this regard the clinician can focus upon the patient's behaviors and style of interaction (clinical signs) or upon the patient's related complaints and history (clinical symptoms). Both areas are rich with implication, providing pertinent clinical signals for any interviewer who cares to read them.

1) SIGNAL BEHAVIORS

Since personality disorders represent long-standing patterns of behavior, it is not unusual for patients to reveal some of their pathologic behaviors during the interview itself. This does not always occur, but it frequently occurs. I am consistently amazed with the frequency of times these signal behaviors occur in the first five to ten minutes of the interview during the scouting period. This early appearance of characteristic defensive behaviors may result from the patient's anxiety stimulated by meeting a clinician. This self system anxiety probably triggers many of the most ingrained defenses of the patient.

Earlier we discussed the mnemonic PACE as representing the mental activities of the clinician during the scouting period. If the reader will recall the "A" stands for an assessment of the patient's mental status and behaviors. An important part of this assessment process is the clinician's careful openness to the presence of signal behaviors. Signal behaviors may also appear during any subsequent phase of the interview as well.

The signal behaviors represent signs suggestive of specific personality disorders that may warrant further investigation. They do not indicate that the patient necessarily has these disorders, for these behaviors may be present in personality disorders other than the ones listed or in people without character pathology at all. But what the signal behaviors do suggest is the increased likelihood that a particular disorder may be present.

Each clinician could probably develop a long list of signal behaviors gleaned from experience. In this chapter I am sharing some of those that have been most useful for me. Many others exist, and I am not attempting an exhaustive study here. The following observations are derived from clinical experience and do not represent research-validated data. Nevertheless, I think they provide a useful jumping off point for clinicians who are attempting to master the fine art of delineating character pathology.

One of the more peculiar signal behaviors is the presence of comments made by the patient during the interview about the interview itself or the interviewer. Most patients do not make such process comments, for they are inhibited by the newness of the situation and do not want to do something that is wrong. I remember a young man who was being interviewed by a student in front of a group of fellow students. The patient had a dramatic intensity and related several times that he was an extremely sensitive individual. It has been said that if one has a good trait, one never needs to tell others about it. Such was the case with this "sensitive" patient, for in the middle of the interview he turned to the obviously struggling interviewer saying, "You sure seem to be having a lot more trouble with this interview than me." If the clinician was not feeling awkward enough already, then this statement certainly pulled out a few more beads of sweat.

This practice of commenting on the process of the interview, frequently in a somewhat caustic fashion, is often a dead give away that the clinician is speaking with one of the following four disorders: an antisocial personality, a histrionic personality, a borderline personality, or a passive-aggressive personality.

A somewhat related signal behavior arises when the patient makes some type of complaint during the interview itself. These complaints may be coupled with demands of a subtle nature and sometimes of a not so subtle nature. For example, a patient may walk in the door for the first appointment announcing that the patient does not intend to sit in the waiting room so long the next time. Or the patient may begin, "You really should get better parking arrangements for your patients, although I'm sure you've already looked into this matter before (topped off with a pleasant smile)." Such behaviors are often the window dressings of disorders such as the following ones: a passive-aggressive personality, a borderline personality, a narcissistic personality, a paranoid personality, or an antisocial personality.

At the other extreme one may encounter the patient who seems a little too pleased with the clinician. These are the patients who drop gentle sexual innuendoes during the interview. This may consist of overly frank discussions of sexual adventures or may be more blunt, such as overt offers for a date or the request of a telephone number. In other instances the patient may turn on the charm with phrases such as, "Well, I've always seemed to be fairly attractive to the opposite sex, as I'm sure you have found to be true for yourself." These types of comments represent signal behaviors for disorders such as the following: an antisocial personality, a histrionic personality, and a narcissistic personality. If the innuendoes become more lewd or intrusive, one should become even more alert to the possible presence of an antisocial personality.

This type of behavior is similar to the patient who presents with a dramatic bravado. The patient may be boldly dressed in bright colors or a sinewy scarf. Breasts may be nearly bursting from tight sweaters or legs may be sensually wrapped about each other. The patient is frequently quite enthralled with the very act of talking about the history of the present illness while animatedly gesturing. Frequently the patient may rapidly become tearful and even more rapidly shut off the tears when the clinician asks a new line of questioning. These types of behaviors should serve as an indication that one may be in the presence of a histrionic personality or a borderline personality.

Another type of signal behavior consists of the patient who appears childlike and helpless. These patients may speak with a quiet meekness, accompanied by an earnest attempt to please the interviewer with statements such as, "Is this what you wanted to hear?" As one would suspect such behaviors are often the trademarks of the dependent personality. Such helplessness is sometimes also seen episodically with histrionic personalities and with borderline personalities.

As a final example of a signal behavior, we can look at those patients who become openly manipulative during the interview itself. They may attempt to make the clinician grant them a request or make a condemnation of another clinician. For instance the patient may say, "My current therapist is very bossy. Don't you think that is strange for a therapist." The patient then waits anxiously for the clinician to make a disparaging comment that will undoubtedly be fired as a verbal salvo at the therapist in question. Other types of manipulations may consist of various methods of controlling the interview or bargaining with the clinician, "Look it's getting late, if we must talk let's do it quickly and I need a cigarette first." Once again we've hit the province of the more primitive disorders such as the borderline personality, the histrionic personality, and the narcissistic personality. Such "sighing compliance" may also mark the passive-aggressive personality (See Figure 9 for a summary of signal behaviors).

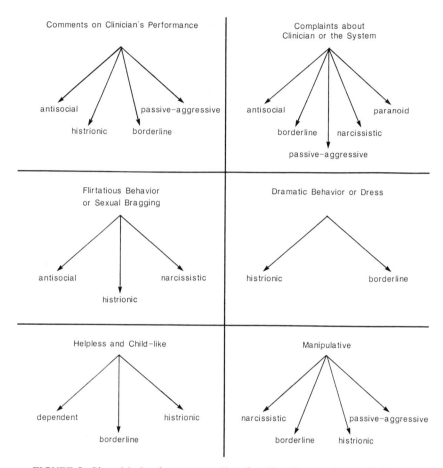

FIGURE 9. *Signal behaviors suggesting fan-like diagnostic possibilities.*

To wrap up this discussion of signal behaviors, an actual clinical example may serve to consolidate some of the ideas. The following activities occurred primarily in the minutes directly preceding the interview and in the first few minutes of the interview itself. The interview was taped for supervision purposes. The patient, who we had discussed earlier in the chapter on nonverbal behavior, had come to the Diagnostic and Evaluation Center because "I'm having problems coping." For the sake of convenience the patient will be called Ms. Dole. Ms. Dole was dressed somewhat shabbily with worn-out corduroy trousers and a faded blouse. Her dull brown hair seemed to "come with the outfit" in the sense that it too had seen better days, as it hung in long folds. Her lengthy hair accented her lanky body.

Both she and the clinician began placing their respective microphones. Ms. Dole fumbled repeatedly with her microphone, until her awkward machinations attracted the eye of the interviewer. Immediately before the clinician looked at Ms. Dole a most curious process unfolded. Ms. Dole had actually managed to get the microphone on, but promptly pulled it off. As the clinician asked if she could manage, Ms. Dole looked up with pleading eyes and nodded her head from side to side, never saying a word. She looked like a three-year-old asking her mother for help. And help was quickly on the way, for the clinician proceeded to attach the microphone for her.

When the interviewer began the actual interview, Ms. Dole quietly handed her some notes, mumbling that these would help the interviewer to understand. "I wrote them a few days ago," she meekly related. At which point the interviewer watched as Ms. Dole fumbled with the papers, taking about a minute to find the passage she wanted read.

Ms. Dole was managing to rapidly gain control of the interview by utilizing a mixture of helpless ineffectuality and manipulative staging. Her helplessness may have represented a signal behavior suggestive of the presence of a borderline personality or a dependent personality. Her manipulative gestures would also be consistent with a histrionic personality, a borderline personality, or a passive-aggressive personality. Subsequent detailed interviewing resulted in a diagnosis of a mixed personality disorder with histrionic, dependent, and passive-aggressive traits. Thus the first three minutes of interaction provided powerful clues as to which diagnostic regions needed further exploration. Sometimes an interviewer's eyes are more useful than his or her questions.

2) SIGNAL SYMPTOMS

As the interview proceeds, the patient frequently relates symptoms or pieces of behavior that may function to guide the clinician towards consideration of specific personality disorders. Once again, as with signal behaviors, the clinician is not actively eliciting these symptoms. Instead, the patient is spontaneously providing them; the clinician needs to only passively recognize their importance.

Some signal symptoms are classic for certain disorders. This does not mean that these symptoms are only seen in these disorders but rather that they are frequently characteristic of these disorders. For instance, the presence of a history of self-mutilation or of frequent suicide gestures should always alert the clinician to the possibility of a borderline personality disorder. People with borderline personalities are notorious for behaviors such as wrist slashing, burning themselves with cigarettes, headbanging, and frequent overdoses.

Another classic signal symptom is the reporting by the patient of an extreme need for perfectionism. This is frequently accompanied by a nagging sensation that the patient has never done enough. It is the mark of a superego run amok and should strongly suggest the presence of an obsessive-compulsive personality or at least some compulsive traits.

A third relatively classic signal symptom is the reporting of a history of run-ins with the law. Repeated arrests, burglary, or frequent fights all strongly suggest the need to expand the antisocial personality region. Other areas to explore include fencing drugs, prostitution, and arrests for disorderly conduct or drunken driving. When asked about arrests, patients frequently conveniently fail to mention the last two types of incidents. It is often best to specifically inquire about disorderly conduct and drunken driving as well as speeding.

Other signal symptoms suggest not just one disorder but a variety of disorders. In a sense these signal symptoms suggest a fanlike differential diagnosis. The presence of frequent feelings of anger, sometimes accompanied by actual physical violence, alerts the clinician to the likely presence of either an antisocial personality or a borderline personality. Other less likely components of the fan include the paranoid personality, the narcissistic personality, and the histrionic personality. The passive aggressive personality is seldom associated with actual violence but frequently complains of angry feelings.

A different signal symptom consists of extreme feeling of low self-esteem. Such intense feelings of worthlessness and inadequacy are frequently seen in the dependent personality, the avoidant personality, the schizotypal personality, and the borderline personality. Figure 10 illustrates some of the various signal symptoms and the possible diagnoses they suggest.

It should be kept in mind that the characteristics that were used earlier to group the various personality disorders may also serve as signal symptoms. Thus the reporting by the patient of powerful and persistent feelings of anxiety should alert the clinician to the possible presence of the obsessive compulsive personality, the dependent personality, the avoidant personality, and the passive-aggressive personality. In a similar fashion the antisocial personality, the histrionic personality, the schizoid personality, and the narcissistic personality are all suggested by a tendency for the patient to demonstrate a poor ability to empathize effectively. Finally, the presence of frequent micropsychotic breaks should alert the clinician to the potential presence of the primitive personality disorders including the borderline personality, the schizotypal personality, and the paranoid personality.

It takes some time for clinicians to begin to routinely recognize the significance of signal behaviors and signal symptoms. But with experience the ability to utilize these invaluable clues becomes almost second

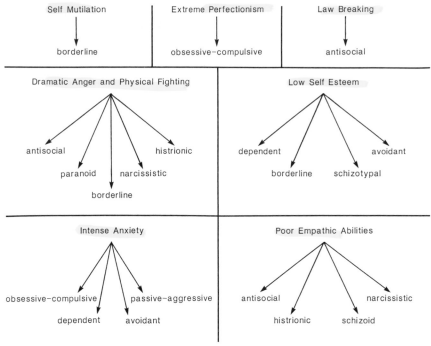

FIGURE 10. Signal symptoms suggesting diagnostic possibilities.

nature. It should be readily apparent that many patients will in the course of thirty minutes practically point the way for the clinician as to the most likely paths to provide concrete evidence of personality psychopathology. The clinician does not have to rely solely upon spontaneous clues by the patient. Instead the interviewer can actively try to draw out evidence of personality dysfunction.

C) Active Scouting and the Finalized Delineation of Specific Personality Disorders

There are two active methods of delineating personality dysfunction. The first technique consists of asking so-called probe questions[10] concerning a specific disorder. If the patient answers negatively to the probe questions, the clinician does not further expand that specific disorder. On the other hand, positive answers suggest that further questioning may uncover a specific disorder. The second technique consists of the further questioning just mentioned. The craft of delicately and thoroughly substantiating a personality diagnosis requires both skill and a sense of timing. The talented interviewer doggedly pursues the evidence needed to make the diagnosis but does so in a manner that fosters both a more powerful blending and an increased understanding of the patient not as a label but as an individual.

First let us examine a list of probe questions for personality disorders, several of which were developed by Jeremy Roberts.

1. Obsessive Compulsive Personality
   a. Do you tend to drive yourself pretty hard, frequently feeling like you need to do just a little more? (yes)
   b. Do you think that most people would view you as witty and light-hearted? (no)
   c. Do you tend towards being perfectionistic? (yes)
   d. Do you tend to keep lists or sometimes feel a need to keep checking things, like is the door locked? (yes)
2. Passive-Aggressive Personality
   a. Do you frequently feel like your friends or employers tend to take you a little too much for granted? (yes)
   b. Sometimes have bosses tended to nag you, you know, ask you to do something a couple of times? (yes)
   c. If your boss asks you to do something that is stupid or that you disagree with, do you sometimes try to make a point by doing it slowly or without your full effort? (yes)
   d. When others are overly optimistic, do you tend to be the one who shows them the problems with their plans? (yes)
3. Dependent Personality
   a. Is it sort of hard for you to argue with your spouse, because you're worried that he or she will really get mad at you and start to dislike you? (yes)
   b. When you wake up in the morning, do you tend to plan your day around the activities of your husband or wife? (yes)
   c. Do you enjoy making most decisions in your house or would you prefer that others make most important decisions? (prefers others to make the decisions)
   d. When you were younger, did you often dream of finding someone who would take care of you and guide you? (yes)
4. Avoidant Personality
   a. Throughout most of your life, have you found yourself being worried that people won't like you? (yes)
   b. Do you often find yourself sort of feeling inadequate and not up to new challenges or tasks? (yes)
   c. Do you tend to be very careful about selecting friends, perhaps only having one or two close friends in your whole life? (yes)
   d. Have you often felt hurt by others, so that you are pretty wary of opening yourself to other people? (yes)

5. Schizoid Personality
   a. Do you tend to really enjoy being around people or do you much prefer being alone? (much prefers being alone)
   b. Do you care a lot about what people think about you as a person? (tends not to care)
   c. Are you a real emotional person? (no, feels strongly that he or she is not emotional)
   d. During the course of your life have you had only about one or two friends? (yes)
6. Antisocial Personality
   a. If you felt like the situation really warranted it, do you think that you would find it pretty easy to lie? (yes)
   b. Have you ever been arrested or pulled over by the police? (yes)
   c. Over the years have you found yourself able to take care of yourself in physical fights? (yes)
   d. Do you sometimes find yourself resenting people who give you orders? (yes)
7. Histrionic Personality
   a. Do people of the opposite sex frequently find you attractive? (answered with an unabashed "yes")
   b. Do you frequently find yourself being the center of attention, even if you don't want to? (yes)
   c. Do you view yourself as being a powerfully emotional person? (yes)
   d. Do you think that you'd make a reasonably good actor or actress? (yes)
8. Narcissistic Personality
   a. Do you find that when you really get down to it, most people aren't quite up to your standards? (yes)
   b. If people give you a hard time, do you tend to put them in their place quickly? (yes)
   c. If someone criticizes you, do you find yourself getting angry pretty quickly? (yes)
   d. Do you think that compared to other people you are a very special person? (answered with a self-assured "yes")
9. Borderline Personality
   a. Do you frequently feel let down by people? (yes)
   b. If a friend or a family member hurts you, do you sometimes feel like hurting yourself, perhaps by cutting at yourself or burning yourself? (yes)
   c. Do you find that other people cause you to feel angry a couple of times per week? (yes)
   d. Do you think that your friends would view you as sort of moody? (yes)

10. Schizotypal Personality
    a. Do you tend to stay by yourself, even though you would like to be with others? (yes)
    b. Do you sometimes feel like other people are watching you or have some sort of special interest in you? (yes)
    c. Have you ever felt like you had some special powers like ESP or some sort of magical influence over others? (yes)
    d. Do you feel that people often want to reject you or that they find you odd? (yes)
11. Paranoid Personality
    a. Do you find that people often have a tendency to be disloyal or dishonest? (yes)
    b. Is it fairly easy for you to get jealous, especially if someone is making eyes at your spouse? (yes)
    c. Do you tend to keep things to yourself just to make sure the wrong people don't get the right information? (yes)
    d. Do you feel that other people take advantage of you? (yes)

Responses in the indicated direction to one or two of these questions suggests that it would be worth the clinician's time to pursue the personality disorder in more detail. Some of these questions may overlap, and positive answers may be consistent with several different diagnoses. For example, if the patient responds positively to the probe question for the paranoid personality concerning jealousy, several other disorders may also be worth considering. Jealousy is commonly seen in narcissistic personalities, histrionic personalities, and borderline personalities. But an effort has been made in compiling these questions to list those questions that tend to be more specific for each of the diagnoses for which the question serves as a probe. If the patient responds positively to several or all of the probe questions, then it is significantly more likely that the specific probe diagnosis will eventually prove to be valid.

These probe questions are never used in a checklist fashion, but are quietly woven into the fabric of the natural flow of the interview. The clinician will probably only have time to utilize a few of the specific probes for each diagnosis. Fortunately, in this sense, probe questions can often serve to quickly eliminate certain diagnoses. If one asks the following probe for schizoid qualities, "Do you really enjoy being around people or do you much prefer being alone?" and the patient responds, "Oh I love being around people, I'm a party animal" one can safely assume that a schizoid personality is not in the room. All levity aside the point of the matter is that certain answers are inconsistent with certain diagnoses and no further probing would be required.

In point of fact, the clinician will probably not ask most of these questions, for the passive clues given by the patient as described earlier will automatically eliminate many diagnoses, while pointing the way towards those with more potential. Those areas with more potential can then be actively scouted by using several of the probe questions, and, if the diagnosis appears more likely, the clinician will proceed with a more thorough exploration in order to substantiate it.

One may wonder whether there are regions of the interview where it is best to utilize probe questions and to explore for personality dysfunction. The answer to this question is that the interviewer can utilize these techniques essentially anywhere in the body of the interview, but there is one area, the social history, in which personality pathology virtually leaps out at the interviewer, if it has not already done so in the history of the present illness.

As mentioned before, the social history represents the region of the interview in which patients inadvertently discuss the impact of their personalities on the people and jobs behind them. Many signal symptoms will be given here, and probe questions can be utilized effectively to determine which personality disorders warrant a more thorough exploration. Since the social history frequently is not taken in detail until a later part of the body of the interview, the blending has usually had time to develop strongly, thus allowing the clinician to more effectively explore the sensitive types of material frequently associated with personality disorders.

In the following example we will watch a clinician as he delineates which areas of personality dysfunction warrant more careful exploration. The dialogue occurs during the social history. Some of the clinical thinking that might be guiding such an interview is presented in brackets.

> ***Clin.:*** After you left college what happened?
> ***Pt.:*** Let's see, uh, I think the first job I took was with the electric company, but that job didn't really pan out to be what I was promised.
> ***Clin.:*** In what sort of ways?
> ***Pt.:*** Oh, the job was really boring and the pay wasn't so hot either. So I left after about three months and eventually got a job in sales. I liked that much better. I stayed there for, let me see, maybe a year, and then I had a whole string of jobs.
> ***Clin.:*** In the five years following that time how many jobs do you think you had, a couple, twenty, thirty? [symptom amplification]
> ***Pt.:*** Oh, pretty many, maybe close to twenty jobs. [The large

number of jobs, in a relatively short period of time, certainly suggests that something is up here. An erratic job history is a signal symptom frequently suggesting the presence of an underlying antisocial personality, as well as any personality with a tendency for erratic relationships and impulsivity. Consequently the clinician asks several probes concerning sociopathy.]

Clin.: Did anything ever happen on some of these jobs, like having a problem with the law or an arrest, that made you have to leave, because sometimes that's why people leave jobs quickly?

Pt.: Oh no, not with me boy. I don't like the police. They terrify me. I've never been arrested or even pulled over for running a light.

Clin.: Doesn't sound like you have a very extensive criminal record. (clinician smiles and patient laughs)

Pt.: No, it sure doesn't. I don't break the laws. In that regard I'm a pretty straight arrow.

Clin.: What about things like using drugs or selling drugs.

Pt.: Nope, I wouldn't touch them, never even tried them. I just don't think it's right to use illegal drugs, that may sound sort of corny but it's true. [This patient shows little evidence of sociopathy, in fact he seems to have a fairly strong sense of what is right or wrong. Thus there must be something else going on. The clinician will now switch the focus more towards social interaction and friendships.]

Clin.: What kinds of things do you like to do for fun?

Pt.: Now that's a good question, because I don't have a lot of fun. I'm really pretty much of a loner. Sometimes I think that I just wasn't made to get along well with people, so I keep to myself pretty much. [Here a variety of options are opening up. A schizoid personality classically describes himself or herself as being a "loner," but they frequently hold jobs down well. Moreover, the openness and talkativeness of this patient earlier in the interview are uncharacteristic of the schizoid personality. On the other hand, some of the disorders that are rejection sensitive lead to the avoidance of people as a means of protection. The clinician decides to figure out if the patient shuns people because he does not really want the company of people (as with a schizoid personality) or because he fears the company of people (as with an avoidant personality).]

Clin.:   If you had some better skills at being around people, do you think you would like to do that?

Pt.:   Oh yes, I have always wanted to be popular and sometimes I really do enjoy people. I love to laugh, but somehow I always end up getting hurt. [The schizoid personality has been essentially eliminated, for such patients seldom if ever strive for social interaction in the fashion this patient is describing. The feelings of inferiority and inadequacy expressed by this patient also make it unlikely that we are dealing with an entity like a narcissistic personality.]

Clin.:   Do you frequently feel let down or hurt by people?

Pt.:   Very frequently. And to be quite frank it angers me, and that's why I've basically decided to keep my distance, but that's no fun either. And I resent that. Why should I be the one that suffers, what do they want from me anyway? [Plenty of important data is coming to light now. The patient truly sounds rejection sensitive. Entities come to mind such as the schizotypal personality, the dependent personality, the avoidant personality, the histrionic personality, the passive-aggressive personality, and the borderline personality. That is quite a string of possibilities, but they can be decreased relatively rapidly. First, in an earlier part of the interview, when the region of psychotic material was being reviewed, the patient denied any psychotic material even of a subtle nature. Consequently the schizotypal personality is not worth pursuing. A careful sensitivity to the material already uncovered reveals another interesting point. People with dependent personalities and with avoidant personalities tend to stay in jobs for a long time, because they fear new situations, tending to dislike the process of job interviewing or meeting new coworkers. To sort out this situation better, the clinician refers back to the job history, to see if the erratic history may be related to interpersonal problems with bosses or with coworkers. If frequent angry interactions are uncovered, then one could essentially rule out more timid entities such as the dependent personality and the avoidant personality.]

Clin.:   Earlier you mentioned that you changed jobs frequently. Did you find that some of the people you were around were difficult people to work with? [utilization of shame reversal]

> **Pt.:** As a matter of fact I did, some of them were very difficult.
> **Clin.:** What types of arguments would you get into?
> **Pt.:** The usual kind, you know, a boss who can't let you do your own work and who asks you to do things one way one time and another the next. I hate that. I never know what they want. Now don't get me wrong, I sometimes had something to do with it too, but not usually, at least I don't think so.
> **Clin.:** Did some of the bosses get angry and ask you to leave?
> **Pt.:** Yeah, I've been fired a couple of times if that's what you mean. And I think it's been fifty-fifty.
> **Clin.:** How do you mean?
> **Pt.:** Fifty percent of the time my fault and fifty percent of the time their fault. [The demonstration of open anger, the firings, and the tendency to see a lot of other people at fault all essentially eliminate the dependent personality and the avoidant personality as suggested before. This pattern is also certainly not the job history of a compulsive personality.]

At this point the differential is becoming a good deal more manageable. We are left with the histrionic personality, the passive-aggressive personality, and the borderline personality. The patient's history is thus far consistent with all three, but the histrionic personality seems less likely for several reasons. In the first place, not too many histrionic personalities view themselves as socially inept, and despite repeated painful experiences they seldom become more reclusive. The better bets are probably the borderline personality and the passive-aggressive personality. One thing ruling against the borderline personality is that, thus far, the patient seems to have a reasonably strong ego, in the sense that there is no history of micropsychotic breakdowns or violent outbursts.

Probably the more likely diagnosis is going to be a passive-aggressive personality or perhaps a mixed personality with histrionic, borderline, and passive-aggressive traits. It is also possible that the patient will prove to fit the criteria for both a passive-aggressive personality and a mixed personality with histrionic and borderline traits. Thus, in a relatively short time, the clinician, by utilizing the social history, has narrowed the regions worth exploring in detail to two or three entities. If pressed for time, the clinician would probably choose to thoroughly expand the most likely diagnosis, the passive-aggressive personality.

This example illustrates how quickly the clinician can begin to develop a differential along Axis II, by utilizing passive techniques, such as recognizing signal behaviors and signal symptoms in conjunction with the more active technique of asking probe questions. What remains is for the clinician to skillfully expand the most likely diagnosis in a graceful and noninvasive manner.

To sculpt out the diagnosis in this fashion, the clinician must become intimately familiar with the specific criteria for each diagnosis in the DSM-III-R. Such familiarity comes both from conscientious study and, more powerfully, from experience. The process is greatly enhanced as the clinician develops a more sophisticated feel for the manner in which these diagnoses present and what it is like to be this particular patient with this particular style of "being in the world" in a more phenomenological sense. Once again the skillful blending of empathy, intuition, and analytic reasoning remains critical to the art of crafting a successful interview.

In order to delineate the principles behind performing a sensitive and thorough expansion of a personality disorder, we will focus upon a single example to serve as an illustration. The enigmatic diagnosis of the borderline personality disorder will be examined in more detail. In some respects this diagnosis remains somewhat controversial. But despite its controversy, it stands as one of the diagnoses that in certain instances, may more readily be made in a single interview, for many of its criteria are behavioral in nature. Those criteria, which are of a more subjective nature, tend to be unique enough that they are fairly easy to spot.

Before continuing with an examination of the phenomenology of the disorder, it is of value to look at some of the thoughts regarding its etiology, for here is where much of the controversy resides. In my opinion, the radically unstable nature of the moods and perceptions of these people may truly be multiply determined. Some people who have this behavioral presentation may have developed it more from one etiology in one case and more from another etiology in a different case. Thus, some borderline personalities may represent people with subaffective disorders, whose chaotic emotionality may be intimately related to biological malfunction, much like some major depressions or dysthymias. In this regard, it is not unusual to find patients who fulfill the criteria for dysthymia as well as a borderline personality. Others may represent people with subthreshold seizure activity, which is missed by the equipment currently available to the electroencephalographer. Another percentage of these patients may prove to be people suffering from an unresolved attention deficit disorder as it appears in adulthood. The impulsiveness, moodiness, and inability to achieve stable relationships as seen with the borderline personality is highly reminiscent of the child with an attention deficit disorder with hyperactivity.

There may also be a subgroup of these patients whose problems stem mainly from more purely psychological and environmental difficulties. To me some of these patients are best regarded as having significant developmental delays in their cognitive abilities, much as Piaget would describe cognitive deficits. This view has been championed by Gerald Adler in his book *Borderline Psychopathology and Its Treatment.*[11] For instance, these patients may not have fully developed such basic cognitive skills as being able "to see the grey" in situations as opposed to always seeing black or white, possessing an ability to consider past experiences when evaluating current experiences, or being able to develop a strong sense of object constancy (even with regard to themselves). A more thorough examination of these cognitive deficits will lead us into a richer understanding of the phenomenology of these patients.

Taking just one of these deficits, the inability to see grey, the world of the borderline personality becomes at once more comprehensible and intriguing. If the patient with a borderline personality must always clump experiences into extremes, then the simplest of frustrations or rejections may be interpreted quite naturally as a vicious attack. By way of example, if the clinician must cancel an appointment because of an unexpected meeting, then the borderline personality is limited, by his or her inability to see grey, into hearing from the clinician only one of two things, either "I care about you" or "I don't care about you." In this instance the words of the clinician are more on the unpleasant side than the pleasant, so they are immediately transformed into the latter cognitive interpretation, and it is no wonder that the patient subsequently slams the phone down yelling, "You really are a son of a bitch aren't you?" Such a response is no different than the small child who berates his mother for not buying the toy airplane with an, "I hate you. I hate you!" The child sees the denial as a true rejection, a black act.

Meanwhile, at the other end of the phone, the clinician sits dumbfounded, wondering what went wrong. In actuality, the "irrationally" angry response of the patient is not as irrational as it may seem at first glance. It would be irrational for a person with a normal ability to see grey to respond in such a fashion, for the normal response would be to view this cancellation as disappointing but understandable. On the other hand, if a person simply did not have the cognitive ability to see grey, then the angry response is reasonably appropriate, for this patient literally "heard" the therapist state, rather boldly, that the therapist did not care about the patient. In essence, the psychological deficit is more with the patient's ability to interpret the environment than in the patient's actual display of anger. From this viewpoint, the patient's unsettling rages may be understood from a more compassionate

stance, realizing the tremendously punishing interpersonal environment that these patients must encounter on a daily basis.

This tendency for seeing only the black or the white may tip off
interviewers that they are in the presence of borderline psychopathology. The clinician may even see the patient rapidly change opinions
about the interviewer as the interview unfolds. Such developmentally
delayed manners of cognitively interpreting the world can also be seen
in other primitive personality disorders, including the paranoid personality, the schizotypal personality, and the more regressed forms of
the narcissistic personality. In mild degrees it can be seen in all of us
and can lead to a variety of neurotic tensions.

To illustrate the tendency for the borderline personality to display black or white perception in the course of the interview itself, I am
reminded of a young woman, who I interviewed directly after another
clinician. The patient quickly began, "You know, the person I was just
talking with didn't seem to know what she was doing. I didn't like her.
I'm not going to have to talk with her again, am I?" As our interview
proceeded, the patient seemed to warm to me relatively quickly, eventually stating that she would not mind working with me. She eventually attempted to demand placement on a specific inpatient unit,
which we felt was inappropriate for her. When I told her that she would
not be able to go to that particular unit, she angrily pouted. Later her
boyfriend came up to me privately saying, "My girlfriend is very displeased with you, and frankly so am I." More classic borderline behavior could not be found. I jumped from Prince Charming to Idi Amin in a
single bound. This type of rapid idealization-devaluation is a classic
signal behavior suggestive of borderline psychopathology or some
other primitive personality.

This patient also displayed a trait, commonly seen with borderline
personalities, loosely known as "splitting," in which the patient attempts to pit one person against another. This was demonstrated when
she told me her complaints about the previous interviewer. It was also
demonstrated by her ability to eventually pit her boyfriend against me.

In considering a different cognitive delay seen with borderline
patients, one can also imagine the havoc that the lack of an ability to
view objects as stable could have on an individual. In this regard, being
a borderline personality is a little like being a toddler who rolls a ball
under a couch and believes the ball to have literally vanished into
nonexistence. A good cry will soon follow as the child finds that its
favorite playtoy has disappeared. People with borderline development
may have problems believing in the constancy of those who love them.
Consequently, these patients may frequently feel abandoned. Even
more curious is the disturbing quality of the borderline personality to
feel almost empty inside, as if his own sense of self were mercurial.

They may become very dependent upon the presence of others for a sense of security, frequently going to frantic efforts to avoid being alone, a condition in which they feel that they risk the same annihilation that the errant rubber ball encountered. For people with a normal cognitive development, this type of world view is very difficult to empathize with, but it occurs nevertheless. I have never seen it quite so elegantly described as by D. H. Lawrence in his novel *Women in Love*.

And yet her soul was tortured, exposed. Even walking up the path of the church, confident as she was that in every respect she stood beyond all vulgar judgment, knowing perfectly that her appearance was complete and perfect, according to the first standards, yet she suffered a torture, under her confidence and her pride, feeling herself exposed to wounds and to mockery and to despite. She always felt vulnerable, vulnerable, there was always a secret chink in her armour. She did not know herself what it was. It was a lack of robust self, she had no natural sufficiency, there was a terrible void, a lack, a deficiency of being within her.

And she wanted someone to close up this deficiency, to close it up for ever. She craved for Rupert Birkin. When he was there, she felt complete, she was sufficient, whole. For the rest of time she was established on the sand, built over a chasm, and, in spite of all her vanity and securities, any common maid-servant of positive, robust temper could fling her down this bottomless pit of insufficiency, by the slightest movement of jeering or contempt. And all the while the pensive, tortured woman piled up her own defences of aesthetic knowledge, and culture, and world-visions, and disinterestedness. Yet she could never stop up the terrible gap of insufficiency.[12]

This particular character may or may not completely fit the designation of a borderline personality, but this description of the hollowness experienced by the borderline could not be more convincing.

Returning to an actual patient, I remember a woman who described feeling intensely angry at her partner anytime her partner would roll over to fall asleep. Suddenly the patient was left with herself and experienced a disquieting sense of panic, like a lost child, who suddenly realizes that a parent is not nearby in a department store. At these moments she would feel acutely abandoned by her partner, deeply resenting her partner's need for sleep.

With these ideas in mind let us watch a clinician expanding the diagnostic region of a borderline personality. The patient was a casually dressed woman with dark brown hair that was somewhat unkempt. She spoke with a curious blandness, as if commenting upon a character viewed from afar as opposed to her own life. She tended to have poor eye contact, which seemed purposeful, as if she would look at you if she felt moved to do so. Earlier aspects of the interview had demonstrated that the patient had experienced, besides her current episode, only a single bout of major depression in her life. She also denied a history of manic episodes. The immediate reason for her presentation involved her transfer from another hospital. Apparently she had been doing reasonably well, but when she went down to the patient store, she bought a bottle of aspirin and promptly ingested all twenty-four tablets. She conveniently waited awhile before presenting to her physician's secretary at a time when he was out. She proceeded to casually inform the secretary that she had just overdosed. We will join the conversation roughly midway in the body of the interview:

Clin.: Mrs. Jacobs, tell me a little more about what led up to your overdose?

Pt.: In the first place, I told him I was going to do it. I really did, but I guess nobody wanted to believe me. Now Dr. Johnson claims I said that I was all done hurting myself, maybe I did, but I sure don't remember telling him that. In fact, I told him I was feeling impulsive like I might overdose, maybe he was just thinking differently, I don't know. But my husband thinks he blew it, and he's real mad that Dr. Johnson let me go down to that store. And it was so easy, I just cut off my patient wrist band and they sold me a bottle of aspirin (patient smiles).

Clin.: You seem to have some mixed feelings for Dr. Johnson.

Pt.: Do I? . . . Well I suppose I do. I really like him but I think he's dumping me by sending me here. He says he'll take me back, I don't know. You see, I liked my psychologist before Dr. Johnson and I never would have believed I could work with anyone but him, but I got along well eventually with Dr. Johnson too. I guess he'll take me back, but he's mad at me even though I told him.

Clin.: With both Dr. Johnson and your previous therapist you seem to have formed strong relationships. Has that been typical of yourself, say back in junior high and high school?

Pt.: Oh yeah (said in a somewhat disinterested fashion). I always seem to have this thing for an older man who will sort of guide me, help me with my development. That's happened a lot with me, maybe I have a thing for father figures, I don't know. But I had several teachers who I was very close to and there was a minister of our church group who helped a lot too. I'd rather spend my time with these kinds of men.

Clin.: Did you ever find that some of these friends would later let you down and you learned to dislike them?

Pt.: Oh yes, people use me for a doormat. Reverend Jenkins was a good example. I viewed him as very special, like almost a saint or something, but I wasn't special to him. He saw hundreds of other people in his congregation, I mean there I was sharing my deepest feelings and he'd soon be listening to another person's problems, just like I was one of them.

Clin.: Back around that time, during your school years, what were your friendships like?

Pt.: They weren't so hot. My mother always told me I was the most gifted kid, but look how I turned out, I wasn't that popular, and people are all basically bastards, trust me.

Clin.: Did you form any friendships in your life that have lasted for over four or five years?

Pt.: Not really . . . let me . . . no . . . not real friends.

Clin.: What usually happens to your friendships?

Pt.: We end up having an argument or something like that, and I tell them off or they tell me off. For some reason people always seem to take advantage of me and it makes me angry?

Clin.: When you get angry, do you tend to keep your anger bottled up inside or do you tend to let it out, maybe by yelling at the person or throwing something?

Pt.: I keep a lot of it in, but when I let go I can get pretty mean, I mean I have thrown things, I threw a plate at my husband when we were on a pass about two weeks ago.

Clin.: I know you've been feeling pretty depressed recently, how about just when you're feeling your normal self, how many times do you think you've broken things when some one angered you?

Pt.: Oh I've done that, probably more times than I could count easily, I remember throwing down my husband's camera, that set him off.

Clin.: Sounds like it would. What's the biggest thing you've ever broken?

Pt.: My husband's nose (patient smiles and both patient and clinician chuckle).

Clin.: Pretty big nose huh?

Pt.: Yeah and it got bigger.

Clin.: Well, what about when you're feeling very angry, say back in your school days again, did you ever pound your fists into a wall?

Pt.:   Oh yeah, I put my fist in the wall once, my mother almost screamed, but then she needed shaking up a bit.

Clin.:   Some patients tell me that when they get really angry, they might even pound their heads against the wall, just to get the anger out. Have you ever felt that way?

Pt.:   I think I've done that, yeah I think I've done that.

Clin.:   What do you remember?

Pt.:   A long time ago I used to do that, not a lot though, sort of sounds silly, hurt too. You know, I've done this too. (Mrs. Jacobs rolls up her sleeve and reveals some small scars on her wrist, her affect also hardens a bit, with a very mildly angry undertone.)

Clin.:   Looks like you've cut at yourself at times. Is that what these marks are?

Pt.:   Yeah, that's what they are all right.

Clin.:   Did it hurt when you cut at yourself?

Pt.:   Not really, I just sort of like to watch it bleed.

Clin.:   What makes you stop?

Pt.:   I've never figured that one out, somehow it just feels better, I feel like it's all over.

Clin.:   Like what's all over?

Pt.:   The anger, the pain, I don't know, all I know is I'm probably going to do it again, 'cause I like it. And you're not going to stop me.

Clin.:   Are you worried that I'm going to try to stop you?

Pt.:   No I'm not, 'cause I know you can't.

Clin.:   I think you're right about the fact that I can't ultimately stop you, only you would be able to do that and right now you don't want to. So let's not focus on that right now, we'll come back to it a little later on. With all these tough times you've had, and you've had some tough ones, do you feel that your moods change pretty rapidly?

Pt.:   Yeah that's something I don't like. And if you could help me with that, I'd appreciate it.

Clin.:   Do your moods ever change rapidly in a single day, you know, you might wake up in one mood and somebody says something and boom you're in a bad mood and three hours later you're O.K. again.

Pt.:   Oh yeah, I'm moody, just like that.

Clin.:   Do you think your parents or friends in high school viewed you as moody?

Pt.:   Sure, I've always been a moody person and people just have to learn to live with my moods. I don't try to be irritable, but sometimes I can't help it.

Clin.: What about when you're alone, what is your mood like for you when you are all by yourself, say back in your apartment?

Pt.: Sometimes I like it and sometimes I don't.

Clin.: When you don't like it, what does it feel like?

Pt.: I just don't like it, I get depressed.

Clin.: Say a friend of yours just left for the evening. As the door shuts and you suddenly find yourself alone, does your mood ever change as that door shuts?

Pt.: Yes it does, sometimes I feel really bad, like a piece of me has been torn away, and sometimes I get angry, sometimes that's when I cut myself. I really am a moody person, and I don't know what to do about it. I guess that's why Dr. Johnson hates me now (Mrs. Jacobs becomes quietly sadder).

Clin.: When you feel depressed like that, do you ever start to feel almost empty inside, like a piece of you is missing?

Pt.: Sort of, I don't know if I would phrase it that way.

Clin.: What does it feel like to you, that's what I'm most interested in understanding.

Pt.: Dead. I feel dead.

Clin.: With the deadness, do you frequently feel bored?

Pt.: No, not really. But it's as if a part of me were not in the room, it's very hard to explain, but it is very unpleasant. My husband just simply can't understand it. He can be such a mean person, but then I guess I've let him down. I let all the people down at the hospital.

Clin.: How do you mean?

Pt.: I think my friends back at the hospital were disappointed that I tried to hurt myself. Maybe they're worried I might lose control. Will I be on a locked ward?

Clin.: Yes the ward will be locked. I guess that can be sort of scary, are you worried about it?

Pt.: Yeah, but I guess they better lock me up.

Although this illustration is somewhat lengthy, it probably only required around fifteen minutes of interviewing time. In this relatively short period of time, the clinician has uncovered a variety of characteristics seen in the borderline personality, including mood instability, chronic feelings of emptiness, tendencies for idealization alternating with devaluation (as seen with her minister), inappropriate outbursts of anger, tendencies for self-damaging acts, and a general dislike of being alone. In fact, the clinician has probably already gathered close to enough data to fulfill the criteria for a borderline personality disorder by DSM-III-R standards, all in a matter of fifteen minutes. In addition, the blending seemed reasonably high as indicated by shared periods of levity and a report by the patient, when the interview actually ended, that she liked this clinician.

What is of particular note is the fashion in which the clinician gently and persistently pursued the criteria needed for the diagnosis. The clinician tended to carefully search for historical data by utilizing focusing statements such as, "back in your high school years do you think you felt . . ." or "Do you think that your parents or school-friend's would have viewed you as. . . ." In the process of unraveling the complexities surrounding a specific personality disorder, once the interviewer has uncovered a particular trait, it is critical to search for evidence that the trait is long-standing in nature. Thus, if a patient brings up many angry periods as an adolescent, then the clinician will need to eventually guide the conversation to a point in which an exploration can be made of angry feelings during the subsequent periods of the patient's life or vice versa.

This clinician was also careful to not assume that behavior occurring during an actual episode of major depression was related to the presence of character pathology, as shown by the following excerpt:

Clin.: When you get angry, do you tend to keep your anger bottled up inside or do you tend to let it out, maybe by yelling at the person or throwing something?

Pt.: I keep a lot of it in, but when I let go I can get pretty mean, I mean I have thrown things, I threw a plate at my husband when we were on a pass about two weeks ago.

Clin.: I know you've been feeling pretty depressed recently, how about just when you're feeling your normal self, how many times do you think you've broken things when someone angered you?

In this fashion the clinician is trying to uncover episodes of impulsive anger that are not related to Axis I psychopathology. Sure enough, Mrs. Jacobs proceeds to describe a long-standing pattern of angry and hostile feelings. If the interviewer does not frequently make it explicit to the patient which areas of time are being discussed, then patients almost invariably begin to merge time periods. Once this inadvertent blurring occurs, the clinician is destined to gather a history that may be considerably distorted.

I have seen clinicians interview patients who acted impulsively, with angry outbursts and suicidal threats or gestures, during episodes of hypomania or mania. Sometimes these patients were subsequently inappropriately labeled as borderline personality disorders. Certainly the behavior of these patients was consistent with a borderline personality during the manic periods, but it was the underlying mania that was causing the impulsive behavior. Careful interviewing of the patient and/or collaborative sources would have shown that these impulsive behaviors were not present outside of periods of acute Axis I psychopathology.

Another secret to structuring the interview effectively is remaining flexible, demonstrating an ability to side-track when the patient has a need to side-track. For instance, this clinician spent some well-used time when he joked with the patient about her husband's nose. This brief interlude helped the patient to feel more at ease, while also conveying to her the clinician's own sense of humor. This clinician was truly listening with the patient, not just attempting to complete a checklist.

Even when Mrs. Jacobs begins to turn-on the so-called borderline charm with the interviewer, the interviewer does not over-react. For example, when she challenges the interviewer concerning the issue of wrist cutting with, "I don't know, all I know is I'm probably going to do it again, 'cause I like it. And you're not going to stop me," the interviewer does not reflexively counterattack, immediately telling the patient of the need not to undertake such activity. Such a display of clinician fear would be"just what the chef ordered" for a borderline personality. Soon the patient would begin to push the clinician in a tug of war and nerves. Instead, this clinician calmly acknowledged the dilemma, agreed with Mrs. Jacobs' impression, and gracefully proceeded with the pertinent exploration of diagnostic information. At a later point in the interview the issue of lethality would be more thoroughly explored.

Besides demonstrating a method of unobtrusively expanding a specific diagnostic region, this excerpt serves to remind us of the intensely unsettling world of people with the personality structure we refer to as a borderline personality. Mrs. Jacobs' world is one of ceaselessly circular contradictions. Her husband is at one moment the good guy who will protect her from the carelessness of Dr. Johnson; at another moment, he has been transformed by her tendency to see only black or white into "such a mean person." Her minister is transmuted from a saint into a demon merely because he does not devote all of his attention to her.

She is truly frightened of the world, for she battles back an insistent feeling of "deadness," which threatens to swallow her and those around her for all she knows. Consequently she resorts to the age-old axiom of the best defense is an offense. She attacks. Even during this first encounter with a new clinician, she quickly challenges him to a duel of sorts over the issue of who will rule her wrists. Wisely he declined the verbal glove that so unexpectedly slapped his face. Even at a subtle level, she antagonizes because of her unpredictability. By way of illustration, at the end of the excerpt she suggests a fear of being placed on a locked ward. The clinician attempts to calm this fear with an empathic inquiry. No sooner does the clinician extend his concern than Mrs. Jacobs coolly responds, "Yeah, but I guess they better lock me up." This type of inconsistent interaction is what clinicians frequently report as being "jerked around" by borderline patients. Just as the clinician tries to be nice, the patient conveys a cool nonchalance.

The compassionate interviewer tries to see beneath this type of anger, realizing that the patient is coping with an ominous sense of impending doom and cannot find anything to hold on to to prevent a lethal plummet. In this sense Mrs. Jacobs represents a child trapped in an adult's body, and no one wants to play her game. The art is for the clinician to understand both the child and the adult, helping the patient to recognize that they do not need to be enemies.

Perhaps this is a good time to close this chapter. An attempt has been made to examine many of the core principles and intrigues surrounding the issues of character psychopathology. Hopefully the reader has come away with a variety of new perspectives and specific techniques that can be of immediate practical use. In the last analysis, the ability to readily recognize the presence of these disorders is probably one of the most difficult tasks facing the initial interviewer. The ability to not only recognize them, but to see the person beneath them is an even greater challenge. Without the latter skill, the former pales considerably in significance.

References

1. American Psychiatric Association: *Diagnostic and Statistical Manual of Mental Disorders.* Third edition, revised. Washington, D.C., APA, 1987, p. 335.
2. Siever, L. J., Insel, T. R., and Uhde, T. W.: Biogenetic factors in personalities. In *Personality Disorders*, edited by J. P. Frosch, Washington, D.C., APA, 1983, pp. 42–65.
3. DSM-III-R, 1987, 349.
4. Gunderson, J. G.: DSM-III diagnosis of personality disorders. In *Personality Disorders*, edited by J. P. Frosch, Washington, D.C., APA, 1983, pp. 20–39.
5. American Psychiatric Association: *Diagnostic and Statistical Manual of Mental Disorders,* Third edition, revised. Washington, D.C., APA, 1987, p. 335.
6. Vaillant, G.: Sociopathy as a human process. In *Major Psychiatric Disorders*, edited by F. Guggenhehim and C. Nadelson. New York, Elsevier Biomedical, 1982, pp. 179–188.
7. DSM-III-R, 1987, p. 349.
8. Hammacher A. M.: *Phantoms of the Imagination.* New York, Harry N. Abrams, 1981, p. 17.

9. Pomeroy, W. B., Flax, C. C., and Wheeler, C. C.: *Taking a Sex History*. New York, The Free Press, 1982.
10. Roberts, J. K. A.: *Differential Diagnosis in Neuropsychiatry*. New York, John Wiley and Sons, 1984, p. 26.
11. Adler, G.: *Borderline Psychopathology and Its Treatment*. New York, Jason Aronson, 1985.
12. Lawrence, D. H.: *Women In Love*. Franklin Center, Pennsylvania, The Franklin Library, 1979, p. 12.

III

Advanced Techniques of Interviewing

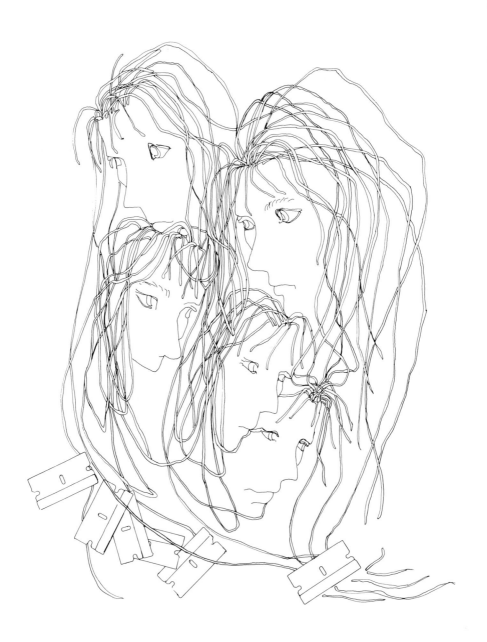

8

Exploring Suicidal and Homicidal Ideation

Dying
Is an art, like everything else.
I do it exceptionally well.

I do it so it feels like hell.
I do it so it feels real.
I guess you could say I've a call.
> *Sylvia Plath*, Lady Lazarus

These words written by Sylvia Plath invoke the coolness of death. They appear even more unsettling when one realizes that their author would eventually go on to kill herself, her words acting not so much as art but as prophecy. Her death added one more digit to the frightening statistic of 22,000 suicides per year in the United States, with the rate of 11 deaths per 100,000.[1] Moreover, these values probably represent conservative estimates, since they exclude dubious accidents, such as one-driver auto fatalities, which may actually represent masked suicides. In any case, with suicide representing the ninth leading cause of death in the United States, the determination of suicidality represents a daily task for many mental health professionals.

It is a task that requires a gentle sensitivity and a tenacious persistence. All of the interviewing skills previously discussed are put to their most rigorous test. If ever there was a moment of critical importance in interviewing, it is the moment when one listens for the harbingers of death. This arena is not a place for haphazard approaches or reliance solely on intuitive skills. Instead, interviewers possess two major tools that can assist their intuition in the determination of lethality. First, there exists a wealth of knowledge concerning statistical indicators of suicide potential that may help the clinician to predict increased suicide potential. Second, one can utilize interviewing techniques that may enhance the clinician's ability to elicit suicidal ideation itself.

In this chapter, we will examine the first tool by reviewing the many risk factors that may lead to increased lethality. A review will be generated by the use of two mock case histories, which illustrate many of the facets of suicide assessment. We will approach the second tool by looking, in depth, at a three-step method of probing for suicidal ideation. I doubt that one can overemphasize the importance of technique in the craft of eliciting suicidal ideation. In my opinion it is important for an interviewer to both develop and practice a consistent style of questioning.

A consistent approach provides the interviewer with a chance to become familiar with responses to specific questions from both suicidal and nonsuicidal patients. Such a familiarity with responses offers the experiential framework from which the most subtle of nuances indicating lethality can be picked up. The same interviewing principles are also useful in delineating homicidal ideation. Consequently homicidal ideation is discussed briefly at the end of the chapter. At this junction, it seems expedient to begin a review of risk factors by meeting our first patient.

SECTION I: SUICIDAL RISK FACTORS

CASE ONE: MR. JAMISON

Mr. Jamison is a twenty-one-year-old male who comes to the emergency room at 1:00 A.M. accompanied by a male friend. Mr. Jamison's shaggy hair hangs to his large shoulders, which cap a body obviously shaped by the rigors of a weight lifting room. Mr. Jamison reports feeling "odd" for months, with frequent ideas of reference. He also displays a loosening of associations sporadically. He relates, "It all comes down to the way the clouds kiss the moon." Other than this sentence, he demonstrates no illogical thoughts, tangential thought, or thought blocking, and he denies hallucinations. His speech has a gentle quality to it, with a peculiarly long latency before responses, as if preoccupied with a disturbing decision. His affect is guarded with periods of unusual intensity.

He denies feeling depressed and reports few neurovegetative symptoms of depression. He claims to have felt "upset" since he witnessed the brutal slaying of a friend by a motorcycle gang member. As he warms to the interviewer, he admits to recent abuse of alcohol, speed, LSD, and marijuana. When asked about whether he wants to kill himself, he replies testily, "I've no intention of killing myself . . . (pause) that's what I'm fighting for." He refuses to elaborate. At the end of the interview he refuses admission.

At this point, the clinician is faced with a formidable disposition problem. Does the suicide risk of this patient warrant hospitalization, or can he be treated as an outpatient? A second consideration is the fact that even if admission is warranted, the patient is refusing such treatment. Inadequate grounds for commitment are present. Can the interviewer discover adequate grounds if necessary? With these issues in mind, we can begin an examination of risk factors.

In the first place, Mr. Jamison's sex and age are consistent with an increased suicide risk. With regard to sex, males more frequently successfully commit suicide at a three to one ratio when compared to females. On the other hand, females attempt suicide three times more frequently than males.[2] Perhaps this increased "suicide efficiency" in males relates to the choice of the means of suicide. Males more frequently choose violent methods, such as guns, which provide a surer means of death.

With regard to age, in general, suicide risk is greater for both sexes with increasing age. In women the greatest number of completed suicides occur after age 55. In men it tends to peak around age 65. In males the curve is complicated by a bimodal tendency, with a second peak occurring in late adolescence,[3] a point of special significance with regard to Mr. Jamison. Unfortunately, in recent years there has been a disturbing rise in the frequency of adolescent suicide attempts, with suicide representing the third highest cause of death among teenagers.[4] Moreover, a clinician should always keep in mind that even a child can commit suicide.

But there is more to worry about with Mr. Jamison than the implications of his sex and age, for the interviewer left the encounter feeling that Mr. Jamison might be psychotic. The presence of psychosis, with or without depression, should nag an initial interviewer when evaluating suicide potential. Psychosis should be considered a potentially major suicide risk factor, for rational thought often acts as the final obstacle to self-destruction. In particular, three psychotic processes should be carefully evaluated when the clinician is suspicious of suicide: (1) command hallucinations, (2) feelings of alien control, and (3) religious preoccupation.

Command hallucinations represent auditory commands to perform a specific act. Such commands may be egging on patients to harm themselves or others. Their presence in some instances should strongly lean the evaluator towards immediate hospitalization. Many times they are not volunteered by the patient. Consequently they require active inquiry by the clinician.

During the inquiry several phenomenological considerations merit the attention of the clinician. Command hallucinations are not black or white phenomena in the sense that the patient either has them or does not. In actuality command hallucinations can vary in numerous fashions. Some of the defining characteristics include emotional impact on the patient, loudness, frequency, duration, content, degree of hostility, and the degree with which the patient feels driven to follow them.

With these variables in mind, command hallucinations can vary from relatively innocuous phenomena with little frequency and impact on the patient to dangerous phenomena in which the voices incessantly hammer at the patient in an effort to provoke violence. Some chronic schizophrenic patients have literally adapted to their voices and pay them little heed. This type of command hallucination is probably of minimal concern. At the other end of the continuum, command hallucinations can become acutely harassing, loud, and insistent. In such cases the clinician should always ask to what degree the patient feels in control. Sometimes patients may even feel unable to resist soft yet persistent voices. These types of acutely dystonic command hallucinations generally indicate the need for acute hospitalization. In order to determine the dangerousness of the command hallucination the clinician must take the time to explore the numerous pertinent variables.

In recent years several papers have purported that there is little or no statistical correlation between command hallucinations and suicide.[5-9] But if one looks at these papers, it becomes evident that none of the research carefully categorized the hallucinatory phenomena along the critical variables listed above. Indeed, the research is generally based upon hospital charts, which are notorious for poor reporting of the nuances of patient phenomenology. No one knows whether these voices were at one end or the other end of the continuum of dangerousness. Consequently, the statistical analyses are essentially meaningless.

To date I have not seen a prospective study that carefully operationalized the phenomenological data in such a way that the data are appropriate for statistical analysis in a valid sense. Until such a paper exists, it remains necessary for clinicians to carefully consider the fact that some patients definitely do act violently upon command hallucinations. The question is what type of patient and which phenomenological experiences result in such actions.

At present, the only method available for this decision remains the detailed exploration of the variables discussed above. It is hoped that future research, well grounded in phenomenology, will provide better guidelines. But even if better statistics become available, it is crucial to remember that the suicide of a given patient is not a statistical phenomenon. More specifically, a patient may kill himself whether the statistics suggest he is at risk or not at risk. Apparently patients are not always aware of the statistical rules they are meant to follow.

In a similar sense, alien control as evidenced by the feeling that one is being controlled by an outside agent, may represent a second dangerous psychotic process if this "other agent" becomes suicidally or homicidally oriented. It is not uncommon for a patient to literally battle off such potentially lethal urges on a minute-by-minute basis.

A third significant concern arises when the patient exhibits a specific type of excessive religious preoccupation. This type of rumination centers upon ideas that God wants the patient to perform certain acts in order to prove the patient's love for God. These acts may include suicide, homicide, or self-mutilation. Such concerns may be associated with command hallucinations as described above. Only this time, the commands originate from figures as ultimately persuasive as God. Patients may feel that their faith is being tested, perhaps comparing themselves with Abraham, who was commanded by God to sacrifice his own son, Isaac. This Abraham syndrome can prove fatal. At other times patients may feel that Satan is pushing them towards violence.

In a related fashion, the patient may be preoccupied with specific verses from the Bible that suggest violent action. Such a biblical injunction may be interpreted from Matthew 5:29, where lustful wanderings of the eye are handled in a rather absolute fashion, "If your right eye causes you to sin, pluck it out . . ."[10] Obviously, psychotic process can provide ample reasons for acting on such phrases. Bizarre methods of self-mutilation, such as autocastration and removal of the tongue, may result when verses such as this one are twisted by psychotic thought.[11] If religious preoccupation is found, it may be very useful to ask simple questions, such as, "What are some of the parts of the Bible that seem particularly important to you?"

Before leaving the topic of psychotic process and its relation to suicide, an important and easily overlooked consideration should be mentioned. Patients with schizophrenia probably more frequently attempt suicide, not in relation to psychotic processes but in relation to depression occurring in response to their acute psychotic breaks.[5,8] The core pains of losing a sense of internal control and subsequently a loss of meaning in life can represent a devastating combination for some patients. As the patients perceive themselves as being hopelessly damaged, then reasons for living are gradually extinguished. It has been postulated that patients with the following characteristics may be most at risk: young age, chronic relapses, good educational backgrounds, high performance expectations, painful awareness of the illness, fears of further mental deterioration, suicidal ideation or threats, and hopelessness.[12] Mr. Jamison illustrates yet another important factor in the determination of lethality. He is a heavy drug abuser. The presence of chronic alcohol abuse or other drug abuse should be viewed as another risk factor, since these agents may decrease impulse control or precipitate psychotic process.

The acutely intoxicated patient presents a particular problem, for the intoxication predisposes the patient towards a suicide attempt in two fashions. First, impulse control may be significantly lowered. Second, because of cognitive impairment, the patient may inadvertently commit suicide in a variety of fashions, such as forgetting that a large number of pills were taken earlier in an evening and subsequently proceeding to ingest "just a few more." Such miscalculations can result in a fatal overdose. Because of these factors, even chronic emergency room abusers who present with serious suicidal ideation while acutely intoxicated should be observed until they sober up. Frequently, as the alcohol wears off, the suicidal ideation disappears and may not even be remembered.

These points also highlight the fact that significant organic impairment of the sensorium can also increase risk. Thus, fluctuating levels of consciousness or impaired concentration warrants careful attention during the mental status. At this juncture, Mr. Jamison presents a disturbing clinical dilemma. Too many gaps exist in the knowledge base to enable a sound decision to be made. To clarify the issue an interview with Mr. Jamison's friend unearthed the following material:

Mr. Jamison had not been himself since the murder of his friend, who was, indeed, shot. Recently Mr. Jamison had seemed more distant than usual and was using a "load of uppers." He had been discharged about three weeks ago from some type of psychiatric hospital. Unfortunately Mr. Jamison was at odds with his family and was living by himself, currently in a dingy apartment, subsisting on food stamps. The friend knew of no previous suicide attempts.

When asked whether he had seen Mr. Jamison with any type of potential weapon, he remarked, "I hadn't really thought about it, but he does carry a hunting knife he got after he left the hospital. But he's had hunting knives before." Mr. Jamison lost his girlfriend about a month after the murder. When asked if he could stay with Mr. Jamison until he had an outpatient appointment, the friend quietly replied "No way."

In the first place, the above data illustrate the important principle of interviewing appropriate friends or family members, for they may provide invaluable information. In general, they should be asked if they have seen anything that suggests possible suicide intent. After such a general inquiry, specific questions such as the following may be useful:

a. Has he made any comments about being "better off dead?"
b. Has he joked about killing himself?
c. Have there been any statements about "things being better soon?"
d. Does he have any potential weapons in the house such as guns or knives?
e. Has he ever tried to hurt himself before, even in small ways like taking a few pills too many?
f. Has he appeared depressed or tearful?
g. Is he spending more time alone than usual?

In this type of questioning, besides determining lethality, one is also searching for information that would fulfill involuntary commitment criteria. Specifically, using Pennsylvania criteria, one checks to see if the patient has participated in behavior that is a clear danger to himself or to others. The criteria are also met if the patient has expressed a desire to harm himself or others while taking some steps (such as purchasing a weapon) to fulfill this desire. In the case of Mr. Jamison, his friend knew of no such behavior.

The collateral interview also provides a chance to determine stressors and social supports. With regard to stress the clinician should search for situations such as unemployment, family disruption, abrupt changes in career responsibilities, or a recent catastrophic stress (such as witnessing a murder in Mr. Jamison's case). Concerning supports, a lack of friends, family, or societal supports, such as church organizations, has often been reported as a risk factor. In particular, one should be looking for evidence of recent losses, such as Mr. Jamison's estrangement from his girlfriend and his family.

Probably one of the most striking statistical correlations with suicide remains the increased risk associated with the absence of a spouse. As compared with the rate of 11 per 100,000 in married individuals, single, never married patients show double this rate. Widowed individuals show 24 per 100,000. Divorced women show an increased rate of 18 per 100,000, while divorced men show a startling rate of 69 per 100,000.[13]

Immediately available supports are particularly important, when postponing a triage decision until a more thorough evaluation can be done the next day. Such a situation may arise when the clinician is ambivalent about the seriousness of the lethality while simultaneously confronted with a "stacked up" emergency room. If a friend or family member can stay with the patient constantly until the scheduled appointment, then such a plan may be feasible.

In such cases it is critical that the family members thoroughly understand that the patient is not to be alone. Moreover, I generally find it useful to also have a discussion with the patient and the family together, talking openly about suicidal concerns and the designated treatment plan. Such a procedure helps to teach the patient and the family that it is both safe and appropriate to discuss suicidal ideation frankly. To the contrary, it is the ideation not talked about that may prove more deadly.

With regard to the items discussed above, including long-term supports, immediate supports, and recent stressors, Mr. Jamison looks more and more worrisome. The risk is further heightened by the relatively recent discharge of Mr. Jamison from a psychiatric hospital (which could provide "no information at this time because medical records is closed"). In particular, the first month following discharge represents a particularly high-risk period.[14] As a further point, Mr. Jamison has no known suicide history. With regard to previous attempts, collateral informants often provide information withheld by the patients. Previous attempts are clearly associated with increased risk, as evidenced by a recent study in which over 46 per cent of the successful suicides had previously attempted suicide.[14]

With regard to Mr. Jamison's clinical disposition, the interviewer investigated one more pertinent system of support, the mental health system itself. The charge nurse, when queried, related that the outpatient department was flooded with appointments and backlogged for several weeks. She felt it highly unlikely that Mr. Jamison could be seen the next day. Thus, because of a lack of immediate social support, and a lack of professional support, the clinician felt very uneasy about outpatient triage. But at this point, despite many statistical risk factors, it remains unclear how lethal a risk Mr. Jamison presents. It must be remembered that he denied suicidal intent, albeit in a somewhat quizzical fashion. Furthermore, at present, good grounds for commitment are lacking.

At this point the interviewer made a wise, but often underused decision. He decided to re-interview the patient. This time an even more concerted effort would be made to bring psychotic ideation to the surface, while persistently listening for adequate grounds for commitment, if indeed Mr. Jamison appeared more imminently suicidal. The following dialogue evolved after about 10 minutes:

> ***Pt.:*** I don't think there's anything that could have been done. Peace is what is needed. Peaceful mankind . . . but it all seems so weird and I try to stop them.

Clin.: To stop who?

Pt.: Bad people . . . bad people who push me and make me do things, make me watch things.

Clin.: Have you ever felt like someone or something was really trying to take you over?

Pt.: Oh . . . they take me over, or try to, but I don't let them.

Clin.: Who are you talking about?

Pt.: Something inside me, something about my heart, scratching at my heart, my muscle.

Clin.: It sounds very frightening.

Pt.: Very frightening, but I won't do it.

Clin.: What do they want you to do?

Pt.: To cut it out, to cut the scratching out of my heart, to bring peace to mankind, to wipe off the pain. But I won't do it unless I see the sign. The clouds will kiss the moon, you'll see.

Clin.: What do they want you to use to cut yourself?

Pt.: My knife.

Clin.: Have they ever made you hold the knife in your hands?

Pt.: Oh yes . . . one night, I think it was last night, they put it in my hand. I told them I didn't want it, but they made me hold it with the point pressing on my chest, just waiting.

Clin.: And what did they want you to do?

Pt.: To thrust it deep inside my heart, to let my scratching out, to let my God in, to thrust steel truth into God.

The interviewer has succeeded. He has been granted access to the patient's inner world, which proves to be grossly psychotic, as was initially suspected. By probing along the lines of alien control the interviewer has skillfully uncovered both suicidal ideation and action. In the earlier interview, Mr. Jamison had denied suicidal ideation probably because he felt that an alien force wanted him to die, not his own will. In his mind this was murder not suicide. Clearly, Mr. Jamison warrants hospitalization, and adequate grounds for commitment are now available if necessary. It should be noted that the interviewer had gently guided Mr. Jamison towards a concrete description of his suicidal actions in the hope that grounds for commitment would emerge. Many times a patient will not grant such information unless sensitively guided towards it.

Perhaps a review of some basic principles illustrated by Mr. Jamison may be of value here:

1. A significant number of people who attempt suicide are psychotic.

2. Any evidence of psychosis warrants a thorough evaluation of lethality.

3. Three particularly dangerous areas of psychotic process are command hallucinations, feelings of alien control, and hyper-religiosity. These areas should be actively probed by the interviewer if not elicited spontaneously.

4. Recent evidence suggests that many suicides in schizophrenia occur in response to depressive episodes while the patient is relatively nonpsychotic.

5. Demographic material such as age, sex, and marital status may indicate risk factors for suicide.

6. Recent losses and poor social support systems also represent risk factors for suicide.

7. Alcohol, drugs, or any physiologic insult to the central nervous system may increase the likelihood of suicide or homicide.

8. When evaluating systems of immediate outpatient support, one should carefully consider whether the mental health system itself is prepared to offer adequate support.

9. Interviews with collateral informants may yield valuable information.

At this point, it may be best to move on to our second patient, who presents some new areas of concern, when considering lethality.

CASE TWO: MRS. KELLY

Mrs. Kelly, a fifty-year-old married mother of three, has arrived for an outpatient initial assessment, accompanied by her eldest daughter. Mrs. Kelly appears frail, walking as if each step presented a personal challenge. There remains a glint to her eye, but it is a weary one. Her hands are grossly deformed by the ravages of rheumatoid arthritis. She reports feeling very depressed, her speech punctuated by heavy sighs. She complains of many neurovegetative symptoms of depression. They have persisted for over six months, "although I've not felt normal since the arthritis began over seven years ago." She continues tearfully, "I'm not the same woman my husband married." She manages to smile as she wryly adds, "You know, if my memory serves me right, I used to move a little faster."

When asked about suicide, she admits to having thought of it occasionally but denies any intention of pursuing it. She has no organized plan. She relates an increasing sense of hopelessness, adding, "I think I'm starting to lose my fight. I think my husband would be better off with me dead, at least he says so." She is without evidence of psychosis and does remarkably well when tested for cognitive dysfunction.

Her daughter relates that her mother used to be a real fighter. At one time she was "the belle of the ball." With the onset of the arthritis, she had been forced into a strikingly more sedate lifestyle. Her illness has greatly affected her husband, who always wants to be on the go socially. They bicker constantly. Her daughter has seen no evidence of suicidal behavior in her mother, but is frightened of what her mother will do when she becomes bedridden.

Mrs. Kelly certainly presents a picture that raises different concerns than those encountered with Mr. Jamison. In the first place, she appears significantly depressed. As expected, depression represents one of the suicide risk factors. It is important to keep in mind the possibility of atypical depression. Indeed, various somatoform disorders, such as the psychogenic pain syndrome, may be accompanied by depression. With such an atypical presentation an interviewer can be lulled into a feeling of false security concerning suicide potential.

With regard to physical illness, Mrs. Kelly highlights the fact that severe illnesses are often associated with increased suicide risk. The clinician should pay particular attention to illnesses that result in markedly decreased mobility, disfigurement, and chronic pain.[16] Mrs. Kelly's rheumatoid arthritis unfortunately creates all three of these burdens. The interviewer should also keep in mind the impact of illnesses in which the patient perceives a horrifying demise. Such illnesses as Huntington's chorea, multiple sclerosis, severe diabetes, and severe chronic obstructive pulmonary disease may present more suffering than the patient is willing to accept. The interaction of these illnesses with the patient's underlying personality structure also warrants attention. Put simply, some people handle illness much better than others.

Leonard had described three personality types who may be predisposed to suicide when stressed.[17] The first type is a controlling personality in which patients tend to constantly manipulate their environment. They are often hard-driven and feel a need to be on top of things. They frequently pilot their way into roles of power and authority. When such people are suddenly struck by the loss of control caused by a crippling illness, they may attempt escape through death. Mrs. Kelly certainly may possess some of these dynamics, for she had always been an "on the go" person. Her daughter's fear of what will happen when her mother becomes bedridden represents a well-founded concern.

A second personality type is exemplified by a dependent-dissatisfied approach to life, a common element of borderline personality disorders. Such people often leave a long line of exasperated caretakers in their wake. When the last source of aid finally closes the door, these people are suddenly without any means of emotional support. Suicide may loom as the only viable option. And, finally, a third predisposing characterological type involves people who have evolved a truly symbiotic relationship with a significant other. These people are at high risk if their sustaining support dies or abandons them.

All of these examples emphasize one of the most important characteristics of suicide. Suicide is an interpersonal phenomenon. As such, an evaluation of suicide potential not only involves consideration of the identified patient. It requires an evaluation of the interpersonal systems surrounding that patient. At times, this evaluation proceeds through the use of collateral interviews. At other times, the interviewer must depend on information provided solely by the patient. In either case, a careful consideration of interpersonal factors is warranted.

In a simplistic but practical approach, the interviewer should attempt to determine whether the patient is returning to a supportive or hostile environment. If the patient's family and/or friends provide a caring milieu, this fact bodes well for the patient. Even in this situation, a paradoxical problem can arise if the patient begins to feel guilty "about being a burden to everyone." Phrases such as Mrs. Kelly's, "I think my husband will be better off with me dead," should perk the ears of the interviewer. In this vein of reasoning, after suicide has been broached as a topic, questions such as the following two can be revealing:

a. If you would kill yourself, how do you think that would affect your family?
b. What do you think your spouse would feel if you killed yourself?

Such questioning may lead directly to evidence of an interpersonal maelstrom. As the evaluation proceeds, the interviewer seeks for clues that suggest that a supposed support system, in reality, may wish at some level that the patient were dead. A death wish may be unconscious or conscious, innocuous or sinister. The clinician's recognition of such death wishes is not a moral judgment passed upon a potential support system but rather an objective attempt to see the potentially lethal ramifications stemming from such situations. A premature dismissal of such factors may represent a dangerous naivete on the part of the interviewer. Certainly, in the case of Mrs. Kelly, one wonders to what degree the marital alliance has been severely strained. At some level, does Mr. Kelly "want out?"

An unconscious death wish may show itself by a lax attitude of the family towards appropriate precautions against suicide. The clinician may discover that the suggestions of previous mental health professionals, such as removing a firearm, have not been followed by the family. On another plane, there may be resistance to hospitalizing a seriously lethal patient. Considering the perspective of psychological defense mechanisms, family members may see a falsely rosy picture because of denial or repression.

At a more disturbing level, clinicians will undoubtedly encounter, at some point in their practice, a death wish laced with true malice. Perhaps it will be a spouse who has long been denied a divorce or a battered wife unable to retaliate. These family members may consciously wish the patient dead. It is not known how many times people have waited a few hours before contacting help when they have happened upon a "sleeping" family member surrounded by empty pill bottles.

In this regard, I remember one patient I hospitalized whose spouse literally yelled at her "to take the damn pills, in fact I'll stuff them down your throat, and trust me I won't call a soul." The uncovering of such vicious interaction should serve as a warning to the clinician. It may lean the clinician towards hospitalizing a patient who otherwise might have been safely discharged to a more supportive environment.

Another aspect of the hostile environment may be the fact that the patient might be equally angry with family members. With revenge in mind, the patients may kill themselves, hoping "to show them they'll be sorry when I'm gone." Questions such as, "What have you pictured your funeral being like?" may provide revealing insights into the patient's motive for suicide. It is not at all unusual to receive answers such as, "They will all be really hurt, realizing at last what they've done to me." In a similar vein, some authors have viewed suicide as the result of a murderous impulse turned inward, a symbolic murder with an ironic satisfaction.[18]

Reasoning of the types described above emphasizes the importance of determining whether the patient is developing powerful interpersonal excuses for suicide. The more rational the suicide appears to the patient, the more concerned the interviewer should become. It becomes particularly ominous when the excuse has a humanistic flavor to it, as with "it's the only way I can really help my family." Such thinking may be the first note in a death toll.

Leaving the interpersonal realm and returning to Mrs. Kelly, there appear several indicators suggesting lowered suicide risk. In the first place, she denies immediate hopelessness. Aaron Beck's work with the cognitive aspects of suicide has suggested that the presence of hopelessness may be an ominous sign. In fact, hopelessness may even be a better indicator of lethality than the severity of depressive mood.[19] Viewed from a logical perspective, suicide usually represents a last option taken when no other alternatives are apparent to the patient. Moreover, a sense of helplessness is often coupled to this state of despair. Patients generally kill themselves for one major reason, to escape what appears to them an inescapable pain.

Further questioning also revealed that Mrs. Kelly was not only raised a Catholic, she strongly practiced her faith, believing that suicide was a mortal sin punishable by eternal damnation. At this intensity, religion is probably acting as a major framework for meaning that precludes the suicide option. Other patients may have different frameworks for meaning, such as caring for their children or fulfilling other important societal roles. In any case, the clinician should seek out evidence of such powerful deterrents.

A peculiar and unsettling twist can enter the picture with regards to children. Some patients may decide that their children would be even worse off after the patient's suicide. For instance, the patient's spouse may be an alcoholic or child abuser. In these instances the patient may be contemplating taking the lives of the children before killing himself or herself. Although rare, one only needs to read the newspaper in order to learn about such tragedies. If suspected, a natural gate may be of use in moving unobtrusively into this extremely sensitive area.

> **Pt.:** I am a total failure, a miserable mother, and I now realize that my only option is death . . . I intend to take that option.
>
> **Clin.:** You know, sometimes when people feel really angry at themselves, they also find themselves turning the anger outwards onto others. Have you felt like hurting anyone else?
>
> **Pt.:** (pause) Yes I have. I don't think I'd do it, but maybe it would be better anyway.
>
> **Clin.:** What are you referring to?
>
> **Pt.:** I've thought of killing my husband.
>
> **Clin.:** Anyone else? Such as your children?

At other times the following type of approach may be useful:

> **Pt.:** My husband will never change. He likes to hurt us. We have no future and I now realize that suicide is my only option.

Clin.:   You mentioned "we." What do you think is going to happen to your children after you kill yourself?

Pt.:   (long pause) I don't really know.

Clin.:   Sometimes parents consider taking the lives of their children. Has that thought ever crossed your mind?

Pt.:   Yes, it has . . . it's a terrible thought but it has.

Clin.:   What have you thought of doing?

Another positive note in Mrs. Kelly's presentation is the lack of a recent, abrupt change in clinical condition in either direction. The sudden onset of severe sleeplessness, agitation, or marked dysphoria may indicate that patients are rapidly approaching a pain level they cannot tolerate. On the other hand, one hears of the often quoted clinical observation that an unexpected improvement in clinical condition may be masking a sinister outcome. The patient's peace may be secondary to the patient's decision to commit suicide. Suddenly, the patient senses a perceivable end to the suffering. The most upsetting decision of the patient's life is over.

Another problem concerning "improvement" surfaces from the fact that depressed patients appear more likely to attempt suicide as they begin to improve. Suicide is less common while they are in the troughs of their depression. This curious finding is probably related to the fact that as they initially improve, they regain initiative and energy, even though their dysphoric mood may remain severely intense. The clinician should keep this fact in mind when encountering a patient recently started on an antidepressant.

Finally, further interviewing revealed that Mrs. Kelly has no immediate models for suicide. Neither friends nor family members have ever attempted suicide. If one discovers a legacy of suicide in a family tree, this should arouse concern on the part of the interviewer.

At this point a summary of issues illustrated by Mrs. Kelly may clarify some principles.

1. The presence of disease may increase suicide risk, especially if it leads to immobility, disfigurement, or severe pain.

2. The interviewer should search for evidence of hopelessness or helplessness.

3. A hostile interpersonal environment may substantially increase suicide risk.

4. A strong framework for meaning, such as a deeply held religious conviction, may decrease risk. It should be sought for by the clinician.

5. Sudden changes in clinical condition, either positive or negative, may indicate an increased risk.

6. Rational excuses for committing suicide may indicate increased intention.

7. The presence of a positive family history of suicide should be actively looked into by the clinician.

Chronic Versus Immediate Risk of Suicide: The Triad of Lethality

Perhaps the most important indicator that Mrs. Kelly is not imminently suicidal is the fact that she denies current suicidal intent and has no organized plan to harm herself. This point illustrates the usefulness of making a distinction between chronic suicide potential and immediate suicide potential. If a patient presents with a variety of risk factors present over a significant period of time, then the patient may well represent a chronic risk for suicide. Such is the case with Mrs. Kelly, who presents with the following risk factors: increasing age, debilitating illness, increasing sense of hopelessness, a strained marital alliance which may actually represent a hostile environment, and the slow evolution of a rational excuse for suicide.

But the presence of numerous risk factors does not necessarily indicate an immediate risk of suicide. More importantly, the absence of most risk factors does not necessarily indicate the lack of a serious risk if certain critical factors are present. By way of example, concerning the first point, Mrs. Kelly most likely could be safely triaged to an outpatient therapist despite her substantial list of risk factors (although she would probably benefit from hospitalization). Thus, the pressing question facing the clinician is to determine what factors would have suggested that she was in immediate danger of suicide.

In my opinion, the three most useful indicators, which form a lethal triad of sorts include: (1) recent history of a serious suicidal attempt, (2) the presence of acutely disturbing psychotic processes suggestive of lethality, and (3) indication from the interview that the patient seriously intends self-harm. The presence of any one of these factors should warn the clinician that suicide may be imminent. With respect to triage, the clinician should strongly consider hospitalization, even if opposed by patient.

In my opinion, the last element of the triad represents the single most important indication of suicide potential. The major factor determining a sensitivity to it is the skill of the interviewer. So important is this interviewing process that we will spend an entire section of this chapter reviewing its subtleties.

In the meantime, as we look back at the first element of the triad of lethality, the presence of a recent serious attempt, certain points may help in the determination of the significance of the attempt. First, the clinician wants to get an idea of the potential dangerousness of the method used. For example, taking a few extra aspirin is a great deal less disconcerting than shooting oneself or ingesting lye. Moreover, the threat of overdosage in a physician, who understands the use of medications, is more worrisome than the same threat in a nonmedical person.

Secondly, the clinician wants to determine whether the patient appeared to really want to die or not. Looked at differently, did the patient leave much room for rescue? The interviewer should search for factors such as the following: Did the patient choose a "death spot" where the patient could easily be discovered? Did the patient choose a spot where help was nearby? Did the patient leave any hints of suicidal intention that could have brought help, such as an easily accessible suicide note? Did the patient contact someone after the suicide attempt.?[20] The absence of the previous findings may indicate that the patient was frighteningly serious.

At this point I would like to refocus on the general issue of chronic versus immediate suicide potential. By way of illustration, Mr. Jamison and Mrs. Kelly appear to represent two ends of this continuum. Mrs. Kelly lacks all the elements of the triad of lethality. Specifically, she has no recent history of an attempt, she has no evidence of psychosis, and she gives no feeling from the interview of current suicidal ideation. Thus, despite the fact she has numerous risk factors, she is probably not in immediate danger. On the other hand, Mr. Jamison possessed all three elements of the triad, and hence, was worrisome indeed. These two cases highlight the point that there is no mechanical formula one can use for determining suicidal potential. Instead, clinicians utilize a craft in which they carefully weigh various risk factors, historical elements, and pieces of information gleaned from the interview. Perhaps a summary of these factors and their interplay would be helpful at this time.

Statistical and Clinical Risk Factors: Summary and Use

Through the examination of the two case studies, the risk factors most often cited in the literature have been surveyed. When pressured by time constraints, clinical demands, and the other standard pressures of being a mental health professional, it is sometimes difficult to remember all these issues. To facilitate their recall and use, the following two acronyms can provide some reassuring structure in the most chaotic of situations. The first acronym, the SAD PERSONS Scale, was developed by Patterson, Dohn, Bird, and Patterson.[21] It serves as a useful checklist of pertinent risk factors. The second acronym, NO HOPE, developed by the author, adds further depth to the evaluation of suicide potential

The SAD PERSONS Scale	The NO HOPE Scale
Sex	No framework for meaning
Age	Overt change in clinical condition
Depression	Hostile interpersonal environment
Previous attempt	Out of hospital recently
Ethanol abuse	Predisposing personality factors
Rational thinking loss	Excuses for dying are present and
Social supports lacking	strongly believed
Organized plan	
No spouse	
Sickness	

Needless to say, the acronym NO HOPE itself emphasizes the need to inquire about feelings of hopelessness.

If clinicians routinely explore the ramifications of these factors before making a triage decision, they can be assured they are utilizing a sound knowledge base. Moreover, the presence of a large number of these factors should increase clinicians' suspicions of suicide potential. And, as mentioned earlier, the presence of any one of the factors assumed under the triad of lethality should strongly lean clinicians towards hospitalization even if few of the other risk factors are present. In the final analysis, despite an extensive knowledge of risk factors, it is the clinician's impression of imminent suicidal intent, garnered from the interview, that remains the cornerstone of intervention. It is to this process that we now turn our attention.

SECTION II: THE ELICITATION OF SUICIDAL IDEATION

There exists little doubt that as mental health professionals we will all be interviewing a patient at some point in our careers who has decided to commit suicide. As we talk, the patient will have already accepted an invitation to die. The question becomes whether the patient will decide to share this decision with us.

At such a moment, the interviewer, as a measuring instrument, should be set at the highest pitch of sensitivity. The clinician essentially wants to elicit even the smallest of suicidal intentions, for such ideations suggest important implications for disposition and treatment. In the following pages, an attempt is made to offer various principles that may significantly increase the likelihood that suicidal ideation will be shared. As usual, each interviewer must ultimately develop an individually tailored style, but these suggestions may serve as useful stimulants for thought. They are discussed within a framework built of three steps. These three steps are (1) setting the appropriate stage, (2) asking the specific question, "Are you having thoughts of killing yourself," and (3) carefully exploring the extent of the suicidal ideation. Thus, the query for suicidal ideation presents not as a single question but as a meticulously developed process, gently guided by the interviewer.

Step One

With regard to the first step, setting the stage, the interviewer attempts to create an atmosphere in which the patient is most likely to share suicidal ideation. If one reflects upon it, the most effective atmosphere is probably a rather unusual state. In it, the patient should feel maximally safe with the interviewer while being intensively involved, psychologically, with the painful emotion that is pushing the patient towards suicide. I have found that intense emotional involvement usually tends to lower conscious defenses, thus increasing the likelihood that suicidal ideation will be shared.

Many times, patients will spontaneously enter these areas of intense involvement, but at other times, the interviewer must skillfully lead them there. In our previous example of Mr. Jamison, the utility of leading the patient towards intense affective involvement was elegantly illustrated.

In the first interview with Mr. Jamison, he essentially denied suicidal ideation, refusing to elaborate. Perhaps the stage for sharing had not been adequately set. To the contrary, in the second interview, the clinician quietly entered the actively psychotic world of the patient, sensitively leading him into a discussion of his psychotic concerns. As Mr. Jamison entered this world of emotional pain his affective involvement became more intense, leading to an increased desire to relieve his pain by sharing his burdens with a compassionate listener. Obviously, to be effective this process is predicated on the fact that the interviewer has previously decreased the patient's initial paranoia. Consequently, at this delicate point where secrets are shared, the interviewer will be perceived as an ally worthy of such trust.

With regard to psychosis, such well-timed focusing upon affectively charged content may lead the patient into a mildly dissociated state, in which conscious and unconscious defenses may be diminished, direct questions often yielding direct answers. Processes mentioned earlier, such as command hallucinations, alien control, and hyper-religiosity may be described more openly by the patient at these times. In essence, the interviewer has created a gate with which to enter the realm of suicidal ideation.

At this junction, it may be of benefit to look at the various gates that can provide more effective access to suicidal ideation. There appear to be three primary gates that lead people towards sharing their thoughts of suicide. These gates are (1) psychotic process, (2) depression and hopelessness, and (3) a sense of crisis, anger, or confusion. Generally speaking, it pays the interviewer to refrain from asking about suicidal ideation until the patient is obviously emotionally involved in one of these three areas. The clinician does not pop the question to the patient; the clinician leads up to it.

If the interviewer suspects the patient has been depressed, then the interviewer may wait to inquire about suicide until the patient gives evidence of being involved in depressive affect. In some cases, the interviewer may need to gently lead the patient into these areas, for the patient may be using denial or other mechanisms to avoid such painful affect. This principle of guiding the patient towards emotional involvement also applies to the third gate, in which the patient contemplates suicide secondary to some specific emotional turmoil. Sensitively setting the stage in such a manner as described above also provides the interviewer with the time needed to have established a sound degree of blending with the patient, further enhancing the likelihood of eliciting suicidal intent. Generally this evolving process reaches a peak somewhere in the middle of the interview.

On the other hand, not infrequently, the interviewee will hint at suicidal ideation earlier. Such hints suggest that the stage may already be set and that the patient is ready to share. If spontaneous gates appear, they should generally be pursued quickly by the interviewer, as follows:

Pt.: My life is very different for me now. Over the past several years it seems to have gone empty.

Clin.: How do you mean?

Pt.: After the divorce, I was on automatic pilot, but eventually it all sunk in, it all seemed horribly empty, not worth continuing, much as it seems now. But I have managed, and have had some brighter days.

Clin.: When you say, it seemed not worth continuing, had you thought of ending your life?

>   ***Pt.:***   Oh yes . . . and I still do.
> ***Clin.:***   What kinds of things have you thought of doing?
>   ***Pt.:***   I thought of taking pills and I did that once . . .

If the clinician does not pick up on such nuances by referring to them directly, the conversation can quickly move to new topics. If this movement occurs, the clinician may have missed the most opportune spot for inquiry. By bringing up such thoughts, the metacommunication of the patient seems to be a simple one, "Ask me about suicide." When given such an open gate, it seems unwise to walk by it. By not following up, the interviewer may discover that later on, due to an unexpected problem with engagement, the interviewee will no longer feel comfortable about sharing. The suicidal ideation will remain silent, a most deadly situation.

Before leaving the process of setting the stage two other technical points bear mentioning. First, if one gate fails, then the interviewer can try a different gate. For instance the evaluation may hit a denial of suicidal intent when flowing with depressive ideation in a man with a psychotic depression. Approached by the gate of psychosis, this same man may admit to suicidal ideation.

Some interviewers may initially approach suicidality with a mildly ambiguous question, which essentially invites the interviewee to discuss suicidal ideation without spelling it out. Such questions may provide back doors through which the patient may feel more comfortable about entering a discussion of suicide, as follows:

>   ***Pt.:***   Nothing seems to matter much anymore and everything seems wrong.
> ***Clin.:***   How do you mean?
>   ***Pt.:***   I can't sleep, I can't eat, and every minute seems worse than the one before. I'm not kidding when I say I feel miserable.
> ***Clin.:***   Have you ever thought of a way of ending your pain?
>   ***Pt.:***   Yes, yes I have . . . I thought of blowing my brains out (nervous laughter) but that's a little messy.
> ***Clin.:***   Sounds scary.
>   ***Pt.:***   Yes it is.
> ***Clin.:***   Do you have a gun in the house?
>   ***Pt.:***   Yes I do . . . beside my bed.

If the patient does not pick up on the interviewer's more subtle invitation to discuss suicide, then it is imperative to proceed to step two.

Step Two

The second step, asking specifically whether patients have had thoughts of killing themselves, appears deceptively simple. It is not. Asking the question raises many factors pertaining to issues such as metacommunication, resistance, validity, and reliability.

In the first place, I have made it a habit to always ask about lethality, at some point, using specific words such as "kill yourself," "commit suicide," or "take your life." I do not think lethality inquiries are any place to risk misunderstandings. The patient needs to know exactly what the clinician is talking about. Such calm frankness on the part of the interviewer provides a powerful metacommunication to the patient. This metacommunication states, "It is okay to discuss thoughts of suicide with me." In an immediate sense, this implied reassurance may relax the patient, increasing the patient's sense of safety. In a long-term sense, it may be the single action that brings a potentially suicidal patient to help. Several months down the road, if the patient becomes seriously suicidal, the patient may remember that there was one place where the patient's "horrible secret" could be shared. Such knowledge could literally save a life.

A trainee related a relevant vignette concerning the specific words chosen during the suicide inquiry. The interviewer had asked an adolescent girl, "Have you had any thoughts of wanting to hurt yourself?" The girl assuredly answered no. Because of a large number of suicide risk factors, the clinician readdressed the issue later, asking, "Have you had any thoughts of wanting to kill yourself?" To the clinician's surprise the girl matter of factly responded, "Oh yes, I've thought about it a lot. I've stored up a lot of pills, and I may really try it someday." The clinician asked the girl why she had denied suicide earlier and she replied, "You didn't ask me about suicide. You asked if I wanted to hurt myself, and I hate pain. Even the method I have chosen for suicide is not going to be painful."

The above discussions also bring up several other interesting points concerning patient resistance to discussing suicidal ideation. Several resistances come to mind:

a. The patient feels that suicide is a sign of weakness and feels shame.
b. The patient feels that suicide is immoral or a sin.
c. The patient feels that discussion of suicide is a taboo subject.
d. The patient is worried that the interviewer will perceive the patient as crazy.
e. The patient fears that the patient will be "locked up" if suicidal ideation is discussed.

f. The patient truly wants to die and does not want anybody to know.

This is quite a formidable list. It re-emphasizes the importance of effective engagement and appropriate setting of the stage. It also brings up issues of how to approach navigating some of these potential resistances.

To begin with, the clinician may attempt to dissipate patients' fears that they will be perceived as bizarre or unusual. A simple lead-in, as follows, is often helpful, "Frequently, when people are feeling very upset, they have thoughts of killing themselves. Have you had any thoughts of wanting to hurt yourself?" Said matter-of-factly and sensitively, this lead-in can be significantly reassuring to patients, indicating that they are not being viewed as odd or deviant by the interviewer.

The clinician must also be concerned that clinician anxiety over suicidal issues is not conveyed to the patient. Such anxiety may be misinterpreted as a forewarning of moral disapproval. If, indeed, the patient picks up evidence of moral condemnation through tone of voice or body language, the patient may shut up like a frightened child before an unforgiving parent. With this problem in mind, it becomes important for interviewers to be keenly aware of countertransference issues. An awareness of such issues may surface by asking questions of oneself such as:

a. What are my beliefs about suicide?
b. Do I feel that suicide is sinful or unnatural?
c. Do I feel that people who commit suicide are weak?
d. Do I ever picture myself as capable of taking my own life?
e. Have I known anyone in my family or friends who killed themselves? And how does this fact affect the way I approach the issue in my interviews?

The answers to such questions may help the interviewer to notice stylistic elements that may increase patient resistance.

It also seems pertinent to raise a countertransference issue that many interviewers do not like to admit, but one that I think is present in most of us. Namely, if we uncover serious suicidal ideation, we are potentially creating a mess for ourselves. For instance, if suicidal plans emerge, we may need to greatly prolong our assessment when we are already strapped for time. Family members may need to be involved. We may have to deal with an irate patient or equally irate family member if we need to proceed with involuntary commitment. And, finally, we may have to spend a day in court if commitment occurs. The bottom line is, if we do our job well, we may have to pay a not so insignificant price. This process can definitely emerge as counter-transference in the guise of such processes as not even inquiring about suicide, waiting until the end of the interview to ask about it, poorly setting the stage, hurrying the assessment, and asking questions in a manner that decreases the sensitivity of the questions themselves.

With regard to the last concern, it is important to avoid type A validity errors such as asking questions with a negative, as follows:

> **Pt.:** Sometimes things are simply too much. My husband can't stop yelling, the dog is barking, kids screaming, too much, just too much.
>
> **Clin.:** You've *not* thought of hurting yourself, have you?
>
> **Pt.:** Why no, I haven't thought of that really.

Such a leading question, which is actually a statement of inquiry containing a "negative," may suggest to the patient that the interviewer does not morally approve of suicide and may be judgmental if told of suicidal ideation. In reality, it may merely represent the hassled interviewer's unconscious prayer that nothing serious comes up. Unfortunately, to the interviewee, it clearly indicates that this interviewer wants "no" for an answer. As a general rule, interviewees try to please interviewers. Validity clearly becomes an issue here. I watched such an interaction in which the patient denied suicidal ideation to an initial interviewer. A second interviewer reapproached the same patient at the end of the first clinician's interview. This time the second interviewer avoided the question begun with a negative. He subsequently discovered that the patient had overdosed on aspirin about five days earlier. Technique counts.

Concerning the issue of resistance, a second general principle comes to mind that can be simply stated: Do not accept the first "no."

I am consistently amazed at how many people flatly deny suicidal ideation when first asked despite the presence of such ideation. The clinician should seldom, if ever, leave the topic after a single denial. As noted earlier, all sorts of resistance issues may be at work. And I generally re-approach the topic with a statement that decreases the risk of patient shame, as follows:

> **Pt.:** . . . but I never bought cyanide, or even looked into buying it.
>
> **Clin.:** What other ways have you thought about killing yourself?
>
> **Pt.:** I haven't. I would never hang myself or shoot myself. That would be silly and I'd never do it.

Clin.: Well, have you ever had thoughts of maybe hanging yourself, even if only fleeting thoughts?

Pt.: I might have thought about it.

Clin.: Have you ever actually gotten a rope or a belt out to try it?

Pt.: I actually did get a rope out once.

Clin.: Did you put it around your neck?

Pt.: Yes I did.

Clin.: What did you do then?

Pt.: I wanted to see what it would feel like, to see if I could do it.

Clin.: And?

Pt.: It hurt too much as I began kicking out the stool, so I stopped.

Clearly, this man initially denied even having thoughts of hanging himself. To my surprise, he had actually progressed to the point of kicking the stool out. In this excerpt the use of words such as "have you had even fleeting thoughts" may have decreased the shame component for the patient. After the first denial, I frequently use such phrases. It is the atypical patient, indeed, who in the midst of a severe depression has not had at least some fleeting thoughts of suicide. Total denial in response to this question should stir some suspicion in the interviewer about the validity of the information base.

Another point illustrated by this dialogue can be stated as follows. If a patient spontaneously brings up a specific method of suicide, then the patient has probably given it some thought. Even if arising as a denial, as it did with this patient, it demands further exploration.

Sometimes a patient who is quite resistant to sharing suicidal ideation may hint at it. When such hints are made, it may not be best to simply ask, "Have you had any thoughts of wanting to kill yourself?" This closed-ended question can easily be answered with a quick "no." Instead, the likelihood of the patient answering openly may increase if the inquiry is made as a gentle assumption, as discussed in Chapter 7. The gentle assumption may decrease the patient's fear of being viewed as sick or odd and is also more difficult to answer with a denial. The technique is illustrated below:

Pt.: I've been feeling really low. I don't know what to do with myself and my husband is really worried.

Clin.: It sounds like a really painful time for you.

Pt.: It sure is. I cry all the time, just like a little kid. It's so embarrassing. I'm not going to do anything crazy, but sometimes I just wish I didn't have to wake up.

> ***Clin.:*** What kinds of thoughts have you had, if any, about kill-
> ing yourself?
> ***Pt.:*** (pause) I've thought about it, yes, I have. But I don't know
> what I'd do.
> ***Clin.:*** What ways have you actually thought about?
> ***Pt.:*** Well, I've thought of over-dosing on aspirin. I have
> thought of that.
> ***Clin.:*** What other ways have you thought about?
> ***Pt.:*** Last week I though of cutting my wrist and running out
> into the woods where nobody could find me in a million
> years.

Several other points come to mind concerning lethality questioning. They can be summarized as follows:

1. The least hesitancy of patient response may suggest that the
patient has had such thoughts, even if he or she proceeds to deny them.
2. Answers such as "no, not really," often indicate that there has
been concrete suicidal ideation. The interviewer can often break the
resistance with a concerned tone of voice and a question such as,
"What kind of thoughts have you had?"
3. The interviewer should carefully look for any body language
clues that the patient is being deceptive or feels anxious.
4. To increase clinician awareness of such clues, there is probably
no excuse for note taking during the elicitation of suicidal ideation.
5. Avoid nonverbal evidence that one might be conveying anxiety, such as increased displacement activities or looking away from the
patient.

As we near the end of our discussion of the second step, it seems
advisable to look at a common myth concerning the search for suicidal
ideation. Simply stated, the myth reads: "I might give patients the idea
to kill themselves if I talk about it."

In the first place, to my knowledge, there is not a single case
example of such a process unfolding. In the second place, the idea of
suicide is no secret. A patient would have to be unusually backward to
have never heard of suicide before encountering the clinician. And
thirdly, and probably most importantly, suicide is extremely hard to
do. It will take a lot more than a single interviewer's discussion of the
topic to lead someone to make the decision.

To the contrary, as discussed earlier, the clinician's frank discussion allows the patient to share a heavy burden, made much heavier by
the isolation imposed by silence. Moreover, the demonstration that
suicidal ideation can be openly discussed conveys that help may only

be a spoken word away. Suddenly, suicidal ideation is no longer a sin to be hidden, but rather a problem to be solved.

In closing our discussion of the second step, it seems appropriate to add that sometimes, later in the interview, it may be worthwhile to repeat the inquiry. Sometimes resistance varies with time. If the interviewer is not satisfied with the first inquiry, a second one may yield some surprises.

The Third Step

The final step in the elicitation of suicidal ideation concerns the exploration of the extent of the lethality. There exists a long continuum, ranging from mild suicidal ideation to concrete plans that may have already been acted upon at some level. Depending upon where the patient is situated on this continuum, the degree of immediate risk increases. It is the role of the interviewer to determine the patient's position. The key to this process is the clarification as to whether the patient has developed an organized plan. If they have such a plan, then how far has the patient carried it out.

There are four issues that concern the interviewer: (1) frequency of suicidal ideation, (2) duration of ideation, (3) concreteness of the suicidal plan, and (4) extent of action taken with regard to the plan. Although bits of information concerning these items are generally spontaneously related by the patient, these issues are often not adequately addressed. Consequently, it is up to the interviewer to make thorough inquiries. To this end, the skilled interviewer displays the persistent tenacity of an expert detective. It is sobering to see the differences in validity that result from differences in interviewers' skill displayed during this third step.

In the first place, if the patient denies suicidal ideation when asked in step two, it sometimes helps to become more specific. By offering concrete examples of what the clinician is asking about, confusion may be decreased. Moreover, it is more difficult to be deceitful when asked about a specific issue than when asked about a general issue. Persistence can provide big dividends. This principle is illustrated below where both behavioral incidents and the use of gentle assumption is once again employed to increase validity:

> **Pt.:** After I left the police force, things started downhill. I guess I didn't retire very gracefully. Sometimes it doesn't seem worth the effort to continue.
>
> **Clin.:** Have you had any thoughts of wanting to kill yourself?

Pt.: No, not really.
Clin.: What have you thought of doing?
Pt.: Nothing that's worth mentioning.
Clin.: Have you ever thought of taking an overdose of pills?
Pt.: No, I haven't.
Clin.: What about cutting yourself or jumping off a bridge?
Pt.: No, those options aren't very good. You might not die.
Clin.: Have you thought of a way you think might be more certain, perhaps like using a gun?
Pt.: (long pause) I have thought of shooting myself.

At this point, the interviewer has broken the initial resistance, uncovering some concrete ideation. The trick now depends upon delineating the concreteness of the plan by gently pushing for more and more detail.

Clin.: What have you thought of doing with the gun?
Pt.: I pictured myself going off to the woods north of town and putting it up to my head and then . . . it's all over.
Clin.: Do you own a gun?
Pt.: Yes I do.
Clin.: Have you ever held it in your hand while thinking about killing yourself?
Pt.: Yes I have.
Clin.: Have you ever put it to your head, John?
Pt.: Yes.
Clin.: And what happened? (said very gently).
Pt.: And I didn't pull the damn trigger . . . (suddenly sobbing) I didn't have the guts. I've never had the guts to do anything. I can't even kill myself.

The interviewer has obviously helped the patient to share very painful material that also suggests serious dangerousness. But the interviewer is not done. It is important to determine even more accurately how serious the patient's intent has been.

Clin.: John, how frequently have you put the gun to your head?
Pt.: I'm not certain (more composed now), maybe ten, fifteen times.
Clin.: When was the last time you did this?
Pt.: Last night, and I really thought I'd do it.
Clin.: How long did you think about it?
Pt.: Probably over an hour. I just sat there in my car with the gun in my hand. It was very cold and the snow was coming

down. I pictured what it would look like with me on the snow.

Clin.: John, do you want to die right now?

Pt.: Yes I do . . . I really do (tearful).

With careful questioning, the interviewer has discovered a man at high risk for suicide. The ideation has been concrete, with extensive actions taken upon a well-organized plan. Even if the number of risk factors discussed earlier was quite low, this type of interchange demands grave concern.

In summary, several important points to consider are as follows:

1. After beginning with general questions, it is often useful to ask quite specific questions.
2. Be persistent.
3. Carefully probe for the specific actions taken on the plan.
4. Do not forget to assess frequency and duration of suicidal ideation.

The search for suicidal ideation described here is used to complement a careful search for the risk factors described earlier. Using these combined approaches, the clinician can begin to gain a deeper understanding of the potential suicide risk of the patient. In the process the interviewer has helped the patient to share painful information, which the patient often has shouldered alone for too long a time. At a different level, perhaps the thoughtfulness and thoroughness of the questioning have conveyed that a fellow human cares. To the patient, such caring may represent the first realization of hope.

A FEW NOTES ON HOMICIDAL IDEATION

The approach to homicidal ideation is a good deal foggier than the approach to suicidal ideation. The reason for this problem is the fact that the risk factors for homicide are not as well delineated. In fact, to my knowledge, no study has indicated an effective way of accurately predicting homicide. Generally, the factor considered most worrisome is a previous history of violence, poor impulse control, or attempted homicide. Certainly, if these factors are present, then one should more aggressively explore for homicidal ideation. But without a long list of risk factors, interviewers become even more dependent upon their interviewing skills. Fortunately, most of the principles discussed with regard to eliciting suicidal ideation are equally applicable to eliciting homicidal ideation.

With these reservations in mind, let us begin by looking at a theoretical triad of lethality for homicide. These three factors tend to arouse the highest concern for homicidal potential:

1. A history of recent violent or homicidal behavior.
2. The presence of psychotic process predisposing to violence or other acute loss of impulse control.
3. Evidence from the interview of significant concrete homicidal plans and intent.

The reader probably recognizes that this homicidal triad looks very similar to the triad of lethality for suicide.

With regard to the first element, a history of violence, the clinician feels more concerned when the frequency or severity of these episodes is significant. To this purpose, the interviewer needs to probe persistently, once again asking specific questions. Questions such as, "During that fight, did your opponent need stitches or have to go to the hospital?" or "Have you ever killed a man?" may be very revealing. An interviewer should not be afraid to ask such questions because of social decorum. When asked in a calm, straightforward manner such questions often get straightforward answers.

Another important aspect of history concerns the issue of whether the intended victim has been an object of the patient's violence before. If so, this fact should be disconcerting, for the risk of violence may increase in such a "powder keg" environment. Keep in mind that most homicides occur between people well known to each other.

A powder keg environment may also develop when the potentially homicidal patient is placed around other people who have poor impulse control. In short, anger may beget anger. And violence may breed violence. Furthermore, the presence of alcohol abuse or drug abuse, in either the patient or the companions, may increase the risk of violence as well. It is important for the interviewer to actively hunt for evidence of such powder keg environments. As with suicide, collateral interviews may be revealing in this regard.

Concerning the second element, psychosis, the same three processes are very concerning. Once again, the interviewer should actively pursue evidence of (1) imperative commands, (2) alien control, and (3) hyper-religiosity. With regard to the latter, the clinician wants to pay particular attention to "missions from God to rid the earth of some evil." Such an intense preoccupation with right and wrong may be signaling underlying homicidal ideation. Once again, the search for specifics may be rewarding, as follows:

Pt.: The world is filled with scum. Derelicts and bums. I hate them all. God wants them gone.

Clin.: How do you mean?

Pt.:	God has his ways.
Clin.:	Has he given you any ideas of how to get rid of them?
Pt.:	Yes he has. He wants me to slit their eyes out. And I might do just that.
Clin.:	Have you thought of anyone in particular you've thought of hurting?
Pt.:	Sammy . . . what a scum life. I've thought of him.
Clin.:	What have you thought of doing to him?

In talking about psychosis, another important avenue to pursue is the presence of paranoia. In particular, the interviewer wants to search for evidence that the patient so believes in the delusional material that methods of acting upon it have been pursued as illustrated below:

Pt.:	The neighbors know everything, I can't keep their eyes out of my brain.
Clin.:	What are they planning on doing to you?
Pt.:	They're going to cut off my feet but I'm not going to let them.
Clin.:	What have you thought about doing to protect yourself?
Pt.:	I'm going to scissor them.
Clin.:	How do you mean?
Pt.:	I'll stick a scissor in their spines.
Clin.:	Have you armed yourself with scissors or some other weapon at home?
Pt.:	Yes I have. Last night I patrolled my house with a pair of scissors and a butcher knife.

This degree of acting on the premise that the delusion is a real threat should strongly suggest hospitalization. Any neighbor of this man may be in serious danger for merely accidentally crossing his path. But the point is, it is not enough to find out if a paranoid delusion is present. The clinician needs to find out what the patient intends to do about it.

With regard to the third element of the triad, evidence of significant homicidal intent from the interview, the principles discussed under suicide elicitation are equally useful here. Once again, the major goal consists of determining whether a concrete homicidal plan has been reached and whether any actions have been taken on it. A point to keep in mind is that if the interviewer suspects that the patient truly intends to kill a specific person, the clinician may have the legal responsibility to warn that potential victim promptly, as mandated by the Tarasoff decision.

One aspect to consider in setting the stage for asking, "Have you had any thoughts of killing someone?" remains the variety of gates available. Homicide has more than the three gates useful in suicidal ideation. Some of these homicidal gates include (1) psychosis, (2) interpersonal conflict, (3) need for money and other practical concerns, (4) revenge, (5) political concerns, (6) organized crime, and (7) pathological murder for pleasure. Naturally, any of these gates could be used to form a window with which to look upon homicidal ideation.

The clinician should also keep in mind that rape should be approached with the same practical and thorough approach as shown with suicide or homicide. It is important to carefully explore for evidence that the patient is moving closer to the actual crime. Questions such as "In the past month have you actually followed anyone with the intention of raping them?" or "How much of your day is spent thinking about rape?" can be very useful. A past history of rape should also be asked for in a nonjudgmental tone of voice.

In closing, with regard to the elicitation of homicidal and violent ideation, the major limiting factor for the interviewer, as with suicidal ideation, remains the interviewer's own skill, tenacity, and sensitivity.

References

1. Resnik, H. L. P.: Suicide. In *The Comprehensive Textbook of Psychiatry*, edited by H. I. Kaplan, A. M. Freedman, and B. J. Sadock. 3rd edition. Baltimore, Williams and Wilkins, 1980, pp. 2085–2098.
2. Patterson, W. M., Dohn, H. H., Bird, J., and Patterson, G.: Evaluation of suicidal patients: The SAD PERSONS scale. *Psychosomatics* 24:343–349, 1983.
3. Resnik, H.L.P., 1980, pp. 2085–2086.
4. Patterson, W. M. et al., 1983, p. 343.
5. Roy, A.: Depression, attempted suicide, and suicide in patients with chronic schizophrenia. *Psychiatric Clinics of North America* 9:193-206, 1986.
6. Wilkinson, G., and Bacon, N. A.: A clinical and epidemiological survey of parasuicide and suicide in Edinburgh schizophrenics. *Psychological Medicine* 14:899-912, 1984.
7. Breier, A., and Astrachan, B. M.: Characterization of Schizophrenic patients who commit suicide. *American Journal of Psychiatry* 141:206–209, 1984.
8. Drake, R. E., Gates, C., Cotton, P. G., and Whitaker, A.: Suicide among schizophrenics: who is at risk? *The Journal of Nervous and Mental Disease* 172:613–617, 1984.
9. Hellerstein, D., Frosch, W., and Koenigsberg, H. W.: The clinical significance of command hallucinations. *American Journal of Psychiatry* 144(2):219–221, 1987.
10. *The Holy Bible*, Revised Standard Version. New York, Thomas Nelson, Inc., 1971.
11. Lion, J. R., and Conn, L. M.: Self-mutilation: Pathology and treatment. *Psychiatric Annals* 12:782–787, 1982.
12. Drake, R. E. et al., 1984, p. 617.
13. Resnik, H. L. P., 1980, p. 2086.
14. Roy, A: Risk factors for suicide in psychiatric patients. *Archives of General Psychiatry* 39:1089–1095, 1982.
15. Roy, A., 1982, p. 1092
16. Resnik, H. L. P., 1980, p. 2086.
17. Fawcitt, J.: Saving the suicidal patient—The state of the art. In *Mood Disorders: The*

World's Major Public Health Problem, edited by F. Ayd. Ayd Communication Publication, 1978.

18. Everstine, D. S., and Everstine, L.: *People in Crisis: Strategic Therapeutic Interventions.* New York, Brunner/Mazel, 1983.
19. Beck, A.: Hopelessness and suicidal behavior. *Journal of the American Medical Association* 234:1146–1149, 1975.
20. Weisman, A. D., and Worden, J. M.: Risk-Rescue rating in suicide assessment. *Archives of General Psychiatry* 26:553–560, 1972.
21. Patterson, W. M. et al., 1983, pp. 343–349.

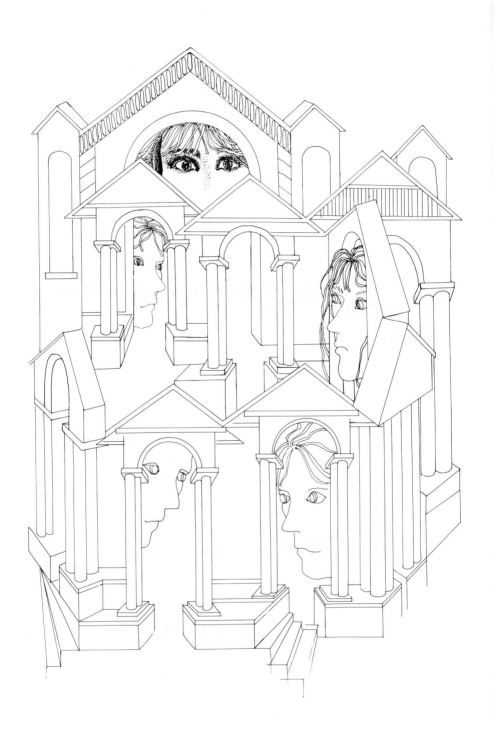

9

Vantage Points: Bridges to Psychotherapy

Man designs for himself a garden with a hundred kinds of trees, a thousand kinds of flowers, a hundred kinds of fruit and vegetables. Suppose, then, that the gardener of this garden knew no other distinction than between edible and inedible, nine-tenths of this garden would be useless to him. He would pull up the most enchanting flowers and hew down the noblest trees and even regard them with a loathing and envious eye.

Herman Hesse, Steppenwolf

During the initial years of training and, indeed, during the remaining course of the clinician's career, the clinician cultivates a garden of sorts. In this garden, the clinician attempts to develop a variety of perspectives or vantage points from which to gain an increased understanding of the patient. There exists no rational reason for the clinician to become fixated upon one viewpoint. Such a narrowing of perspective is suggestive of the gardener, described by Hesse above, who does not comprehend the beauty inherent in each flower, heedlessly discarding that which may be of most value.

Instead, like the gardener, who realizes that a rose delights the eye but a lowly tomato more suitably satisfies the stomach, the maturing clinician begins to understand the advantages of differing viewpoints and schools of thought. Moreover, the maturing clinician avoids overinvestment in personal beliefs, always allotting ample time for a good laugh at himself or herself, for taking oneself too seriously is perhaps one of the most common and treacherous traps awaiting the budding clinician.

Consequently, it seems appropriate as the close of this book approaches to examine at least a few of the many vantage points available to clinicians. By vantage point we are referring to the idea that during any specific moment of the interview, the clinician can consciously concentrate upon different aspects of the ongoing interview process.

443

These viewpoints can be broadly classified into two clusters, attentional vantage points and conceptual vantage points.

For instance, four common attentional vantage points consist of the following: (1) the clinician attempts to listen *with the patient*, seeing the world through the patient's eyes, (2) the clinician attempts to look *at the patient*, as if the patient were an organism to be studied, (3) the clinician attempts to look *at himself or herself*, in order to understand the manner in which the clinician may appear to the patient, and (4) the clinician attempts to look *within himself or herself*, in order to gain an understanding of the patient from the clinician's own emotional responses. These four attentional vantage points may be viewed as forming two axes upon which the clinician may rapidly and flexibly move during the course of the interview (see Figure 11). Each vantage point can provide information that the others may easily miss or may literally prevent from being accessible to the clinician.

Beside these four attentional vantage points, numerous conceptual vantage points can be utilized. Indeed, the number of conceptual vantage points is at least as large as the number of differing theories of counseling and psychotherapy, hardly a small dinner party. In this chapter, three of these conceptual vantage points will be explored, including the perspective concerned with attempting to evaluate the patient's suitability for dynamic psychotherapy, the perspective concerned with deciphering the underlying personality structure of the patient using Kernberg's structural interviewing, and the clinician's ongoing use of intuition and spontaneity. Earlier, in Chapter 2 we examined in detail a fourth conceptual vantage point, facilics, which represents an attempt by the clinician to focus attention on the structuring of the interview as it actively unfolds.

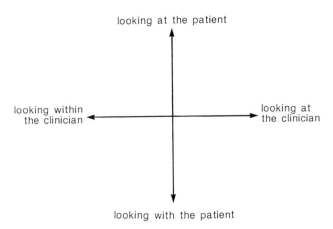

looking at the patient

looking within
the clinician

looking at
the clinician

looking with the patient

FIGURE 11. *Clinician vantage points.*

Each of these conceptual vantage points represents a rich new vista from which the clinician may gain fresh insights. The more of these perspectives in which the clinician feels at home, the more flexible the clinician's style and the more fascinating the art of interviewing become. The clinician becomes constantly surprised by new pathways to follow suggested by the developing characteristics in the immediate interview.

Some clinicians seem to move effortlessly among these various vantage points with little or no conscious awareness that such movements are being made. Such a natural gift for utilizing varying perspectives is not typical. The more natural course consists of slowly learning about the advantages of each perspective, first in a didactic sense and subsequently through experience. As clinicians consciously employ differing vantage points, these clinical perspectives gradually become increasingly more natural, eventually becoming integrated aspects of the interviewer's style. As more experience is gained, frequently the shifts become spontaneous and more intuitive, leading to the sense of surprise, mentioned above, as the clinician happens upon an insight that was not viewable from a previous perspective. As this stage of integration occurs, clinicians frequently report experiencing more vivid feelings while interviewing, and, indeed, the practice of interviewing is never the same again. Clinical challenges, such as encountering resistance, evoke more excitement than they do fear. In this regard, talented interviewers enjoy their work, as evidenced by the spontaneity of their mannerisms and wit.

The question becomes one of discovering a practical method of incorporating the ability to change vantage points into the development of the clinician. Towards this end we will briefly wander into a somewhat enigmatic realm, the world of the "philosopher" G. I. Gurdjieff.[1]

Gurdjieff was born in the Caucasus region of what is now Russia in the 1870's. He would eventually find his way to Europe, where he established the Institute for the Harmonious Development of Man in Fontainebleau, France. Controversy and fanatic fervor were destined to follow Gurdjieff throughout his career more dependably than his own shadow. He would be called everything from a philosopher and sage to a charlatan and fraud. In the last analysis, there may have been a good deal of truth in all of these attributions. No doubt exists that Gurdjieff, at a minimum, was gifted with both creativity and wit. We turn to a study of him, not because of his more occult and suspect beliefs, but because Gurdjieff developed a remarkably modern view of human psychology, much of his thinking focusing upon the interpersonal matrix as well as man's abilities to develop increased self-awareness.

He felt that most people operated, during their moment by moment existence, in a habitual fashion, seldom "awake" to both what they were doing and why they were doing it. In such a state, he postulated that it was impossible to effectively alter behavior or patterns of thought, habit acting as a protective shell against self-growth. Consequently, Gurdjieff attempted to help people gain an awareness of their spontaneous thoughts, emotions, and body movements.

In one famous exercise, as his dancing troop performed a strenuous routine, he would intermittently clap his hands. At the sound of the clap, all dancers were to hold their positions no matter how complex. With this exercise Gurdjieff attempted to instill in his dancers an immediate awareness of the normally unconscious movements and positionings of their bodies.

Although quite serious about his beliefs, Gurdjieff had a knack for making sure that neither his students nor those who came to observe his training programs took themselves too seriously. With regard to the above exercise, it is said that during one performance, he sent his dancers racing towards the audience. Gurdjieff clapped, rather late it would seem, and his dancers froze into human statuettes as they soared into the front rows of the audience. The startled audience had clearly expected the dancers to be halted before take-off, as did the dancers. But then Gurdjieff did not generally work from the realm of the expected.

Of more importance to us, Gurdjieff further developed his idea of increasing self-awareness into the concept of self-remembering, a phrase ideally suited for application to the arena of clinical interviewing, as we shall soon see. Periods of self-remembering occur when people suddenly become aware of their own immediate activity and existence. These periods represent the breakdown of mere habit and are frequently accompanied by a sense of awe or wonderment. For interviewers it is that moment when they become aware of their own participation in the interviewing process. An important distinction must be made here. At these moments of self-remembering, clinicians are not just listening to the patient, they are aware that they are listening to the patient. This ability to step outside of the process itself is similar to the analytic concept of developing an observing ego, the ability to look at one's own actions as they are unfolding.

Now we can see why it is worthwhile examining the beliefs of Gurdjieff, for during periods of self-remembering, the clinician can consciously choose varying vantage points, at times with an amazing rapidity. The ability to insert periods of self-remembering into the interview itself provides the solvent that loosens the ties of habit binding many untrained interviewers. In this regard, several times during the scouting period, the clinician should consciously move into interludes of self-remembering during which various vantage points may be explored. During the remainder of the interview it is wise to insert at least two or three other periods of self-remembering.

In the early stages of training, clinicians generally must consciously insert periods of self-remembering while consciously utilizing differing vantage points. Eventually interviewers become adept at entering them facilely. Soon enough, these periods of increased awareness appear spontaneously as well. For skilled interviewers, there is a feeling of being at home during these periods, as if all their resources were suddenly at hand, which is indeed the case. It is a moment of balance, the natural poise that marks the style of a veteran clinician.

These moments of self-remembering are at the very heart of psychotherapy. Through them the therapist changes vantage points, utilizing various conceptual frameworks or shifting into a purely intuitive mode. At these interludes the therapist's own fantasies are transformed from distractions into avenues of insight. These interludes of self-remembering, through which the clinician flexibly adopts various vantage points, represent true bridges into the psychotherapeutic process itself. To the degree that the clinician can develop an ability to frequently experience periods of self-remembering this will, in some respects, determine the clinician's ultimate potential as an interviewer or a psychotherapist.

It sounds simple, but this ability remains one of the most elusive skills for the beginning clinician. Some clinicians never obtain it. To further our understanding of the uses of self-remembering, in the remaining sections of this chapter we shall examine in detail the four attentional vantage points and the three conceptual ones mentioned earlier. With these discussions providing an operational framework, it is hoped that the reader will then apply these vantage points in the actual interview situation during periods of self-remembering, for only experience can act as the real mentor at this stage of development.

EXPLORATION OF THE ATTENTIONAL VANTAGE POINTS

Looking at the Patient

We will begin by examining the vantage point that some may view as the most obvious and simplistic, looking at the patient. But this vantage point is deceptively simple. It requires a true discipline in order to utilize it effectively. Sensitive clinicians are frequently drawn towards the vantage point of looking with the patient in an empathic sense. Naturally this empathic perspective is extremely valuable and, in a sense, is critical for success. But it can be a trap if the clinician overutilizes it to the detriment of other vantage points, such as looking at the patient. In this context I observed a clinician empathizing with a subtly psychotic patient to the point that the clinician did not recognize that the patient was displaying a loosening of associations and other soft signs of psychosis. In this instance sole reliance upon empathic listening blocked the clinician from establishing enough distance to observe with an objective compassion. The clinician was drawn into the patient's world view, with the result that the patient did not receive the appropriate recommendation for antipsychotic medication.

Two slightly different approaches are useful when attempting to observe the patient with a sensitive eye, the "impact status" and the mental status. The impact status refers to the immediate behavior and affect of the patient at any single moment of the interview. Thus, the impact status represents a quick mental snapshot of the patient, in which the clinician focuses upon the immediate impact on the patient of both the patient's inner world and of the behaviors of the clinician. In contrast, the mental status is a composite of all the observations or "snapshots" made during the course of the interview. It is more a time-lapse film as opposed to a single exposure.

In many respects the impact status was discussed in length in the chapter on nonverbal behavior, but this area is worth a second look. The skilled clinician keenly observes all aspects of the patient's behavior, including mode of dress, hygiene, motor activity, affect and facial expression, mannerisms, and attitude. It is valuable, during the course of the interview, to periodically note the immediate affect of the patient, while asking oneself whether one's own behavior may be affecting the patient negatively, as evidenced by a decrease in the blending process. If such negative interactions are recognized early, one can quickly act to alleviate the stress before significant disengagement has occurred. At other times one may opt to explore with the patient the reasons behind the change in affect. In this fashion the clinician may uncover projective defenses or parataxic distortion, as described by Harry Stack Sullivan.

The clinician may also uncover significant unconscious material or attitudes betrayed by the patient's mannerisms. In this regard it is also useful to consciously make a note of the baseline nonverbal activity of the patient, so that subtle variations can be reflected upon. I am reminded of a young woman who had been in psychotherapy for roughly a year and a half. In one of her sessions she described an upcoming meeting with a supervisor in her graduate program. While she commented, "I guess I better go in and find out what my future is gonna be," she gave a childlike grin, accompanied by a helpless tone of voice. Apparently, at that moment in time, the thought of meeting her supervisor produced an attitude of childlike subservience. This impact status observation could be immediately put to use. I asked her what she had been feeling while discussing her upcoming supervision. I also shared some of my observations on her appearance at that time. This led to a rich exploration of her tendency to not take herself seriously. As she became more aware of her facial expressions, she was also able to successfully role-play meeting this supervisor while displaying an adult affect and attitude.

Throughout the book much has already been discussed with regard to nonverbal behavior, the behavioral indicators of blending, and other aspects key to the concept of the impact status. Consequently, it may be of value to shift our emphasis to the numerous considerations involved in uncovering a sound mental status.

The mental status represents an attempt to objectively describe the behaviors, thoughts, feelings, and perceptions of the patient during the course of the interview itself. These observations are usually written as a separate section of the patient's evaluation. The general topics covered by the mental status are categorized as follows: appearance and behavior, speech characteristics and thought process, thought content, perception, mood and affect, sensorium, cognitive ability, and insight.[2] Clinicians may vary on the exact categories that are used, and some clinicians collect all of these observations into a single narrative paragraph (although I find this somewhat confusing). In any case the clinician attempts to convey the state of the patient during the interview itself, as if a cross-section was being taken of the patient's behavior for sixty minutes.

Here an intriguing phenomenon is encountered, for it is difficult to discuss the gathering of the mental status without carefully considering the process of preparing the written evaluation. The written document frequently reflects the clinician's activities during the interview itself. For example, if the clinician has a difficult time moving into a relatively pure vantage point of observing the patient, then the mental status frequently reflects this inability with omissions, premature assessment opinions, or misplaced bits of the history of the present illness that "explain the patient's psychopathology." In this light a disorganized or confusing written document is usually a reflection of an equally disorganized interview.

Assessment opinions and other conceptual perspectives do not belong in the mental status. They represent contaminants of this vantage point that were probably also present during the interview itself and may have hindered the clinician's ability to observe accurately. The mental status should represent an earnest attempt to describe objectively what is being encountered during the actual clinical interview. It therefore represents a unique and highly valuable aspect of the psychiatric record, for it serves as an area in which the clinician can read about the appearance of the patient, as recorded by a fellow mental health professional at a given point in time. The clinician can then compare the patient's current presentation with the past in an effort to determine evidence of improvement or decline. The use of the mental status in this more disciplined fashion trains clinicians to effectively utilize the vantage point of looking at the patient with as clear an eye as is possible.

The mental status complements other aspects of the written evaluation and is relatively distinct from them. By way of example, the history of the present illness (HPI) describes the pertinent historical aspects of the patient's behavior up until the interview itself. The HPI is frequently a compilation of reports from the patient, the patient's family, previous clinicians, written documents, and other sources of information. The mental status only includes information gathered from the patient, in the same sense that the physical exam only includes the immediate blood pressure reading of the patient, not the history of blood pressure readings taken by previous clinicians.

In a similar vein the narrative assessment, a different section of the written document, allows the clinician to piece together the patient's history and immediate presentation into a cohesive whole, utilizing the added perspective of the clinician's opinions and knowledge base. Neither the history of the present illness or the mental status should include the clinician's assessment opinions, for these are confined primarily to the narrative assessment. On a practical level, one of the reasons it is important to emphasize these distinctions is the fact that clinicians frequently waste an inordinate amount of time repeating themselves in the written document. If a good description of the patient's delusions appears in the history of the present illness, then the mental status need only refer to this material as opposed to repeating it, for the focus should be the current thought content of the patient as illustrated below.

Thought Content

Patient has a history of an extensive delusional system regarding communist infiltration (see HPI). In the interview itself he continues to believe that his place of work is teeming with communists. He even believed that the psychiatric nurse he had just met was also a communist. Upon asking whether his mind might be playing tricks on him, he reported, "I'm not crazy. I know for a fact that the invasion has begun, will you help me?" He denied the belief in an alien invasion reported in the HPI.

Note that the clinician does not go into detail about the specifics of the delusional system for those details had already been related in the HPI. Moreover, the clinician does not discuss his assessment of the patient's distance from his delusion with a statement such as, "This patient clearly remains very delusional and psychotic," for such an appraisal is most effectively made in the narrative assessment, where the clinician provides clinical opinions. Instead, the clinician carefully records the exact words of the patient, which demonstrate the patient's adamant belief in his delusional system. The focus is once again where it belongs in the mental status, on the actual behaviors and thoughts of the patient during the interview itself.

To become an accurate observer, the clinician must learn how to look, in a relative sense, without the contamination of previous beliefs and theoretical assessment issues. This objective stance represents one of the prerequisites of a sound mental status and of the vantage point of looking at the patient. To convey one's observations accurately, it becomes critical for clinicians to utilize a common language. There is no room for a sloppy use of terminology, for such a practice can clearly confuse other clinicians, potentially biasing them towards faulty observations themselves.

Consequently, we shall now examine each segment of the mental status as it might appear in a standard written evaluation. An effort will be made to summarize commonly utilized descriptive terms, to clarify confusing terms, to point out common mistakes, and to provide an example of a well-written mental status. As the clinician becomes adept at writing the mental status, the clinician will also be developing improved skills at using the vantage point of looking at the patient with a highly skilled focus and increased awareness.

Appearance and Behavior

In this section the clinician attempts to accurately describe the patient's outward behavior and presentation. One place to start is with a description of the patient's clothes and self-care. As Wallace suggests, it is probably best to avoid interpretations when describing the patient's clothing and presentation. Instead the clinician records the exact data that ultimately led to the opinions written in the subsequent narrative assessment. In this regard the clinician should describe the patient's apparel as opposed to relying solely upon subjective terms such as "stylish," for not everyone would agree upon the meaning of the word "stylish."[3] Striking characteristics such as scars and deformities should be noted, as well as any tendencies for the patient to look older or younger than his or her chronological age. Eye contact is usually mentioned. Any peculiar mannerisms are noted, such as twitches or the patient's apparent responses to hallucinations, which may be evident through tracking movements of the eyes or a shaking of the head as if shutting out an unwanted voice. The clinician should note the patient's motor behavior; common descriptive terms include restless, agitated, subdued, shaking, tremulous, rigid, pacing, and withdrawn. Displacement activities such as picking at a cup or chain smoking are frequently mentioned. An important, and frequently forgotten characteristic, is the patient's apparent attitude towards the interviewer. With these ideas in mind, let us first take a look at a relatively poor description.

> Clinician A: The patient appeared disheveled. Her behavior was somewhat odd and her eye contact didn't seem right. She appeared restless and her clothing seemed inappropriate.

Although this selection gives some idea of the patient's appearance, one does not come away with a feeling for what it would be like to meet this patient. Generalities are used instead of specifics. Let us look at a description of the same patient that captures her presence more aptly.

> Clinician B: The patient presents in tattered clothes, all of which appear filthy. Her nails are laden with dirt, and she literally has her soiled wig on backwards. She is wearing two wrist watches on her left wrist and tightly grasps a third watch in her right hand, which she will not open to shake hands. Her arms and knees moved restlessly throughout the interview, and she stood up to pace on a few occasions. She did not give any evidence of active response to hallucinations. She smelled badly, but did not smell of alcohol. At times she seemed mildly uncooperative.

This passage clearly presents a more vivid picture of her behavior. The reader now has an idea of what her odd behaviors consist of. The clinician has included pertinent negatives, indicating that she shows no immediate evidence of hallucinating, as might be seen in a delirium. In this example one can almost intuit some of the thinking processes of the clinician with regard to the development of a differential diagnosis. This is a hallmark of a well-organized mental status. Each section adds a new series of pieces to the puzzle, suggesting certain diagnoses and making others less likely. For instance, this patient's agitation may be suggestive of a manic picture.

Speech Characteristics and Thought Process
The clinician can address various aspects of the patient's speech, including the speech rate, volume, and tone of voice. At the same time

the clinician attempts to describe the thought process of the patient, as it is reflected in the manner with which the patient's words are organized. The term "formal thought disorder" is utilized to suggest the presence of abnormalities in the form and organization of the patient's thought, as discussed in this section of the mental status. The less commonly used term, "content thought disorder," refers specifically to the presence of delusions, and it is addressed in a different section of the discussion of mental status. The more generic term "thought disorder" includes both the concept of a formal thought disorder and of a content thought disorder. In this section the emphasis is on the process of the thought (presence of a formal thought disorder), not the content of the speech. Frequently used terms by clinicians include the following:

Pressured speech: Refers to an increased rate of speech, which may possibly best be described as a "speech sans punctuation." Sometimes it is only mildly pressured, whereas at other times, the patient's speech may virtually gush forth in an endless stream. It is commonly seen in mania, agitated psychotic states, or during extreme anxiety or anger.

Tangential thought: The patient's thoughts tend to wander off the subject as the patient proceeds to take tangents off his or her own statements. There tends to be some connection between the preceding thought and the subsequent statement. An example of fairly striking tangential thought would be as follows, "I really have not felt very good recently. My mood is shot, sort of like it was back in Kansas. Oh boy, those were bad days back in Kansas. I'd just come up from the Army and I was really homesick. Nothing can really beat home if you know what I mean. I vividly remember my mother's hot cherry tarts. Boy, they were good. Home cooking just can't be beat." "Circumstantial thought" is identical in nature but differs in the fact that the patient returns to the original topic at hand.

Loosening of associations: The patient's thoughts at times appear unconnected. Of course, to the patient, there may be obvious connections, but a normal listener would have trouble seeing them. In mild forms, loosening of associations may represent severe anxiety or evidence of a schizotypal character structure. In moderate or severe degrees, it is generally an indicator of psychosis. An example of a moderate degree of loosening would look like this: "I haven't felt good recently. My mood is shot, fluid like a waterfall that's black, back home I felt much better, cherry tarts and Mom's

hot breath keeps you going and rolling along life's high-
ways." If loosening becomes extremely severe it is sometimes referred to as a "word salad."

Flight of ideas: In my opinion this is a relatively weak
term, for it essentially represents combinations of the above
terms, which is why most trainees find it confusing. For
flight of ideas to occur, the patient must demonstrate tangential thought or a loosening of associations in conjunction
with a significantly pressured speech. Usually there are connections between the thoughts but, at times, a true loosening
of associations is seen. A frequently but not always seen
characteristic of flight of ideas is the tendency for the patient's speech to be triggered by distracting stimuli or to
demonstrate plays on words. When present, these features
represent more distinguishing hallmarks of a flight of ideas.
Flight of ideas is commonly seen in mania, but certainly can
appear in any severely agitated or psychotic state.

Thought blocking: The patient stops in mid sentence
and never returns to the original idea. These patients appear
as if something had abruptly interrupted their train of
thought and, indeed, usually something has, such as a hallucination or an influx of confusing ideation. Thought blocking is very frequently a sign of psychosis. It is not the same as
exhibiting long periods of silence before answering questions. Some dynamic theorists believe it can also be seen in
neurotic conditions, when a repressed impulse is threatening to break into consciousness.

Illogical thought: The patient displays illogical conclusions. This is different from a delusion, which represents a
false belief but generally has logical reasoning behind it. An
example of a mildly illogical thought follows: "My brother
has spent a lot of time with his income taxes so he must be
extremely wealthy. And everyone knows this as a fact because I see a lot of people deferring to him." These conclusions may be true, but they do not necessarily logically follow. Of course, in a more severe form, the illogical pattern
may be quite striking as with, "I went to Mass every Sunday,
so my boss should have given me a raise. That bum didn't
even recognize my religious commitment."

Let us take a look again at the woman we have already begun to
describe. The first example once again could use some improvement.

Clinician A: Patient positive for loosening of associations
and tangential thought. Otherwise grossly within normal
limits.

This clinician has made no reference to the degree of severity of the formal thought disorder. Specifically, does this patient have a mild loosening of associations or does she verge upon a word salad? Moreover, the clinician makes no reference to her speech rate and volume, characteristics that are frequently abnormal in manic patients. The following brief description supplies a significantly richer data base:

> Clinician B: The patient demonstrates a moderate pressure to her speech accompanied at times by loud outbursts. Even her baseline speech is slightly louder than normal. Her speech is moderately tangential, with rare instances of a mild loosening of associations. Without thought blocking or illogical thought.

Slowly one is beginning to develop a clearer picture of the degree of this patient's psychopathology. More evidence is mounting that there may be both a manic-like appearance and a psychotic process. In any case, coupled with her strikingly disheveled appearance, the clinician may be increasingly suspicious that the patient is having trouble managing herself.

Thought Content
This section refers primarily to four broad issues: ruminations, obsessions, delusions, and the presence of suicidal or homicidal ideation. Ruminations are frequently seen in a variety of anxiety states and are particularly common in depressed patients. Significantly depressed patients will tend to be preoccupied with worries and feelings of guilt, constantly turning the thoughts over in their minds. The thinking process itself does not appear strange to these patients, and they do not generally try to stop it. Instead, they are too caught up in the process to do much other than talk about their problems. In contrast, obsessions have a different flavor to them, although they may overlap with ruminations at times.

An obsession is a specific thought that is repeated over and over by the patient as if seeking an answer to some question. Indeed, the patient frequently obsesses over a question and its answer. As soon as the question is answered, the patient feels an intense need to ask it again, as if some process had been left undone. The patient may repeat this process hundreds of times in a row until it "feels right." If one interrupts the patient while this process is occurring, the patient will frequently feel a need to start the whole process again. Unlike the case with ruminations, patients find these obsessive thought processes to be both odd and painful. They frequently have tried various techniques to interrupt the process. Common themes for obsessions include thoughts of committing violence, homosexual fears, issues of right and wrong, and worries concerning dirt or filth. Obsessions may consist of recurrent ideas, thoughts, fantasies, images, or impulses. If one takes the time to listen carefully to the patient, bearing the above phenomenological issues in mind, the clinician can usually differentiate between ruminations and obsessions.

Delusions represent strongly held beliefs that are not correct or held to be true by the vast majority of the patient's culture, as described in detail in the chapter on psychotic process.

The fourth issue consists of statements concerning lethality. This is a complex area, as noted in Chapter 8. Since all patients should be asked about current lethality issues, these issues should always be addressed in the mental status write-up. In general, the clinician should make some statement regarding the presence of suicidal wishes, plans, and degree of intent to follow the plans in an immediate sense. If a plan is mentioned, the clinician should state to what degree any action has been taken on it. It should also be noted whether any homicidal ideation is present and to what degree, in the same fashion as with suicidal ideation.

Let us return to our patient with two sample excerpts concerning thought content.

Clinician A: The patient is psychotic and can't take care of herself. She seems delusional.

This excerpt is just simply sloppy. The first statement has no place in mental status, for it is the beginning of the clinician's clinical assessment. The description of the delusion is threadbare and unrevealing. The clinician has also omitted the questioning concerning lethality. Assuming the clinician asked but forgot to record this information, the clinician may sorely regret this omission if this patient were to kill herself and the clinician was taken to court. A more useful description is given below.

Clinician B: The patient appears convinced that if the watch is removed from her right hand, the world will come to an end. She proceeds to relate that consequently she has not bathed for three weeks. She also feels that an army of rats is following her and is intending to enter her intestines to destroy "my vital essence." She denies current suicidal ideation or plans. She denies homicidal ideation. Without ruminations or obsessions.

Now we have evidence of someone who is clearly psychotic with concrete delusions. The next question is whether hallucinations play a role in her psychotic process.

Perception

This section refers to the presence or absence of hallucinations or illusions, which were described in detail in Chapter 6. It is of value to note that there sometimes exists a close relationship between delusions and hallucinations. It is not uncommon for the presence of hallucinations to eventually trigger the development of delusional thinking, but the two should not be confused. Let us assume that a patient is being hounded by a voice screaming, "You are possessed. You are a worthless demon." If the patient refuses to believe in the reality of the voice, then one would say that the patient is hearing voices but is not delusional. If on the other hand the patient eventually begins to believe in the existence of the voice and feels that the devil is planning her death, then the patient is said to have developed a delusion as well as to be experiencing auditory hallucinations. We can now turn to our two clinicians.

Clinician A: Without abnormal perceptions.

The question arises as to whether it is appropriate in the mental status to use phrases such as, "grossly within normal limits" or "without abnormality." Generally speaking the mental status is improved by the use of more precise and specific descriptions, but sometimes clinical situations require flexibility. For example, if the clinician is working under extreme time constraints, then such global statements may be appropriate, but in most situations it is preferable to state specifically the main entities that were ruled out, for this essentially relays to the reader that the clinician actually looked for these specific processes. Stated differently, with these global phrases, the reader does not know whether they are accurate or the end result of a sloppy exam. If one has performed a careful exam, it seems best to let the reader know this fact.

Another problem with the phrasing used by Clinician A is the fact that he has stated that the patient does not, in actuality, have hallucinations, but perhaps this patient is simply withholding information for she fears that the voices represent a sickness. Numerous reasons exist for a patient to not share the presence of hallucinations with a clinician, including the fact that the voices may have told the patient not to speak to them. Thus, it may be more accurate to state that the patient denied having hallucinations rather than stating categorically that the patient is without them. With these ideas in mind a slightly more sophisticated report would be as follows:

Clinician B: The patient denied both visual and auditory hallucinations and any other perceptual abnormality.

Mood and Affect

Mood is a symptom, reported by the patient, as to how the patient has been feeling recently in general and tends to be relatively persistent. Affect is a physical indicator noted by the clinician, as to the immediate feelings of the patient. It is demonstrated by the patient's facial expressions and other nonverbal clues during the interview itself and frequently is of a transient nature. Mood is a self-reported symptom; affect is a physical sign. If a patient refuses to talk, then the clinician can say essentially nothing about mood in the mental status itself, except that the patient refused to comment on mood. Later, in the narrative assessment, the clinician will have ample space to describe the clinician's impressions of what the patient's actual mood has been. In contrast to mood, in which the clinician is dependent upon the patient's self-report, the clinician can always say something about the patient's affect.

Thus it is conceivable that a patient who is quite depressed could deny his or her depression, while still appearing sad during the interview. Such a situation would be reported as follows, "The patient demonstrated a sad affect throughout most of the interview, including several short episodes of tearfulness. However, when questioned as to her mood she reported, 'I'm feeling just fine, really I am.'" Later, in the narrative assessment, the clinician would note that the patient's reported mood was inconsistent with both the history and the mental status, perhaps suggesting the presence of active mechanisms of denial or repression. In this situation, some clinicians are tempted to ignore what the patient states, persisting in relaying in the mental status that the patient is depressed. But this prevents the reader from seeing the patient's denial mechanisms. It is far better to let the story speak for itself, while providing one's final assessment in the proper section of the written report. Let us now return to our patient.

Clinician A: The patient's mood is fine and her affect is appropriate but angry at times.

This statement is somewhat confusing. In which sense is her affect appropriate? Is it appropriately fearful for a person who believes that rats are invading her intestines, or does the clinician mean that her affect is appropriate for a person without a delusional system? The clinician should always first state what the patient's affect is and then comment upon its appropriateness. Typical terms used to describe affect include normal (broad) affect with full range of expression, restricted affect (some decrease in facial animation), blunted affect (fairly striking decrease in facial animation), a flat affect (essentially no sign of spontaneous facial expression), bouyant affect, angry affect, suspicious affect, frightened affect, flirtatious affect, silly affect, threatening affect, labile affect, and edgy affect. The following description gives a much clearer feeling for this patient's presentation:

Clinician B: When asked about her mood, the patient angrily retorted, "My mood is just fine, thank-you!" Throughout much of the interview she presented a guarded and mildly hostile affect, frequently clipping off her answers tersely. When talking about the nurse in the waiting area she became particularly suspicious and seemed genuinely frightened. Without tearfulness or a lability of affect.

Sensorium, Cognitive Functioning, and Insight
In this section the clinician attempts to convey a sense of the patient's basic level of functioning with regard to the level of consciousness, intellectual functioning, insight, and motivation. It is always important to note whether a patient presents with a normal level of consciousness, using phrases such as "the patient appeared alert with a stable level of consciousness" or "the patient's consciousness fluctuated rapidly from somnolence to agitation."

It should be noted that this section may have evolved from two processes, the informal cognitive exam and the formal cognitive exam. The informal cognitive exam is artfully performed throughout the interview in a noninvasive fashion. The clinician essentially "eyeballs" the patient's concentration and memory by noting the method by which the patient responds to questions. If the clinician chooses to perform a more formal cognitive exam, it can range from a brief survey of orientation, digit spans, and short-term memory to a much more comprehensive examination, perhaps lasting twenty minutes or so. Clinical considerations will determine which approach is most appropriate. Let us examine the report, which could use some polishing, by Clinician A:

Clinician A: The patient seemed alert. She was oriented. Memory seemed fine and cognitive functioning was grossly within normal limits.

Once again this clinician's report remains vague. Most importantly the reader has no idea exactly how much cognitive testing was performed. No mention has been made regarding the patient's insight or motivation as well. The following excerpt provides a more clarifying picture:

Clinician B: The patient appeared alert with a stable level of consciousness throughout the interview. Indeed, at times, she seemed hyperalert and overly aware of her environment.

She was oriented to person, place, and time. She could repeat six digits forwards and four backwards. She accurately recalled three objects after five minutes. Other formal testing was not performed. Her insight was very poor as was her judgment. She does not want help at this time and flatly refuses the use of any medication.

At this point we are nearing the end of our discussion on the mental status. A simple exercise can demonstrate the power of a well-written mental status. Simply go back and read in a consecutive fashion the excerpts written by Clinician A. One is left with a rather bland and nebulous picture of the woman in question. Afterwards, read the model excerpts in succession by Clinician B. A strikingly more vivid picture of the woman appears. She suddenly seems more human, and the reader can easily picture her warily stalking the room. This then is the goal of the mental status, to ultimately provide a fellow clinician with a reliable image of the patient's actual presentation over the course of the interview.

It should be openly acknowledged that, in actual practice, the written mental status may need to be significantly briefer, but the principles outlined above remain important and can help prevent the briefer mental status from being transformed into an inept mental status.

Even more importantly, the mental status and the impact status create in the clinician a sharpening of the mind's eye. With time these observational skills become more and more keenly honed, allowing the clinician to quickly and gracefully learn from observing the patient, to successfully utilize the vantage point of looking at the patient. The slightest smile becomes an opening into the world of the patient. Without these observational skills, the clinician may be at the risk of being swallowed by the patient's world as opposed to learning from it. In the next section we shall examine in more detail the methods that help one to see with the patient's eyes.

Looking with the Patient

Looking with the patient, the second attentional vantage point, is frequently viewed by many clinicians as the most natural. It is the perspective of empathic listening. Its importance cannot be overstated. I have never seen an accomplished interviewer who was not adept at it. This vantage point remains so integral to the interviewing process itself that we have already discussed many aspects of it in the previous sections of this book.

Pertinent concepts discussed thus far include the engagement process, blending, unconditional positive regard, empathic statements, the empathy cycle of Barrett-Lennard, the phenomenological perspective, tracking, the use of natural and referred gates, and the numerous nonverbal techniques utilized for conveying empathy to the patient. In this section we will not emphasize these concepts again. Instead we shall look at some new ideas, which provide further avenues for understanding the patient's experience of living. These concepts include somatic empathy, the linguistic techniques of Grinder and Bandler, and counterprojective techniques as described by Leston Havens.

Somatic Empathy. Somatic empathy was alluded to in the chapter on nonverbal techniques. It is based upon the precept that the posturing of the patient's body not only reflects the defenses and feelings of the patient but also serves to foster a way of experiencing the environment itself. For example, a tight-fisted man who sits persistently grinding his jaw will, by the very act of grinding his jaw, experience the world in a "tight-jawed" fashion. One is reminded of the work of Wilhelm Reich, who discussed the term "body armor," a term suggesting that body positioning may itself represent a type of defense mechanism or manner of coping with the stresses of the environment.[4]

In its most effective form, somatic empathy is fostered by literally assuming the position of the patient. Thus, it is usually done not in the presence of the patient but between therapeutic sessions. By assuming the patient's posture or mannerism, the clinician obtains an actual feeling for what the patient was experiencing in the session itself. Clinicians can allow their imaginations to wander freely in the assumed position, noting everything from spontaneous fantasies to muscle tensions. It is sometimes quite surprising to experience the peculiar sensations of rigidity and tension that many patients literally carry around with them. This simple exercise, if carried out in an uninhibited fashion, can provide a powerful experience for the clinician, producing a peculiar sense of closeness with the patient as if suddenly understanding, for the first time, what the patient had been saying.

I am reminded of one woman who spoke with a flutter of gesticulations, as if her wrists were floppy hinges. At times during the initial interview, she would hang her arms down over the arms of the chair. From this position they would jerk around, banging loosely against the arms of the chair as she spoke, a human Raggedy Ann. After the session, when I actually attempted to mimic these movements, I was surprised at the unsettling sensation of being out of control that such posturings could produce. The patient's world was just such a "theater of the helpless." At times during the session itself the clinician may note a small gesture of the patient, perhaps a way of holding his or her hand, that can be mimicked immediately without the patient's awareness. This exercise may help move the clinician into a more empathic understanding of the patient at that moment in time.

Deep and Surface Structure. Leaving the world of nonverbal behavior, the focus can move to a method of increasing an understanding of the patient's world, determined by the patient's language itself. Grinder and Bandler have developed a conceptual model that can help the clinician to move more effectively into the world of the patient. The following description provides a brief introduction to these techniques, and I urge the reader to look at the original work itself.[5]

At one level, language results from the experience of the human organism as it attempts to translate information into a code, which can be immediately understood by other organisms. But the code itself may ultimately begin to determine the manner in which the organism experiences the surrounding world. In a sense, humans begin to limit their interpretations of their experience to those that can be encoded by the language. Unfortunately, as this process unfolds, the language begins to limit experience as opposed to describing it. Stated somewhat differently, the range of actual human feelings and perceptions is vastly more complicated than the language can describe.

For the sake of clarification, if there exist only two words to describe snow, then the person will probably pay little attention to the numerous variations among different types of snow. On the other hand, if there existed ten nouns to represent snow, the human would, by the nature of the language itself, need to pay more attention to what type of snow was encountered in order to communicate the experience clearly. A person armed with ten words may experience the nuances of the snow much more intensely than a companion limited to two words. Experience can literally be determined by language. In this sense it becomes crucial for the clinician to listen to the language utilized by the patient, for the possibility exists that the patient's language may be creating a framework that is detrimental to the patient, for it limits or distorts the patient's view of actual circumstances.

The language used in daily conversation tends to represent a "shorthand" of what the person is actually thinking. Large amounts of the actual message may be left unstated and lost to the receiver of the message, in this case the clinician. Even more disturbing is the possibility that the patient will begin to conceptualize the situation via the limiting framework of this shorthand message. At first, these ideas may appear somewhat abstract, but they become clearer if one views language as having two different levels of meaning, depending upon the completeness of the message communicated. Based upon the study of transformational grammar, Grinder and Bandler describe these two levels as deep structure and surface structure. A very simple and effective method of seeing the world more clearly through the patient's eyes consists of gently probing the patient's surface statements until both the patient and the clinician discover the deleted deep structure.

An example may serve to clarify. Suppose the patient makes the following statement:

People constantly hurt me.

This statement has emerged from a specific substrate that is potentially ripe with powerful information to the clinician but is currently unavailable. There must exist a deep structure, as illustrated below from which the patient's comment was transformed:

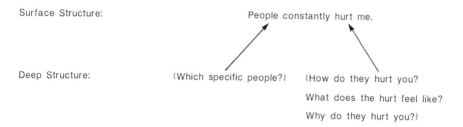

Surface Structure: People constantly hurt me.

Deep Structure: (Which specific people?)   (How do they hurt you?
                                                      What does the hurt feel like?
                                                      Why do they hurt you?)

The deep structure holds many important secrets. Is the patient referring to all people, people at work, his parents, his siblings? Is the pain the "hurt" of rejection, shame, inferiority, abandonment? Grinder and Bandler maintain that by gently seeking answers to such questions, the clinician will gradually uncover progressively more important material, and, at times, the patient may be surprised by the implications of the deep structure. For instance, the patient may have been unaware of feeling rejection or the pain of sibling rivalry. Such discoveries may eventually change the patient's perception of the related experience itself. In any case, at the very least, the clinician gains a better view of what the world looks like to the patient. Let us see the technique in action.

Pt.: People constantly hurt me.
Clin.: Exactly which people are you talking about?
Pt.: Oh, my wife and her brother, I hate him so much.
Clin.: What other people are you referring to?
Pt.: Well I. . . . Let's see, her sister is pretty nasty too.
Clin.: What about your own family?
Pt.: Well, my brother is hard to get along with, but my parents

are actually pretty supportive. (pause) You know, come to think of it, my parents really have been pretty nice to me recently.

Clin.: It sounds like that seems different to you than in the past.

Pt.: (Patient chuckles) To tell you the truth, a year or so ago I'd have been telling you how much I hated my parents, but they really seemed to change back then. (Undoubtedly the patient, either consciously or unconsciously, is referring to a specific time or event by the word "then," so the clinician probes for the deep structure.)

Clin: When did you notice the change?

Pt.: Back when Jan and I moved out of their house. I don't know, maybe living with them was a strain on all of us. It really was too crowded, uh, felt cramped, sort of like a crowded bus station?

Clin.: Do you think your parents realize that you appreciate their new attitude?

Pt.: Hmmm, I really sort of doubt it. Maybe I ought to give them a call sometime, maybe.

Clin.: Let me make sure I have this straight. You're having increased problems with some specific people in your life like your wife. On the other hand your relationship with your parents has matured and is actually stronger?

Pt.: Yes, yes that's it in a nutshell.

But what a different nutshell than the patient began with. By uncovering the deep structure, the patient has come upon information that is both revealing and comforting. The original statement "People constantly hurt me" was a gross distortion caused by generalization. Since the patient came to believe this generalization, the situation seemed worse than it was in reality, for, in truth, some good things were also occurring. By probing for the patient's deep structure the clinician has clearly gained a more accurate perception of what the world looks like to the patient. Yet there is more to the story, for the patient is now viewing the situation in a slightly more positive light. The therapeutic process itself has begun.

These uncovering techniques described by Grinder and Bandler serve as another bridge into the therapeutic process, for the patient may "stumble" upon a more realistic and less threatening perception of reality. These uncovering techniques are similar to the principles behind therapeutic modalities such as cognitive therapy or rational emotive therapy.

In this example the clinician chose to explore the subject of this sentence, but could have just as easily chosen to explore the deep structure beneath the verb or the adverb. In fact by exploring what the patient meant by the word "constantly," the patient may very well have discovered that his wife is not *always* mean to him, a realization that may be of some importance.

Grinder and Bandler state that two of the more frequent transformations that occur between the deep structure and the surface structure are deletions and generalizations, as illustrated in the dialogue above. Although this uncovering technique appears at first glance to be almost too simple, it is remarkably powerful. And to use it well the clinician must be able to switch vantage points.

Counterprojective Statements. The next technique, the use of counterprojective statements, yields another method of improving the blending process, as the clinician attempts to see the world with the patient. Counterprojective techniques were developed by Leston Havens for use in psychotherapy itself as well as during the initial interview.[6] Their use is described in detail in his highly informative and entertaining book *Making Contact.*[7]

Counterprojection is utilized when a guarded or actively paranoid patient is beginning to project hostile impulses onto the clinician. At these moments it is very difficult to view the world through the patient's eyes, for the patient's focus is upon the clinician, who may appear to the patient as representing an antagonistic "other." For blending to proceed, the clinician must switch the focus of the patient off of the clinician and onto a common "screen" that both the clinician and the patient can look at together. Put more colloquially, the clinician wants the heat off himself or herself.

The goal of the counterprojective statement is to deflect the projection off of the clinician before it becomes stabilized and difficult to defuse. In the specific context of the initial interview, the goal is to immediately deflect the patient's suspicion while subsequently sidetracking the patient to a new topic that is away from a focus upon the clinician. It is hoped that this sidetracking will provide the clinician with enough time to shore up the engagement process, resulting in a more trusting alliance. In a simplistic sense the principle works upon the adage that one should not try to stop two people from arguing, for, soon enough, the two will turn on the newcomer as the common enemy. With counterprojection one attempts to find a common antagonist or area on which to focus the attention of both the patient and the clinician. Let us watch the technique in action:

> **Clin.:** What were some of the problems that have been particularly upsetting to you, Mr. Hughlings?
> **Pt.:** They're really quite specific and relate to the needling behavior of my wife, who has to know everything.
> **Clin.:** What are some of the specifics?

> **Pt.:** That's rather difficult to say. She's got her own problems, if you know what I mean.
>
> **Clin.:** What are some of the things that are most unsettling to you, that you came here today about?
>
> **Pt.:** I don't really see why the details should concern you, I don't like it when people ask too many probing questions, if you catch my drift.
>
> **Clin.:** I don't like it when people push me to talk about things that I don't feel like talking about either. Let's back off for a moment. I take it your wife has been pushing and prying recently. Is that correct?
>
> **Pt.:** Yes, she's gone further than she should, if she knows what is good for her.
>
> **Clin.:** She's always on your case then.
>
> **Pt.:** Absolutely, I'm really tired of it.
>
> **Clin.:** Is this a totally new behavior for her or is this sort of a long-standing trait that has gotten worse?
>
> **Pt.:** It's gotten much worse, but I think she's always been part busybody, it's in her genes.
>
> **Clin.:** Her family was also like this?
>
> **Pt.:** You better believe it. In particular her mother was a real busy-body. Right from the start I knew I was heading for some tough times. You know, the problem is that you don't just marry a person, you marry the whole family and this one came from the cheapest level of the bargain basement.

In the beginning of the dialogue, we find the patient answering with the vagueness that frequently typifies a guarded or paranoid patient. As the interviewer attempts to clarify some of the muddy waters, a curious process begins to unfold. The patient's anger towards his wife is beginning to be projected onto the clinician himself. The situation is personalized by the comment "I don't really see why the details should concern you." Immediately the patient and the clinician are becoming two separate worlds oppositionally staring at each other, in contrast to two people jointly observing the world "out there." An antagonism is rapidly brewing as the paranoid attitude begins to solidify a projection onto the clinician. To make matters worse, the patient proceeds to accuse the clinician of the very same behaviors that the patient perceives in his wife with the comment, "I don't like it when people ask too many probing questions, if you catch my drift." At this point the clinician is rapidly becoming enmeshed in a sticky unconscious flypaper. It is time to make a retreat, to deflect the projection.

To accomplish this task the clinician responds, "I don't like it when people push me to talk about things that I don't feel like talking about either." The clinician reports feeling a very similar emotion to what the patient has expressed. Suddenly, the clinician and the patient are part of the same camp, which is looking out at all those people who are "too pushy." It is very difficult for the patient to continue attacking the clinician for a behavior that the clinician also dislikes and claims to be seeing in others. Subsequently, the outside focus is solidified by the clinician identifying a specific new object for the joint focus of the patient and himself. The clinician moves the focus onto the patient's wife with the statement, "I take it your wife has been pushing and prying recently."

At this point the heat is off the clinician, both he and the patient focusing their attention on the patient's wife, a topic that eventually perks the interest of the patient. The follow-up statement, "She's always on your case then," is also a counterprojective technique that further solidifies the patient's attention on an object removed from the clinician. The projection has been successfully deflected. The interview proceeds on course. Note that the clinician does not accuse the wife but merely reflects back the sentiments expressed by the patient himself earlier. Clinicians must be careful not to join the paranoid process, but rather to deflect it away from themselves.

Havens points out that three elements must be present for a counterprojective technique to function effectively. First, the object that is chosen for the new focus of attention must be "out there," thus ensuring that the patient's projection will move to a new focus of attention. Second, a specific object or concept (as opposed to a vague generalization) needs to be mentioned so that the patient's attention will become firmly focused. And third, the clinician relates feeling an emotion similar, if not identical, to that being felt by the patient. In this fashion the clinician and the patient are plopped into the same world view, both of them looking out at those nasty objects that upset them. From this more common ground the clinician can then work to establish a more well-grounded alliance.

Counterprojective statements generally are phrased in the third person, such as "he always seems interested only in himself," or "they never seem to understand you." The third person stance emphasizes the concept of directing the patient's projection away from the interviewer so that there is something "out there" to be discussed and observed by the patient and the clinician. Havens also notes that these statements may convey an empathic quality.

As illustrated above, in some instances, the clinician may opt to utilize first person statements, in which case he or she emphasizes the shared quality of the emotion the patient is experiencing. On a cautionary level, first person statements carry the risk of focusing the patient's attention on the clinician, but in some situations this can be highly effective. For instance, a talented psychiatric resident described the following interaction. An actively paranoid woman interrupted a session with an accusatory tone, "Is this office bugged?" The resident responded, "It would upset me greatly if my office were bugged. No it isn't." The patient accepted this counterprojective deflection readily, and the session continued in a fruitful manner.

We have now reviewed three techniques for enhancing the ability of the clinician to move into the vantage point of "looking with the patient." Essentially the two vantage points explored so far, looking *at* the patient and looking *with* the patient, lie at either ends of an axis whose focus is the patient. The same type of attentional axis can be conceptualized using, not the patient, but the clinician as the focus of attention. Just such an axis is the topic of the next two sections.

Looking at Oneself

This section focuses on the vantage point through which the interviewer attempts to objectively look at himself or herself. The ultimate goal is for clinicians to develop an accurate sense of how they appear to the patient. In this sense clinicians search for their own identifying persona. Naturally, the interviewers cannot know for certain in what ways their persona may be affected by the patient's process of parataxic distortion, but clinicians should possess at least a baseline understanding of their own typical appearance and behavior. From this increased self awareness interviewers may be able to ward off certain aspects of parataxic distortion before significant problems with blending occur. For instance, clinicians who tend to be rather warm and extroverted may purposely tone down their style when initially encountering paranoid patients, for the clinicians are aware that the paranoid processes of the patient may predispose the patients towards distorting the warmth into a sinister attempt to "trick me into trusting you."

Two aspects of this vantage point complement each other. First, during the interview itself the clinician needs to be able to utilize periods of self-remembering, which enable one to ask, "How do I appear to the patient at this moment?" As mentioned in the chapter on nonverbal behavior, this "watching attitude" can be facilitated by imagining a mirror dropping in front of oneself during the interview. This concrete exercise can increase the interviewer's ability to rapidly assume this specific vantage point. The second aspect of this vantage point concerns gaining a knowledge of how one appears, not through imaginative techniques but via feedback provided by outside observers.

In this regard the importance of supervision cannot be overemphasized. Three types of supervision are particularly powerful in helping clinicians to gain an understanding of how they come across to patients. These three types of supervision include videotaped supervision, direct in-the-room observation by a supervisor, and feedback obtained from observing peers (collegial supervision). The numerous advantages offered by videotape supervision are well known, but the latter types of supervision are probably equally of value.

Direct supervision, in which the supervisor sits in on the interview itself, provides a chance for the clinician to be directly observed during actual clinical conditions. The supervisor can also immediately demonstrate techniques as resistances or problems confront the trainee. Despite the naturally occurring hesitancies associated with having a supervisor directly observing, trainees frequently request large amounts of this type of supervision once they have experienced it.

Obtaining feedback from peers provides a third avenue through which a wealth of information can be gained, for each observer tends to notice different aspects of style. Naturally the observers learn as well, for each trainee brings fresh techniques that may be modelled by other trainees.

In this light, it should be emphasized that it is also extremely useful to supervise others. Besides providing an opportunity to observe potentially useful techniques developed by others, the act of supervision trains the clinician to accurately observe the interviewing process. If one cannot first learn to astutely observe the styles of others, then it is highly unlikely that one will be able to effectively study oneself. In this sense it is frequently invaluable to find a peer with whom one switches the supervisory role.

In any case, by utilizing the above techniques clinicians work towards a sophisticated understanding of their own appearances. Interviewers should ultimately be able to describe their styles along a continuum including the following:

$$
\begin{array}{rcl}
\text{responsive} & \longleftrightarrow & \text{not responsive} \\
\text{spontaneous} & \longleftrightarrow & \text{not spontaneous} \\
\text{animated} & \longleftrightarrow & \text{not animated} \\
\text{transparent} & \longleftrightarrow & \text{not transparent}
\end{array}
$$

Each of these four axes focuses upon slightly different aspects of interviewing style. The axis of responsiveness refers to the clinician's tendency to show an affective response to the behaviors or statements of the patient. Thus, a responsive clinician may smile or chuckle if the patient attempts a joke, while the nonresponsive clinician would show no change in affect. The axis of spontaneity represents the degree with which the clinician conveys spontaneous affect and opinion. It may be demonstrated by the clinician's use of humor, for example. The axis of animation delineates the spontaneous baseline of affectivity and body gesturing of the clinician. With large amounts of animation the clinician will be gesturing frequently, while, at the other end, the clinician will seem immobile; occasionally one may even find a clinician remarkably like a stone. The fourth axis, the axis of transparency, is similar to the above axes but refers specifically to the degree with which the clinician consciously reveals emotions or personal thoughts to the patient.

As well as these characteristics the clinician should also be aware of other hallmarks of style, including the following:

1. Tendency to express warmth and/or empathy
2. Displacement activities
3. Self-touching behaviors (such as the hand to the cheek)
4. Use of humor
5. Body language when exploring sensitive areas
6. Body language when confronted with resistance or demands
7. Body language around potentially violent patients
8. Typical distance one sits from patients
9. Frequency and content of notes
10. Rate of speech, tone of voice, and volume of voice
11. Hand gestures and head nodding activity
12. Style of clothing and general appearance (does the clinician look liberal, stylish, establishment, sloppy, preppy, rich, sexy, tired? All of these elements can affect both the engagement process and the development of transference characteristics.)

The ultimate goal is the development of a flexible style in which the clinician feels at ease, while realizing the potential ramifications of the various modes of this style on patients of differing temperaments. Each clinician will develop a distinctive style marked by various aspects of the clinician's own personality.

Once the clinician is aware of stylistic characteristics, flexibility can be achieved. For instance, my own style tends to be mildly animated with a fair amount of spontaneous body language, use of wit, and head nodding. When meeting with a paranoid patient, I consciously tend to decrease all of these elements, arriving at a more low-key style, a style that paranoid patients seem more at ease with initially. Then by following cues given by the patient, I can consciously warm up or further cool down the style as seems appropriate.

In order to gain this type of flexibility, the clinician needs to carefully learn to utilize periods of self-remembering during which the clinician takes advantage of this particular vantage point, a vantage point that is frequently overlooked.

Looking within Oneself

Looking within oneself represents the final attentional vantage point that shall be discussed. Once again the focus is on the clinician as opposed to the patient, only now the clinician attempts to explore his or her own emotions and fantasies. At first glance, it would seem that it should be a relatively easy task to tune into one's own feeling state. The truth of the matter is that many clinicians have more trouble truly understanding what the world looks like through their own eyes than through the eyes of the patient. Many defenses exist that tend to hide emotional responses from the clinician's awareness.

The first step in utilizing this vantage point effectively lies in the ability of the clinician to accurately answer the question, "What am I feeling right now?" It is important that the clinician search for actual feelings, such as sadness, anger, frustration, attraction, excitement, boredom, time pressure, performance anxiety, and fear. One is not hunting for answers such as, "I was feeling that the patient was probably getting upset with me" or "I was feeling that the patient was probably displaying histrionic traits." These statements are not feelings, they are opinions and intellectualizations, and yet most clinicians when asked what they are feeling will offer such answers, just as patients in psychotherapy frequently answer questions concerning feeling in an intellectualized manner. On the contrary, the answers that one is seeking sound like, "I was feeling awkward in there and a little frustrated" or "I was feeling fairly interested, but no more than usual."

As Pilkonis[8] has suggested, one can easily tell when a response is not dealing with a true feeling, for, in such instances, one can use the word "think" as the verb in the clinician's statement. For instance, using the above examples one can replace the statement "I was feeling that the patient was probably displaying histrionic traits" with "I think the patient was probably displaying histrionic traits." This phrase sounds natural and its meaning is essentially unchanged, for the clinician was actually reporting an opinion not an emotion. On the other hand, a statement truly reflecting clinician emotion makes no sense with this substitution, as seen with, "I was thinking awkward in there" or "I was thinking mad." The illogical quality of these transformations suggests that the original statements by the clinician represented true expressions of emotion.

By utilizing periods of self-remembering, through which this vantage point can be entered effectively, clinicians will become progressively more adept at recognizing both subtle and powerful emotional responses in themselves. The next logical question concerns the possible uses of such information. But in order to understand the uses of this perspective, one must also understand from where these clinician emotions originate. Three broad areas come to mind, including (1) naturally intuitive responses, (2) associational responses, and (3) transferential responses. Some clinician responses can fall neatly under one of these headings. Many other responses evolve from two or more of these areas. Each category will be discussed separately, keeping in mind that the separations may be somewhat arbitrary.

Intuitive Responses

Intuitive responses represent emotional states and perceptions arising in the clinician that are both easily accessible to consciousness and frequently represent responses that may be aroused in other people who interact with the patient for any length of time. Intuitive responses are not necessarily indicators of the clinician's own deeper dynamics, but represent naturally occurring and relatively spontaneous responses to the patient. Sometimes these gut-level responses seem quite natural to the clinician and other times they may be somewhat surprising and insightful. For instance, a grossly insulting patient may quickly spark angry feelings in the clinician. Such reactions may be laden with important information, for they may represent mirrors of the patient's psychopathology and/or feelings. In essence, the clinician is being provided with an immediate sample of how this patient may affect other people in his family or on the street. As mentioned before, the interview represents a dyadic interaction, and if the clinician experiences anger, one must wonder what the patient may be doing that creates such a response in the clinician. In this sense the clinician's spontaneously occurring emotional responses may serve as a tip-off to important information that is being overlooked because of a preoccupation with other vantage points.

For purposes of illustration let us look at the development of a feeling of fear in a clinician. Such feelings, if recognized, should be given careful attention, for the clinician's intuitive skills may be recognizing a potentially dangerous situation of which the clinician is not totally aware. I am reminded of a story told to me many years ago by a professor that highlights this point. I have sometimes wondered if the story was more apocryphal than true, but nevertheless it makes the point.

Apparently a clinician had been working with a patient for many months without much difficulty. Unexpectedly the clinician began developing intense feelings of being ill-at-ease and frightened with the patient in a vague manner during the sessions. Convinced that he was suffering from problems with countertransference he sought several consultations all to no avail. One day, to his surprise, the patient began the session with, "Today is your lucky day, Doc." When asked what he meant the patient sported a wry smile, saying, "Today I decided not to kill you." Although not there, I suspect this subtle aside put an end to any note taking on the part of the clinician. It is indeed a novel way of getting the attention of one's therapist. On a more serious note, over the past several weeks the patient had been carefully following the therapist. He proceeded to show the therapist his comprehensive notes concerning the therapist's moment by moment activities. He also provided in detail the method with which the murder was to take place.

Although rather dramatic in nature, the story has a point to convey. Feelings of fear should be taken seriously, especially in settings in which the client is not known to the system, such as when an intake interview is being performed. The fear may represent the fact that the patient is beginning to lose control.

On the other hand, clinician fear may reflect different processes within the patient. For example, it can also be an indication that the patient is demonstrating subtle psychotic signs. In this regard, mild aspects of psychotic process, such as inappropriate affect, may be catching the clinician off-guard leading to an uneasy feeling that has nothing to do with potential violence from the patient but may be the first tip-off that psychotic process is alive and well in the room. At other moments, the clinician's fear can represent an empathic resonance with the fears of a paranoid patient.

Other, less disturbing emotions in the clinician can also represent reflections of patient psychopathology that may be worth examining from other vantage points, demonstrating the fact that vantage points tend to complement one another. For example, if the clinician becomes unusually fascinated by a patient's story, it suggests that the clinician is in the presence of a "gifted storyteller," perhaps a storyteller with underlying histrionic traits. It may be the patient's dramatic flair that is triggering the clinician's fascination. If during such an interview the clinician looks inwards, recognizing the unusual degree of attentiveness caused by the patient, then the clinician can switch to a more revealing vantage point. The vantage point of looking at the patient could provide confirming evidence suggestive of a histronic presentation such as dramatic gesturing or flirtatiousness. Thus one vantage point can suggest the use of other vantage points. The key point remains that interviews represent interactional processes in which clinician responses are evidence of patient attributes and vice versa.

By way of further example, if clinicians find themselves feeling frustrated by the need to constantly repeat questions, this frustration may be the flip side of the presence of either tangential or circumstantial speech in the patient. Feelings of mild confusion in the clinician may suggest the presence of mild forms of loosening of associations or illogical thought in the patient. Boredom in the clinician may reflect the presence of a patient with a blunted affect or monotone voice to whom quite literally it is boring to listen. Boredom may also suggest a variety of other processes that may be occurring within the clinician. For instance, boredom may represent a defense against specific feelings such as anger or erotic arousal.

Associational Responses

At times, the responses generated in the clinician such as boredom or anger may represent, for the most part, normal responses to the behaviors of the patient as discussed above in relation to intuitive responses. But in other circumstances the clinician may begin feeling a response that most people would not feel or perhaps not feel as intensely with a specific patient. Such idiosyncratic feelings bring us to the second category of response etiologies, associational responses. In associational responses the patient is reminding the clinician of some other person in the clinician's past or current history. These feelings are not particularly deep. They are either immediately conscious or easily made conscious. Various aspects of the patient from clothing to demeanor may be associated with important people in the clinician's life, including people whom the clinician either likes or dislikes. Thus the clinician may rapidly develop feelings ranging from sexual attraction to distaste or bitterness. It is important for the clinician to become rapidly aware of such associational responses, for they can significantly affect the clinician's ability to make sound judgments and may also affect the blending process itself.

If aware of one's associational responses and their possible negative ramifications, then these responses can frequently be utilized to the clinician's benefit. Suppose that a clinician was raised by highly domineering parents with the result that the clinician developed an uptight feeling anytime the clinician was near the parental dyad. If this clinician begins to feel this uptightness around a patient, it may be a sensitive barometer that the patient is exhibiting domineering traits, perhaps even in a subtle fashion. If aware of these inner responses, the clinician could then more carefully explore for the presence of domineering character traits in the patient. In fact, this clinician may actually be more sensitive to such traits, recognizing them more readily than other clinicians because of an ability to identify this uptight feeling.

Transferential Responses

Emotional responses in the clinician are not necessarily bad or evidence of psychopathology in the clinician. They are frequently useful both in diagnostic interviewing and in psychotherapy itself. It is more the unawareness of these feelings or an inability to work with them that frequently leads to problems.

The concept of the dangers of unawareness raises the last category, responses created in the therapist through countertransference. Countertransference refers to emotions, associations, and defenses triggered by the patient in the clinician, whose etiologies are in a true sense unconscious or difficult to bring to conscious awareness. When true countertransference feelings have crystallized, the clinician begins to re-experience past relationships in the current relationship with the patient. By way of example, a clinician may have domineering parents but was never fully aware of the impact of this domination. Furthermore, at an unconscious level the clinician dealt with this anxiety by withdrawing from both parents, highlighted by a tendency to display a cool exterior towards them. In this instance, as the clinician encounters the domineering patient, the clinician may begin to handle the patient with an unnecessary curtness and coolness, previously displayed to the clinician's parents.

Probing self-reflection, increased attention to the vantage point of looking within oneself, supervision, and psychotherapy are all mechanisms available to clinicians that will provide awareness of such countertransference reactions and their potential impact. This leads to an important point. Generally speaking true transferential responses are not commonly seen in the initial interview, for it often takes time for the countertransference to crystallize. Instead, in the context of the initial interview, the interviewer is more apt to see the seeds of the countertransference emerging. In actuality, the more typical responses in the initial interview are associational responses and naturally intuitive responses.

I point this out because some clinicians tend to use the term countertransference rather loosely to define almost any response generated in the clinician. This loose interpretation can be somewhat misleading, for true countertransference responses require a more sophisticated exploration and may be considerably more difficult to utilize in a positive sense, although ultimately they too can be of extreme utility in the actual work of psychotherapy. As countertransference issues are made more available to the clinician's awareness, they are essentially transformed into associational responses, which can once again be utilized as sensitive barometers of patient characteristics by the clinician.

Indeed, viewed together, naturally intuitive, associational, and transferential responses can become some of the most valuable tools for the experienced clinician. As they gain experience, clinicians may begin to notice certain types of responses in themselves that typically are generated by specific personality styles in patients or may be relatively field specific to certain clinical situations such as impending suicidal acting out. This vantage point can then point the clinician to hunt for confirmation of these hunches through the use of other vantage points and avenues of interviewing.

Fantasy

Thus far the discussion has focused upon the emotional responses of the clinician. Another viable region for exploration consists of clinician fantasy material. At times it may be important for the clinician to essentially curb such fanciful wanderings, if for instance the patient needs an empathic listener. At such points, the clinician may mentally note the fantasy images for future exploration. On the other hand, frequently the clinician may be at a point in the interview in which a few moments can be productively spent silently exploring fantasy material in an effort to determine its possible relationship to the immediate clinical interaction.

The fantasy may be tied in with associational or transferential responses or may simply represent the active workings of the clinician's own intuition. In any case, interesting insights may be gained. I remember working with a woman who was describing her activities while working in the home as a housewife. She was in her mid-twenties and had entered therapy following an explosive extramarital affair that now jeopardized her marriage. As she was talking about her work and her time spent with her small girl, I began having memories of a previous coworker. It seemed odd to be thinking about this previous colleague, so I decided to play with the fantasy a bit. I remembered disliking my colleague for she always seemed self-centered and complained rather constantly about her job. She simmered with an underlying resentment of her work and wished to be in a different position.

I wondered if I had been unconsciously led to feelings within the patient of discontent and anger. I turned to her and asked, "Although you talk somewhat glowingly about your work at home, I wonder if at times you feel some anger about being cooped up all the time." She seemed caught off guard by the comment and proceeded to enter a long description of her complaints about wishing she was back at her job as a secretary and that, in reality, she just did not know what she wanted to do with her life. Tears welled in her eyes. This vignette represents an instance in which the unconscious of the clinician was productively at work. Fantasies can provide valuable grist for the mill. In this regard, some clinicians jot down fragments of fantasy material and other doodlings as an active aspect of note taking.

Before concluding the discussion of this particular vantage point, it may be of value to make brief mention of a topic that requires a much more in-depth discussion than is appropriate for this book. Specifically, the question arises as to what degree the clinician should share his or her emotions and memories with the patient. To what degree does the clinician display transparency and self-disclosure? Differing schools vary upon this issue, and the answer also varies depending upon the clinical situation. Generally speaking, I do not use self-disclosure much during initial interviews, for patients will handle self-disclosure remarkably differently depending upon their psychopathology. Paranoid patients and borderlines can quickly twist the self-disclosure into damaging distortions or may be frightened by the process of facing a clinician who self-discloses. In a dynamic sense self-disclosure can also disrupt transference development. Moreover, in the initial interview I seldom need self-disclosure in order to powerfully engage the patient. Thus there seems to be little need to use a technique that can backfire in numerous ways.

On the other hand various clinicians may utilize self-disclosure in certain instances in ongoing therapy. Indeed Val Brown[9] has argued convincingly that during periods of intense affect in the clinician, powerful moments of therapeutic change may occur if the clinician and the patient jointly explore how these emotions appeared in the interpersonal context. Frequently the patient gains insight into the effect he or she has upon others. The issue of self-disclosure remains a complex and controversial topic, which the reader is urged to explore in other readings and in the context of supervision.

One point should be made though. Although I tend not to use self-disclosure in initial interviews, it can be useful both with regard to setting limits and with decathecting hostile patients in certain situations. In some instances, comments to a gradually escalating patient such as, "Mr. Jones, I can see that you're feeling pretty angry at me and to be honest you're scaring me a bit, and I know you don't intend to frighten me. Let's sit down and talk some to see if I might be able to understand better what is upsetting you and perhaps do something about it." I have seen this technique work effectively, but one must learn through experience with which patients it is most appropriate.

As we conclude the discussion of the vantage point of looking within oneself, we are also concluding the exploration of the attentional vantage points. It can be readily seen that these vantage points are intimately related to the transition into the psychotherapeutic process itself. Their effectiveness is contingent upon the clinician's ability to "step away" from the interview during periods of self-remembering. These periods of self-remembering allow the clinician to utilize complementary vantage points rapidly and effectively. In the next section we shall begin a study of three different conceptual vantage points: the assessment for psychotherapy, the structural interviewing of Kernberg, and the use of intuition.

EXPLORATION OF THE CONCEPTUAL VANTAGE POINTS

The Assessment for Psychodynamic Psychotherapy

One of the most challenging tasks facing the initial interviewer is the tentative determination of the patient's potential for psychotherapy. In the first place, the clinician needs to possess an operationally sound understanding of the basic types of psychotherapeutic interventions, including counseling techniques, behavioral techniques, crisis intervention techniques, cognitive therapies, short-term dynamic therapies, long-term dynamic therapies, psychoanalysis, couple's therapy, family therapy, and group therapy. Naturally, each clinician will develop biases, hopefully not tunnel-vision biases, as to which therapies are most effective under what circumstances.

It is important to realize that the initial interviewer need not necessarily be adept at each form of therapy, for frequently the interviewer is acting as a triage agent, who will refer the patient to others. Instead, the clinician needs to understand the advantages of each form of therapy, thus enabling a fit to be achieved between the patient's needs, abilities for change, and the appropriateness of the therapy for the tasks at hand. At differing points during the interview the clinician will be entering the conceptual vantage point concerned with determining the suitability of the patient for some type of psychotherapeutic intervention.

It is beyond the scope of this chapter to discuss the assessment techniques needed to determine the appropriateness of the patient for each form of therapy mentioned above. Instead, the focus will be on the delineation of the maturational level of the patient in the sense of the patient's ego development and sense of a stable self. The maturational level of the patient is of profound importance in determining suitability for psychodynamic therapies (those therapies derived from analytic theory dealing with the unconscious and transference) but is also of definite relevance in determining the potential for success in all of the therapeutic categories described above. The focus of this section is upon a common denominator utilized in considering the use of any of the above techniques.

By the maturation level of the patient, we are simply referring to a commonsense concept that patients will be functioning at widely varying degrees of psychological maturity at varying moments of their lives. At one end of the continuum, the patient may be functioning at a severely regressed and psychotic state, in which reality contact itself is compromised. In the middle of the continuum one finds the psychotic prone personalities (primitive personality disorders) described in Chapter 7. These people generally have better reality contact than grossly psychotic patients but tend to interact with people in highly immature fashions, often accompanied by childlike expectations and equally childlike outbursts when such expectations are not met. In the last category we find the more stable character disorders, the neurotic disorders, and those people with healthy functioning.

During periods of stress individuals may move backwards along this continuum. Following an automobile accident resulting in the death of his spouse, a well-functioning individual may experience a brief reactive psychosis. On a more subtle level, a business executive who displays some passive-aggressive and narcissistic traits may, if hospitalized for a serious illness, begin to function as if truly representing an unstable narcissistic personality disorder.

This issue of stress represents a crucial consideration for the clinician as an attempt is made to identify the suitability of the patient for psychotherapeutic intervention. In general, the more immature the patient's level of psychological integration, the less likely he is to tolerate stress, especially on an interpersonal level. Specific therapies vary in the degree to which the patient is stressed by the clinician either emotionally or cognitively. The goal of the interviewer is to determine which therapy will be of most value for this patient at this time.

It is not really a determination of whether the patient needs psychotherapy, but what type will be of most benefit, for even most psychotic patients will benefit from a low-keyed supportive interaction, in which the clinician merely attempts to provide some calming reality contact over time. This same psychotic patient would truly run the risk of therapy-induced damage if the clinician attempted to employ a long-term dynamic approach replete with confrontations and interpretations at the time of the acute psychosis. In a similar fashion a behaviorist would generally not employ a hypnotherapy or relaxation technique at the time of an acute psychotic breakdown, for such techniques may backfire dramatically by furthering the regression of the patient.

Michel Hersen, the noted behavioral therapist, has pointed out that the failures found in patients with certain behavioral techniques may be related to the fact that, in a psychodynamic or maturational sense, the patient or client was not capable of handling the challenges presented by the therapy. For instance, a clinician may encounter a patient who angrily drops out of a homework-utilizing therapy after several sessions. What may have been missed by the therapist is the fact that the patient was presenting with the maturational level of a borderline personality. More specifically, for this particular patient, whose need for approval was pathologically enormous, the tension of having homework reviewed by the clinician was prohibitively anxiety provoking. The anxiety of performing these relatively simple homework assignments literally drove the patient out of therapy. As Hersen states, talented behavioral clinicians attend to the dynamic concerns of the client, tailoring the level of stress in the therapy to the patient's ability to handle stress, as evidenced by the patient's maturational level.[10]

The question becomes one of which techniques allow the initial interviewer to easily assess the immediate maturational level of the patient. Two approaches immediately come to mind. The first approach is the determination of a DSM-III-R diagnosis. Diagnoses such as schizophrenia, borderline personality disorder, and an adjustment disorder with depressed mood all suggest specific levels of maturation. A second technique consists of assessing the degree of functioning of the patient along a series of differing ego functions and defense mechanisms. This technique adds to the approach by the DSM-III-R for it pushes the clinician to assess specific functions, thus allowing the clinician to spot both strengths and weaknesses. Bellak emphasizes this approach and has developed the concept of the Ego-Function Assessment (EFA).[11]

In the EFA, twelve different ego functions are conceptualized by the clinician. These functions include items such as the following: reality testing, practical judgment, impulse control, object relations, strength of psychological defense mechanisms, and the ability to screen out unwanted stimuli and thoughts. This type of approach, coupled with the diagnostic approach of the DSM-III-R, creates a more individualized picture of the patient's current functioning. The first step in assessing the psychotherapeutic fit for the patient is a determination of where the patient sits on the continuum of psychological maturation. It should be noted that these so-called steps actually tend to occur in parallel, the various assessments occurring throughout the interviewing process.

The next step consists of determining the "therapy facilitative" characteristics of the patient. These have been written about and described in great detail by numerous authors. Basically one is referring to those characteristics that bode well for a psychotherapeutic intervention. Once again the search for these qualities represents a no-nonsense practical conceptualization. The three that come to mind as routinely mentioned include (1) motivation, (2) cognitive skills, and (3) psychological mindedness.

In its simplest form the concept of motivation can be summarized as those who want the help the most tend to do the best (although this is not always the case). This motivation tends to arise from two general areas. First, the degree to which patients are experiencing pain certainly influences the degree to which they are invested in seeking help. Second, the patient's drive for help may be strongly influenced by the belief that help is possible. Both of these influences can be more easily ascertained if the clinician, at some point, asks the patient questions such as the following:

a. What made you decide to come here today at this moment as opposed to several weeks ago?
b. What made you decide to see me specifically, in other words, how had you heard about me?
c. What are some of your expectations about whether therapy can help or not?

A patient who responds, "I came here because my wife wants me to be here, and I have no idea how she got your name" is clearly less motivated than a patient who says, "I think I really need some help with the way I handle people, and you really helped a friend of mine."

The degree of pain does not always indicate a readiness for therapeutic intervention. A patient with a paranoid personality may live a miserable existence, constantly alienated from friends and family, but may not view the pain as being related to anything under personal control. In the same vein, psychotic patients may not perceive a need for intervention. Such considerations lead to the associated concept of insight, for insight generally must accompany pain in order for the patient to voluntarily seek help. This insight need not be sophisticated. The patient merely needs to develop an awareness that psychological pain can be causally related to attitudes and behaviors.

The second therapy facilitative characteristic consists of the patient's intellectual abilities and cognitive functioning, including concentration, memory, abstracting ability, baseline intelligence, and creativity. A patient gifted in all of these areas may have a higher chance for success in therapies requiring a sophisticated use of intellect, such as cognitive restructuring or a dynamic based therapy.

The third characteristic is referred to as psychological mindedness, a somewhat diffuse term that overlaps with the above characteristics to some degree. In a more specific sense it may be viewed as the patient's belief that psychological processes can affect happiness, coupled with the patient's ability to assume a more objective view of personal behavior, including the impact of his or her actions on the happiness of himself or herself and others.

If a patient does not show the types of facilitative characteristics described above, it does not necessarily mean that psychotherapy is not indicated. It means that the patient may not do well in specific forms of therapy. In this light, therapies can be clustered into three broad categories, ego stabilizing, ego nurturing, and ego challenging, listed in order from least stressful to most stressful.

Ego stabilizing counseling and therapeutic techniques represent gentle approaches utilized to help severely ill patients regain a sense of safe environment and sound reality contact. They are often used with psychotic patients, and the sessions may be very brief in nature, essentially helping the patient to reintegrate, as medications such as antipsychotics begin to decrease the terror of the psychotic process. The major goal is to help the patient to regain a reasonable sense of self-integration, accompanied by some mild insight into practical considerations of the current clinical condition. In other instances, nonpsychotic patients may not want psychotherapy of a more probing nature, may not have the intelligence to benefit from such therapies, or may not have the money or time to benefit from such approaches. If these patients are receiving medications, then the medication evaluations themselves can include simple ego stabilizing work, aimed at guiding patients toward a useful understanding of the significance of their problems as they relate to medication issues and their daily routine. Simple fears and anxieties are handled with a quiet and calming educational support.

In contrast to ego stabilizing therapies, ego nurturing therapies gently, but persistently, push the patient towards increased understanding, while recognizing that the character structure of the patient will demand a firm and consistent approach towards primitive outbursts of anger and fear towards the clinician. Examples of ego nurturing therapies are the reparenting techniques frequently seen in use with patients suffering from primitive personality disorders. In contrast to the limited goals of the ego stabilizing therapies, the ego nurturing therapies attempt to foster insight, hopefully accompanied by true gains in self-esteem and a maturing individuality.

The third grouping, ego challenging interventions, are most useful in patients who can be both confronted by the therapist as well as asked to reflect upon the ramifications of their thoughts and behaviors. These therapies frequently demand that the patient display the therapy facilitative characteristics outlined above. Of course, at times, a patient may begin with an ego stabilizing approach and if successfully treated with this technique may be able to benefit at a later time from an ego nurturing approach, ultimately moving on towards ego challenging techniques. Ego challenging therapies include techniques such as time-limited psychodynamic therapies, other psychodynamic therapies, psychoanalysis, more complex behavioral therapies, and more sophisticated cognitive therapies. In specified situations, these therapies can also be of benefit with more primitive personalities, but the clinician must always ensure that patients are not pushed beyond their actual capabilities for change.

The following example demonstrates the need for matching the therapeutic intervention to the psychological maturation of the patient. Suppose that the therapist is faced with headbanging behavior in a mildly retarded adolescent. It is doubtful that an ego challenging technique such as a written self-monitoring technique (which requires motivation and a good ability to observe one's actions) will have any chance of success. Even some ego nurturing techniques, such as very simple cognitive techniques, will probably be too demanding for such a patient. On the other hand, an ego stabilizing technique, employing simple principles of positive reinforcement, may be much more promising. In this regard, counseling techniques and dynamic therapies all tend to vary with how much stress they place on the patient for success. The astute clinician considers these variables while working from the vantage point of assessing potential for psychotherapy.

One method of assessing the presence of therapy facilitative characteristics was hinted at in the chapter on the structure of the interview. Specifically, the clinician can choose to enter psychodynamic regions during the course of the intake interview itself. In such regions the clinician focuses upon the manner in which the patient handles interpretive questions and/or statements. In particular, the clinician can purposely ask an interpretive question or two in an effort to observe the method by which the patient handles such questions, which may suggest the ability of the patient to work in more ego challenging therapies. At the same time the clinician will carefully note the patient's motivation to look at psychological material as well as the patient's ability to look inward.

An ideal response to an interpretive question consists of the presence of a probing self-reflection followed by the production of new and spontaneous material from the patient.[12] The material may consist of newly recalled memories, associations with current life situations, associations with the relationship with the therapist, or newly recovered unconscious material such as dreams. If this pattern does not emerge, it suggests either that the patient is not ready to accept the interpretation or is not capable of making the self-reflective connections or that the therapist may have missed the mark, having made an inaccurate interpretation or asked a poorly conceived question.

But the response described above is an ideal one. It does not typically occur in the initial interview, because many patients require more experience in therapy before understanding how to respond to interpretive questions. If a patient does respond in this type of reflective and creative fashion, then the chance that the patient represents an excellent candidate for a more ego challenging therapy is high.

A more typical response in an initial interview, but also a good one, is the tendency for the patient to show a sincere attempt to reflect upon the question, accompanied by some response, albeit one with minimal insight. But at least this type of response suggests that the patient is willing to engage in an active therapeutic exchange. On the other hand, if the patient becomes strikingly defensive, hostile, or markedly anxious, then one can suspect that this patient may benefit from a less threatening approach such as an ego nurturing or ego stabilizing therapy. The clinician is learning about the patient's psychological maturation by the method in which the patient responds to the interpretive question. The clinician is also obtaining an on-the-spot look at the patient's motivation, cognitive functioning, and psychological mindedness.

Let us look at the use of such a question during an initial interview. The patient was a nicely dressed man in his mid-thirties. He had been referred for possible psychotherapy. Upon first presenting he appeared anxious and quite distressed, as well he should be, for he was in the midst of a situational crisis. He was married and had four children, all of whom he loved. He also happened to be homosexual and his long-standing homosexual partner was threatening to leave him if he did not end his marriage.

As he spoke he appeared articulate and seemed to be of above average intelligence. During the later phases of the body of the interview he began describing some of the actions of his partner that he resented. The dialogue unfolded as follows:

Pt.: I don't know, he's just problematic at times but I think all good relations are that way. But I do hate to bicker.

Clin.: Can you give me an example of the type of thing that you bicker about?

Pt.: (pause) Yes, I can. The other day was a perfect example. We were driving out towards the country and I was enjoying the quiet of the countryside. Next thing I knew he plops a tape into the tape deck and nearly blasts me out of the car, really, I mean really. So I reached over and yanked the tape out of the deck. He must have pouted for over an hour. (The patient seems absorbed in his belief that his partner's behaviors are inappropriate. On the contrary, the clinician is struck by the controlling quality of the patient, and the patient's relative inability to empathize with his lover. The question becomes one of determining whether the patient is capable of reflecting upon his own behavior with any degree of objectivity. The clinician sees an ideal opening for an interpretive question.)

Clin.: Do you feel that you are sometimes a fairly controlling person?

> **Pt.:** (Patient looks away for a moment as he frowns) Control-
> ling? I don't think so, uh . . . what do you mean?
>
> **Clin.:** I was just wondering if you viewed your yanking the tape
> out as being somewhat controlling.
>
> **Pt.:** Oh (raises his eyebrows) I don't really know, uh, I mean I
> guess at some level I am. Not all the time mind you. But
> sometimes. (long pause) Hmm, I guess it is sort of con-
> trolling to pull the tape out on him, but he didn't ask me if
> I wanted to listen. (slight smile) Perhaps I was a bit dras-
> tic at that. I do tend to tell him what to do pretty fre-
> quently. For instance, I almost always choose the restau-
> rant that we will go to, yes almost always.

The patient's response bodes well for the use of an ego challenging form of therapy. We see him balking at first in a natural fashion, but he possesses the ego strength to explore further. Upon further exploration he seems to run material through his mind that the clinician has not mentioned. After a moment of reflection he begins to produce new material. This patient went on to benefit from a dynamic based therapy in which issues of control would play a recurring part.

It is important to realize that the initial balking at the clinician's interpretive question represents in many respects a good sign. Most people will balk when first confronted with an aspect of their behavior that is new to their awareness. The patient who immediately nods his or her head in full agreement, adding phrases such as, "Now I never thought of that but it really is true," may not be such a bargain for the would-be ego challenging therapist. These patients may be attempting to please the therapist and can be excruciatingly frustrating. Later in therapy, when it is eventually pointed out by the therapist that the patient seems to have a need to please, one can almost count on the patient to suddenly smile saying, "My goodness, I never thought of that, but you're absolutely right." Therapists are frequently tempted to return to their own therapy at such moments.

We have reviewed some of the basic principles behind assessing those characteristics that may suggest suitability for therapeutic success. Before ending the discussion of psychotherapy assessment a few odds and ends should be addressed, which for want of a better name can be referred to as practical systems issues.

While making an assessment for psychotherapy, the clinician can ill afford to view the patient in a vacuum. The clinician must consider practical, and at times determining factors, such as the patient's financial resources, time availability, and the resources of the mental health system itself. For example, the staff therapists at mental health centers are frequently overwhelmed with case loads. Such loads may preclude the chance for most patients to be seen in more demanding types of therapy that require frequent sessions. In such instances it becomes even more important for the assessment clinician to spot candidates who are more likely to benefit from such ego challenging therapies, so that these patients may come to the attention of the interested clinicians.

In a similar vein, the clinician needs to become aware of the types of therapy available in the area as well as a recognition that some clinicians do well with certain patients and poorly with others. In fact, some clinicians may have relatively serious psychological problems themselves, which may make it less advisable that they work with more severely impaired patients such as schizotypal personalities or borderline personalities. In this sense, before doing a consult, it is often rewarding to obtain an idea of what types of approaches are available and/or popular in the given center. In this sense clinicians can save themselves the embarrassment of suggesting "ivory tower" treatment recommendations that only serve to alienate the consultee.

At this point we can move on to another conceptual vantage point that has some direct connections with our current discussion.

The Structural Interviewing of Kernberg

In the discussion of the vantage point of assessing the patient for psychotherapeutic intervention, it was noted that one of the major tasks was a determination of the patient's maturation and ego strength. Moreover, it was pointed out that two complementary methods of addressing this area included formulating a DSM-III-R diagnosis and assessing ego strengths in a more systematic fashion. Otto Kernberg[13] has developed an interviewing technique that seems to offer another avenue for looking at both the diagnosis of the patient and the degree of ego strength from a slightly different perspective.

Stated in a highly simplified form, Kernberg suggests that each person can be characterized along a maturational continuum, much as we have already described. Depending upon where the person sits on this continuum, the patient will handle stress differently. Specifically, patients will tend to handle questions that challenge them with differing degrees of facility. In this line of thinking the interviewer attempts to delineate the underlying character structure of the patient by noting the process by which the patient handles the interviewer's questions, hence the name "structural interviewing."

Before examining the technique in more detail, several points are worth mentioning. This approach to diagnosis complements the DSM-III-R, for the DSM-III-R approaches diagnosis by looking at the content of the patient's history and presentation in an effort to determine whether specific content-oriented criteria are satisfied. In contrast, structural interviewing attends not so much to what the patient says but how the patient says it. The process of the response, to a large degree, determines the diagnosis as opposed to the content. In particular, the clinician looks for processes such as the degree of anxiety created in the patient by the question or the resulting hostility or cooperativeness. Consequently, this style of interview can be particularly useful if the validity of the patient's answers are in question, perhaps related to guardedness or even purposeful deceit. In such circumstances it may be difficult to uncover DSM-III-R criteria. Another use of the technique is the fact that by utilizing this conceptual vantage point, the clinician may uncover evidence that a more primitive personality style may be present. The clinician can then pursue the expansion of the appropriate diagnostic region by DSM-III-R criteria.

The actual technique of structural interviewing is delineated by Kernberg as a specific format of diagnostic interview. In this more formalized approach, the clinician tends to explore various types of psychopathology starting with neurotic dysfunction and moving progressively through characterological disorders, functional psychoses, and organic brain syndromes. Throughout this process various aspects of the DSM-III-R and the more traditional psychiatric mental status are employed, but the interview continuously swings back to observations concerning the methods by which the patient handles the questions, even if the questions pertain merely to a description of symptomotology.

During this process the clinician utilizes three major types of interactions with the patient: clarification, gentle confrontation, and interpretation. In the last section we have already seen the manner in which a clinician may learn about the patient's level of functioning by the fashion in which the patient responds to an interpretive question. Kernberg adds to this process, suggesting various avenues of understanding the dynamics of the patient even as the patient clarifies the history of the present illness. In a sense the whole interview is transformed into an exploration of the processes by which the patient handles environmental stress as reflected in the manner in which the patient responds to the clinician.

In everyday clinical work, the more formalized structural interview is not particularly effective for gathering large amounts of material within the time constraints facing the clinician functioning as an intake interviewer. But the clinician can utilize this vantage point intermittently throughout the assessment interview as it naturally unfolds. For example, the clinician may consciously utilize clarifications, confrontations, and interpretations during the expansion of what we referred to earlier as psychodynamic regions. Sensitive observation by the clinician of even a few responses by the patient, can provide surprisingly large amounts of data concerning defense mechanisms and the underlying character structure of the patient.

On a cautionary note, I do not believe that one should rely solely on techniques such as the structural interview in order to obtain a diagnosis, for these techniques are far too dependent upon the subjective opinions and skills of the interviewer to provide a reliable system of diagnosis. Instead, used creatively and with good timing, structural interviewing can provide powerful insight into the underlying character structure of the patient in a fashion that complements the DSM-III-R in an immediately practical sense.

With this background, let us look more specifically at the model proposed by Kernberg. Three broad categories of development are delineated, moving from the least stable sense of self to the most stable sense of self. These three categories are the psychotic structure, the borderline structure, and the neurotic structure. Of particular note is the fact that Kernberg's category of the borderline structure is not used in the sense of only including the borderline personality as described by the DSM-III-R. Instead, he seems to be referring to a variety of DSM-III-R disorders, which earlier we had grouped as the psychotic prone or primitive personality disorders. These disorders include the schizotypal personality, the borderline personality, and the paranoid personality. When poorly integrated, the histrionic and narcissistic personalities may also be included.

These three broad categories (neurotic, borderline, and psychotic) are believed to vary with regard to three structural components, which Kernberg refers to as degree of identity integration, level of defensive operations, and reality testing. By way of example, the patient with a neurotic character structure tends to use relatively high-level defenses such as rationalization, intellectualization, reaction formation, and undoing. The more primitive borderline states rely more upon lower-level defenses such as denial, splitting, magical thinking, and inappropriate idealization. Finally, people with a psychotic structure will tend to utilize more psychotic adaptations such as delusions and hallucinations, although higher-level defenses may be intermittently present as well.

Since these different defense mechanisms are at the very core of protecting the patient from anxiety, one would expect each category of patient to respond to stress with the appearance of the structure-specific defenses available to the patient. And here we approach the underlying premise of structural interviewing. The clinician utilizes processes such as clarification, confrontation, and interpretation to trigger various levels of anxiety, noting which style of defenses arises to alleviate the stress. The resulting styles of defense suggest the possible underlying character structure.

For illustrative purposes we shall focus upon the use of mild confrontation. In this technique the clinician looks for an area of self-contradiction made by the patient during the course of the interview. The patient is then presented with the contradiction, not in an accusatory sense, but from the clinician stance that, "I am a little confused by some of your statements for they seem to contradict themselves." Having provided a somewhat stressful situation, the clinician sits back to observe the manner in which the patient handles the stress with regard to the appearance of underlying defensive mechanisms. From the constellation of defenses that appear, the clinician gains an understanding of the patient's core character structure.

The use of gentle confrontation in the context of structural interviewing will be clarified through the use of three examples. In each patient it will be assumed that similar content has been discussed but that the patients differ in the level of their structural development. In each case it will be assumed that the patient is a mid-thirties male who presents feeling dissatisfied with his personal relationships. Earlier in the interview the patient had stressed that, "I'll tell you one thing, I'm sure not a male chauvinist like my brother. Now he and I don't see eye to eye when it comes to the roles of the sexes." In each of the subsequent illustrations we will see the patient eventually contradict this earlier statement, and the clinician will present this discrepancy to the patient. The responses of the patients will then be examined with regard to the underlying structural style that they belie:

ILLUSTRATION I

Pt.:   Things haven't been going all that good at home. I've got some problems with the little woman. She seems to feel that I don't spend enough time with the kids, you know, like I should stop going out for a drink with the guys after work or something like that.

Clin.:   I was just struck by something you said. You referred to your wife as the "little woman" and yet earlier you said that you were a far cry from a chauvinist. I guess what puzzles me is that the term "little woman" would be viewed as quite chauvinistic in most circles, wouldn't it?

Pt.:   Uh (pause) uh (pause) I guess in some circles that would be true. I (pause) I didn't really mean it to be chauvinistic. You see my wife and I joke around a lot and sometimes I call her pet names and she does the same with me. I sort of

> meant that like a pet name. I didn't mean it to be chauvinistic, at least I didn't think I did.
>
> *Clin.:* How do you think you actually view your wife?
>
> *Pt.:* I've always thought that we had a pretty good relationship. And don't get me wrong, I think we do. We have our spats, but we work things out.

Although this patient may not be demonstrating the most profound insight in the world, one would not expect him to exhibit striking insight during an initial interview. But what his answer does suggest is that he possesses an ability to handle the tension of the moment reasonably well. He has been confronted with a contradiction. Like most normal or neurotic people he is disturbed by the apparent contradiction, a contradiction that he admits, albeit reluctantly. The person with a neurotic or normal structure (as this patient represents) will want to resolve this contradiction, for the patient is disturbed by the incongruity, which had been hidden from conscious awareness before. Moreover, the patient does not wish to be viewed as illogical or hypocritical.

In this particular patient, the defense of rationalization has allowed the patient's anxiety to be dissipated, as the patient rationalizes that the term "little woman" was just another example of a pet name, and his wife calls him pet names too. Following his rationalization the patient is then able to proceed with the conversation with relative ease, although one gets the flavor that the point of the clinician was not totally missed. Now let us see how a patient with a different underlying structure might respond.

ILLUSTRATION II

> *Pt.:* Things haven't been going all that good at home. I've got some problems with the little woman. She seems to feel that I don't spend enough time with the kids, you know, like I should stop going out for a drink with the guys after work or something like that.
>
> *Clin.:* You know, I was just struck by something you said. You referred to your wife as the "little woman" and yet earlier you said that you were a far cry from a chauvinist. I guess what puzzles me is that the term "little woman" would be viewed as quite chauvinistic in most circles, wouldn't it?
>
> *Pt.:* So what if it is. I can call my wife anything I feel like calling her.
>
> *Clin.:* I certainly wouldn't challenge your right to refer to your wife in any way you choose. But I was wondering if there was some contradiction between your earlier statement and some of the attitudes you have just talked about?

> **Pt.:** Look, I'm not here to play word games with you. And I
> don't think I like your attitude that you're so goody
> goody, as if you never contradict yourself. And I don't
> particularly appreciate your insinuation that I'm a bad
> husband.

This patient has responded to the confrontation in a strikingly
different manner than the first patient. He has attacked the clinician,
displaying a rather quick-tongued bite at that. The anxiety generated
by the clinician's question is being handled with significantly more
lower-level defenses. The patient rapidly fires off a salvo of entitlement as he tells the clinician, "I can call my wife anything that I want
to." The patient seems to be projecting his angry feelings out onto the
clinician, who is subsequently misperceived as having stated that the
patient is "a bad husband." The projection is accompanied by a tendency to devalue the clinician and see him as all bad, the early buddings
of the primitive defense mechanism of splitting.

In this example the patient has demonstrated a variety of defenses
suggestive of a borderline structure as might be seen in a borderline
personality disorder or a poorly integrated narcissistic personality
disorder. Thus the technique of calmly presenting the patient with one
of the patient's own contradictions has resulted in a rather distinctive
display of primitive defenses.

Not all primitive personalities will necessarily display anger or
projection. In some instances, the patient may almost seem to tran-
siently crumble psychologically as if crushed by a feeling of intense
abandonment or rejection. In such instances the patient may perceive
the clinician as viewing the patient as all bad or inadequate. At other
times the patient's splitting defenses may be so powerful that the
patient sees no problem with the contradiction, thus experiencing
little if any anxiety. I remember pointing out to an adolescent that he
had stated earlier a desperate desire to stay in his current remedial
placement, yet he had just told me that he would continue to break the
rules even if it meant getting thrown out. I pointed this out as appearing somewhat contradictory. He looked me coolly back in the eyes
saying, "I do what I feel like doing. I can say both things if I want to. I
don't see any problem with that."

In all of the above examples, the defenses of the patient suggest
some type of more primitive character structure at the time of the
interview. One does not see the initial anxiety seen in the neurotic, who
feels uncomfortable with the fact that a contradiction has been displayed. Patients with borderline structure do not as frequently attempt to correct the discrepancy with defenses such as rationalization
or intellectualization. Thus we see that the type of response does
indeed seem to belie the underlying dynamic structure. It should be

remembered that these inferences are broad generalities, and any patient may provide a range of defensive styles. What the clinician is looking for is the preferential style of the patient and/or any hints that more primitive processes may be present, perhaps suggesting the need for a more thorough diagnostic expansion of the various primitive personality disorders. In the following example the clinician will see evidence of an even more primitive process in the fashion in which the patient responds:

ILLUSTRATION III

Pt.: Things haven't been going all that good at home. I've got some problems with the little woman. She seems to feel that I don't spend enough time with the kids, you know, like I should stop going out for a drink with the guys after work or something like that.

Clin.: You know, I was just struck by something you said. You referred to your wife as the "little woman" and yet earlier you said that you were a far cry from a chauvinist. I guess what puzzles me is that the term "little woman" would be viewed as quite chauvinistic in most circles, wouldn't it?

Pt.: Oh uh . . . I I don't really know, I guess somewhere someone would say that (patient looks quite flustered and tense). I guess they could get mad at me, I guess they really could get mad, but chauvinists aren't all that bad. My brother is chauvinistic and he's a reasonable guy. I mean we don't see eye to eye but he is reasonable.

Clin.: Well, how do you feel you view women in general?

Pt.: (long pause, as if having a difficult time sorting his thoughts) I view them, let me see. I like women, I do. But sometimes they can be real difficult. But not usually, my mother and my sister are both very nice and very intelligent. I think intelligence is very important in a person. I admire it a lot. One of the things that has always been a strong trait in my family is intelligence. We have always prided ourselves in being up with the times and sometimes ahead of the times.

In this illustration the clinician may find himself experiencing a brief period of confusion, for the patient's answer is somehow lacking in clarity. There are plenty of words, but they seem to have been forged without meaning. This empty quality is the result of a regressive disorganization of the patient, as witnessed by actual problems in organizing his thinking. The thought process seems subtly disturbed with a tangential flow, which eventually allows the patient to not answer the question as to how he actually views women. One can also see the patient's ambivalence as he swings back and forth between viewing women as difficult or "good mothers." In short, the patient's response to the stress of the clinician's question is represented by the surfacing of soft signs of psychotic process. He shifts rather radically from a speech pattern suggestive of a fairly level-headed individual to speech suggestive of someone quite unsure of himself. At the tail end of the dialogue he begins to regain his composure.

This type of pattern is more frequently seen in people with an underlying psychotic process. If the psychosis is closer to the surface, the clinician may find more and more dramatic disorganization as the patient's defenses are overrun by anxiety. Perhaps even harder signs of psychosis may eventually emerge, such as delusions or ideas of reference.

The above illustrations demonstrate the manner in which structural interviewing can provide valuable insights into the level of functioning of the patient at the time of the interview. Of course, to utilize this conceptual vantage point, the clinician must be able to "pull back" from the interview itself, adopting, for a moment, a period of self-remembering. Once again these periods of self-remembering provide the portals through which the clinician can utilize both attentional vantage points and conceptual vantage points, in this case viewing the patient from the theoretical background envisioned by Otto Kernberg.

The Intuitive Vantage Point

In particular he [a medieval alchemist] approached matter with a passionate conviction that it held a mystery, a "mysterium magnum," the nature of which was different in quality and in essence from its material container . . .

A. McGlashan, Savage and Beautiful Country

We have come to the last vantage point to be discussed in this chapter. Curiously, it is a conceptual vantage point that arises without any conscious attempt by the clinician to apply a conceptual framework. It simply happens. To be aware that one is employing intuition would signal an immediate end to its presence. Elusive and difficult to describe, intuition is both a vital and vitalizing ingredient in the clinical interview. In actual practical terms, its worth is essentially impossible to overvalue. Every experienced clinician can relate times that the clinician just "felt something" such as "this patient is contemplating suicide" or "I have a feeling that this child is being abused." These hunches, if listened to, can then be followed by skillfully guided explorations. Indeed, hunches, guesses, and feelings represent the stuff of which intuition is born. Gifted interviewers are at home here.

But the question remains, "What is intuition and can it be taught?" In the first place, intuition remains difficult to define, thus decreasing to some degree the practicality of the first part of the question. Concerning the second part, it is probably next to impossible to teach intuition didactically. With regard to intuition, one then wonders whether clinicians should hopelessly throw up their arms while praying that somehow or other they have been given the gift? I do not think so, for intuition is not really a gift. It is more of a beneficent habit of sorts, a valuable habit that is ironically often ground out of humans by the educational process itself.

Consequently, in this closing section we shall look more closely at this most peculiar and beneficial of habits, in the hope that our explorations will help us to cultivate it, for intuition is not so much something that originates from something gained as it arises from something lost. More specifically, clinicians must lose the enculturated rules and rigid conceptualizations that block intuitive functioning. Most clinicians begin their work with a healthy abundance of intuition. A misguided education can quickly lay this abundance to rest.

Those clinicians who seem to utilize intuition effectively frequently share a triad of qualities. This triad consists of fascination, openness, and playfulness. All of these qualities depend upon the clinician's ability to become involved in the moment at hand while analytical thinking recedes for a moment. The vacuum is replaced by feeling. Clinicians who cannot give way to the moment in this fashion are seldom intuitive. The interview becomes all thought, no feeling, just another matrix to be solved.

But where does the mystery originate that leads the clinician into moments of fascination? Apparently the mystery frequently arises much in the same fashion that it arose for the medieval alchemist, for the clinician realizes that no human can ever be fully fathomed by another human. The clinician's "mysterium magnum" is the innate complexity of the human organism itself. An immersion in this type of wonderment predisposes the clinician to all three of the qualities conducive to the appearance of intuition.

Indeed, this book is an attempt to increase the clinician's sense of wonderment, as the interviewer finds layer after layer of processes at work during any meeting between patient and clinician. A practical knowledge of the principles behind interviewing sets the stage for the birth of intuition. But there exists an even greater bond between intuition and knowledge. Intuition is essentially the spontaneous appearance of past knowledge whose acquisition the student has forgotten. The lessons gained by experience become so ingrained that the student not only consciously evokes them, they unconsciously arise into awareness. In some instances, the student may never have been aware that a lesson was learned in the first place.

For example, an interviewer may suddenly feel that a patient is deeply saddened but have no awareness as to why this empathic realization has occurred. In actuality, as the clinician grew up, he or she probably became aware of numerous facial mannerisms, inflections of voice, and word choices that came to be associated with sadness. It may very well be an unconscious awareness of such nonverbal signals that have resulted in the intuitive feeling of the clinician. It is the subliminal level and the spontaneous application of this knowledge that leads us to call it intuition. But the intuition itself is based on a knowledge base not on an ill-defined emanation. This does not suggest that intuition can fully be explained, but it does suggest that intuition may be more accessible than it is magical.

The explanation advanced thus far has been given to support the notion that one can develop intuitive skills in a positive sense. In this regard, as alluded to in Chapter 2, the principles discussed in this book will, with increased familiarity, begin to spontaneously cue the clinician into numerous subtleties and intuitive flashes. In addition, if one surrounds oneself with enthusiastic clinicians, who share their ideas and observations, one eventually begins to incorporate the material both consciously and unconsciously. The struggle to learn how to tap this conscious reservoir, while not damming up the spontaneous messages of the unconscious reservoir, is a pivotal developmental task facing all clinicians.

On one hand, clinicians can rely far too much upon intuition, feeling, "I already know how to interview. I really have a great feeling for people." As we have clearly seen, such a pompous attitude is the key to ignorance. On the other hand, some students can apply the principles of interviewing in a fashion that can stifle, as opposed to encourage, the growth of intuition. An example will clarify this point and stand as an important process for supervisors to alertly attend to if it appears.

I am reminded of a social work student who was both innately gifted interpersonally and also enthusiastic and dedicated. After about three weeks in our training program, I began to notice a rather disquieting development in her interviewing style. She was becoming progressively cooler during her interviews, with seldom a smile or sign of spontaneity. She did not seem to have a "feel" for the patient. To my surprise, as soon as she was out of the interview situation, she returned to her engaging and pleasant persona.

As this process was discussed with her, she noted that she was feeling very strained during her interviews saying, "I've just got to get better at this. I know I can be a much better interviewer!" When asked what she was thinking about during her interviews, she practically produced the preceding hundreds of pages of information in this book. No wonder her interviewing was deteriorating. She was a "superego junky." Her intensity and zeal for perfection were rapidly destroying her intuitive abilities. The prescription for the illness was simple: "Forget everything you've learned and just go in there and interview." Within a few days she returned with a smile on her face, stating that her interviews were going much better. Much of the material taught in the class was spontaneously becoming available to her during her interviews. She proceeded to develop an engaging and effective style, which reflected both her personality and her prospering knowledge base.

She represented a rather extreme form of intuitive shut-down, but supervisors should carefully look for this type of response in trainees, as well as the trainee looking out for the same process within himself or herself. The surest sign that one is thinking too much or trying too hard is the feeling that the interview is strained. Good interviewing is, for the most part, fun. In an effort to actualize the goal of creatively developing specific techniques while not inhibiting intuitive functioning, it is often useful to pick a single or perhaps a small number of techniques to focus on during any given interview. In this fashion the student's mind does not become cluttered and overwhelmed. Different clinicians can focus upon varying numbers of skills without interference with their natural abilities. In actual practice, we have found that clinicians can frequently monitor and explore around two to five characteristics during an interview.

Gradually the student gains increasing proficiency in numerous techniques. Interviewing becomes progressively more intriguing as a new sense of balance and confidence arises in the clinician. And here we return to the idea of intuition, for as the clinician gains confidence, the appearance of intuitive moments seems to increase. This increase is probably easily explained by the fact that the openness and playfulness, described earlier as prerequisites for intuition, are greatly dependent upon the clinician's level of confidence. Clinicians are willing to be open and flexible if they feel that they will be able to handle whatever situation faces them. In this more indirect fashion, the knowledge gained from a text such as this one should further increase the intuitive skills of the clinician.

This willingness to experience the interview in a spontaneous fashion is pivotal in the clinician's ability to develop an intuitive eye. This type of seeing and experiencing is gracefully described by the writer Annie Dillard as she discusses her wanderings in nature.

But there is another kind of seeing that involves a letting go. When I see this way I sway transfixed and emptied. The difference between the two ways of seeing is the difference between walking with and without a camera. When I walk with a camera, I walk from shot to shot, reading the light on a calibrated meter. When I walk without a camera, my own shutter opens, and the moment's light prints on my own silver gut. When I see this second way I am above all an unscrupulous observer.[14]

It is from just such a mode of seeing, what we can call the intuitive vantage point, that the clinician will be most open to intuitive insights. As the interviewer develops the delicate art of intermixing this vantage point with more theoretical vantage points, the interviewer becomes increasingly more flexible and sensitive. This open fascination with both learning and the clinical interaction itself is an ongoing process for the clinician. Hopefully, the clinician will still possess this sense of creative naiveté, during the last interview of his or her career. Learning becomes not a goal but a way. This approach to learning is powerfully stated by the Zen Master Shunryu Suzuki in his book *Zen Mind, Beginner's Mind.*

So the most difficult thing is always to keep your beginner's mind. There is no need to have a deep understanding of Zen. Even though you read much Zen literature, you must read each sentence with a fresh mind. You should not say, "I know what Zen is," or "I have attained enlightenment." This is also the real secret of the arts: always be a beginner. Be very very careful about this point. If you start to practice zazen, you will begin to appreciate your beginner's mind. It is the secret of Zen practice.[15]

It is also the secret of interviewing.

References

1. Speeth, K. R.: *The Gurdjieff Work.* New York, Pocket Books, 1976.
2. Mezzich, J. E., Dow, J. T., Rich, C. L., Costello, A. J. and Himmelhoch, J. M.: "Developing an efficient clinical information system for a comprehensive psychiatric institute: II. Initial Evaluation Form," Behavior Research Methods and Instrumentation, 16(4), 464-478, 1981.
3. Wallace, E.: *Dynamic Psychiatry in Theory and Practice.* Philadelphia, Lea and Febiger, 1983, p.157.
4. Elkind, D.: Wilhelm Reich. *In Comprehensive Textbook of Psychiatry III,* edited by H. I. Kaplan, A. M. Freedman, and B. J. Sadock, Baltimore, Williams and Wilkins, 1983, pp. 833–838.
5. Bandler, R., and Grinder, J: *The Structure of Magic I.* Palo Alto, California, Science and Behavior Books, Inc., 1975.
6. Havens, L.: Experience in the uses of language in psychotherapy: Counterprojective statements. *Contemporary Psychoanalysis* 16: 53–67, 1980.
7. Havens, L.: *Making Contact.* Cambridge, Massachusetts, Harvard University Press, 1986.
8. Pilkonis, P.: Personal communication.
9. Brown, V.: *Psychotherapists' Strong Reactions: An Empirical, Phenomenological Investigation.* Doctoral dissertation from Duquesne University, 1986.
10. Hersen, M.: Personal communication.
11. Bellak, L. and Small, L.: *Emergency Psychotherapy and Brief Psychotherapy,* 2nd edition, New York, Grune and Stratton, Inc., 1978.
12. Wallace IV, E. R.: Dynamic Psychiatry in Theory and Practice. Philadelphia, Lea and Febiger, 1983.
13. Kernberg, O.: "Structural Interviewing" from *The Psychiatric Clinics of North America, Borderline Disorders* edited by Michael Stone, Vol 4(i), 169-195, April 1981.
14. Dillard, A.: *Pilgrim at Tinker Creek.* New York, Bantam Books, Inc., 1975.
15. Suzuki, Shunryu: *Zen Mind, Beginner's Mind.* New York, Weatherhill, 1984.

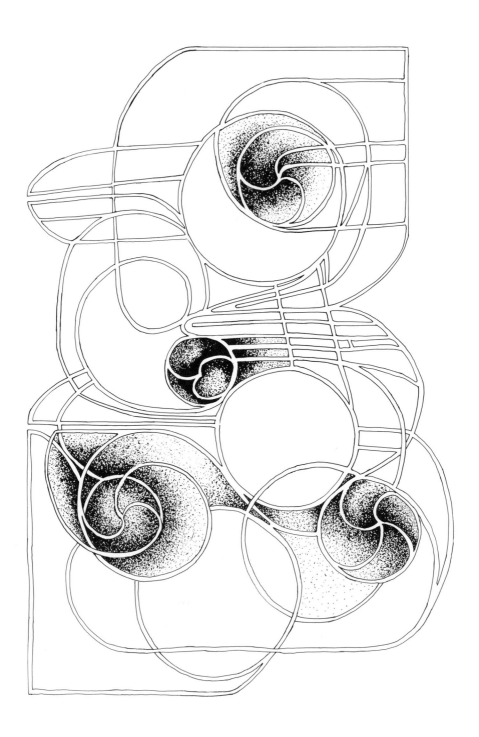

10

The Art of Moving with Resistance

"And how exactly like an egg he is!" she said aloud, standing with her hands ready to catch him, for she was every moment expecting him to fall.

"It's very provoking," Humpty Dumpty said after a long silence, looking away from Alice as he spoke, "to be called an egg — very!"

"I said you looked like an egg, Sir," Alice gently explained. "And some eggs are very pretty, you know," she added, hoping to turn her remark into a sort of compliment.

"Some people," said Humpty Dumpty, looking away from her as usual, "have no more sense than a baby!"

Alice didn't know what to say to this.

Lewis Carroll, Through the Looking Glass

One can easily empathize with the plight of young Alice. She is encountering the unpleasant slap of resistance, and she does not know where to move next. She is probably wondering if she should rebuff the cantankerous egg or politely retreat, admitting her gaffe. The answer, ironically, is that there is no single correct answer.

Clinicians will frequently meet resistance during the initial interview, and indeed throughout the course of therapy itself. Attempts have been made to provide steadfast rules with which to handle these resistances, such as "Always address process" or "Never answer directly." Such statements may provide valuable suggestions for action, but when they become rules, they become traps. These traps are littered with the remains of frustrated interviewers. As opposed to rigidity, creativity and flexibility represent the keys to handling resistance.

More specifically, in this chapter, the focus will not be upon rules; it will be upon the development of a language with which to discuss resistance as it occurs in a clinical setting. This language will provide a clarifying foundation for understanding the underlying principles at work during periods of resistance. By understanding these principles a variety of methods of handling resistance will suggest themselves.

499

In a practical sense, an appreciation of the language of resistance can help an interviewer review a problematic interview with the hope of figuring out what happened in the interview while discovering methods of handling the situation differently the next time it presents itself. At other times the clinician may actually be helped during the interview itself, for specific principles may be recognized and possible courses of action immediately undertaken.

As the clinician becomes more adept at handling resistance, it becomes correspondingly less threatening. Indeed, a seasoned clinician eventually recognizes resistance not as a demon but as an odd ally of sorts, offering an opportunity for insight. The presence of resistance serves to alert the clinician to the fact that the anxieties and defenses of the patient are near the surface. If attended to sensitively, resistance is a pathway to understanding.

During the moments of interpersonal tension stoked by resistance, a curious process frequently occurs. The clinician's own defenses and insecurities are triggered. In this sense few areas of the initial interview provide a better window into the psyche of the clinician than watching the clinician's natural responses to resistance. As Harry Stack Sullivan has suggested, the self system of the therapist quickly comes to the fore, staunchly defending the therapist from the affronts cast by the patient. This point brings us back to Alice, who has clearly been insulted by Mr. Dumpty. The rest of this chapter will attempt to show that Alice has a variety of viable pathways to follow, any one of which may help her to both engage and understand her would-be antagonist. Even for Alice, innocence and good intentions are not enough.

In order to accomplish this task, the chapter is divided into two sections. In Part One, the language of resistance is examined. In Part Two, common types of resistances encountered in the initial interview are discussed, providing a variety of different approaches that can be utilized.

As a last note before beginning, it should be remembered that the goal is not to remove resistance. The goal is to make use of it.

PART I: THE LANGUAGE OF RESISTANCE

In this section we shall attempt to delineate a method of examining resistance as it unfolds. As has been the case in the past, one of the best ways to begin the exploration is to look at a piece of dialogue itself.

In this particular situation, a woman in her mid-thirties had been brought to the evaluation center by the police. Apparently her neighbors had become concerned when they heard angry screams pouring out of the screened windows of her living room. When the police arrived, they found the patient, whom we shall call Mrs. Weston, savagely destroying her furniture. She claimed that, "the witches have my furniture, it's no longer mine!" She was brought to the center on an involuntary commitment.

Mrs. Weston was somewhat unkempt and a little rotund. She frequently looked away with an air of disgust. She adamantly claimed that nothing was wrong with her, but that her neighborhood was teeming with witches and warlocks. These people had been invading her house, planting evil things in her furniture. She was also very proud that she had joined a Pentecostal religion, and she did not want any of those "bad drugs" that were given to her in the past during a hospitalization.

She had been treated for schizophrenia for about ten years but had not taken any medications or been seen for follow-up in the last two years. She also admitted to hearing voices and being "hit by demons." She vehemently denied homicidal or suicidal plans. The clinician was about to explore her psychotic ideation, in an effort to determine whether potentially dangerous psychotic processes such as alien control or command hallucinations were present.

It was at this point that the interviewer made a rather significant error, for which I take full credit, since I happened to be the unfortunate clinician. The error consisted of relaying a subtle self-disclosure, which was said with the intention that the patient might take an interest in educating me about her experiences with demons. To my surprise, the plan resoundingly backfired, plopping me smack into Wonderland, as Alice might say. Let us look at both this point of disengagement and the resulting attempts to rekindle the blending process.

> **Pt.:** I don't know what I'm gonna do about those people, disgusting that's what they are. No right being in my living room, no right at all ruining my furniture, giving it to the devil, his dues alright!
>
> **Clin.:** Mrs. Weston, one thing that you could help me to understand a little better is what it's like to be hit by a demon. I've never had that experience and I'm wondering what it feels like to you.
>
> **Pt.:** You never been hit by a demon? (said with surprised indignation)
>
> **Clin.:** Well . . . I've never had that exact experience.
>
> **Pt.:** Then what are you doing talking to me! (She sits bolt upright, shaking her finger brusquely.) You ought to know all about this stuff, and you're telling me you ain't been

hit by a demon. Who are you anyway? I ain't talking to
you no more (mumbled angrily beneath her breath).

Clin.: Mrs. Weston, it looks like you're concerned about my
lack of knowledge about being hit by demons. What specifically about that is upsetting you?

Pt.: It would mean you ain't no doctor, that's what it would
mean.

Clin.: And how would it mean that I wasn't a doctor?

Pt.: Because to be a doctor you got to deal with demons all the
time, any idiot knows that . . . I just don't know what is
going on here, I just want help with these demons, and
they send me to a moron.

Clin.: I'm going to be honest with you because I think that is
very important. I must admit I may not know everything
about things that are important to you, but I am honestly
trying to understand better, and you can help me to do
that. And I didn't mean to upset you. If other things I say
upset you, please let me know. I'm wondering if the
demons have tried to hurt or enter your daughter?

Pt.: Yes they have, and I ain't gonna let it happen.

Clin.: What have you done to protect her?

Pt.: I put extra locks on her doors.

Clin.: And where does she live?

Pt.: She lives down on the East Side.

Clin.: Roughly how far away from you?

Pt.: Too far for her own good.

Clin.: In what way?

Pt.: She doesn't have a good head on her shoulders, she thinks
she knows everything, but she'll learn, she'll learn the
hard way. She's just growing up and don't know no better.

Clin.: What are some of the things you've been trying to teach
her?

Pt.: To learn to be more careful with men. She don't know
what is going on. They're with the devil I tell her. She's
been hit, that I know.

Clin.: How does she act when she's been hit?

Pt.: She gets that dazed look in her eyes, talks real funny. A
mother can tell she can, and I know she's got demons in
her.

Clin.: Have you thought of any ways to get them out?

Pt.: Praying with the lord, that's all I know.

Clin.: Do the demons in her ever ask you to hurt her or try to
trick you into killing her?

Pt.: They ask me to do things like that. They told me to cut off

her eyelids, but I know that's the devil talking. And I seen
him in her eyes. Somehow I've got to get him out.

At this point it looks as if the interview is back on track. The
blending, although still tenuous, is certainly a good deal better than it
was when the patient mumbled, "I ain't talking to you no more."
Besides the improvement in the blending, the patient is providing the
exact type of lethality material that is of interest.

In this interaction, I made the mistake of sharing personal material with a paranoid patient when I related that I had never been
possessed. I would never have thought that the patient would find this
fact unsettling or odd. But it goes to show that paranoid patients can
frequently twist any personal piece of information. Consequently, it is
generally best to not self-disclose to such patients. The subsequent
situation was a little bit like Alice referring to Humpty Dumpty as an
egg. She had no idea she was putting her foot in her mouth, but somehow it found its way there. Resistances may stem from such awkward
clinician maneuvers, or they may arise spontaneously without any
error on the part of the clinician.

Recognizing Observable Resistance

In order to analyze the appearance and handling of a resistance,
the clinician must first determine the observable form with which the
resistance manifests itself. This observable resistance may appear
with a verbal, nonverbal, or a mixed presentation. The latter form
appears the most frequently. In this example the resistance was mixed.
The patient verbally resisted by challenging my identity as a doctor,
culminating in a statement of her intention to no longer talk. I had, in a
sense, been dismissed.

The patient made her point nonverbally as well. For instance, her
tone of voice became undeniably irritated, and she wagged her hand
with the unmistakable gusto of an Inquisitor General. In this case, the
nonverbal resistances were quite obvious, complementing her blatant
verbal resistance.

Unfortunately, spotting resistance is not always this easy. A
problem may arise if the patient conveys resistance only through subtle nonverbal cues. Clinicians can easily miss these unintentional
messages. To avoid missing such cues, it pays the clinician to develop a
habit of periodically reviewing the blending of the interview. A sudden
drop in the blending process is usually indicative of resistance and can
be picked up during periods of self-remembering.

Here we have stumbled upon one of the major principles of working with resistance. If resistance is building, it is generally best to deal with it. If it is not dealt with during the interview, the patient may never return.

It is also worth keeping in mind that in the same sense that a patient may demonstrate resistance both verbally and nonverbally, the clinician may choose to respond, utilizing either or both of these channels. For example, in the above interview, as the patient became more hostile, the clinician could nonobtrusively push his chair further away, so as to provide the patient with more interpersonal space. Small changes, like this one, can sometimes have surprisingly powerful effects on an interview. Similarly, an interviewer may choose not to take notes if a patient appears guarded or paranoid.

Recognizing Seed Resistances

After noting the observable resistance, it is worth considering the possible presence of nonobservable resistances or what can be called "seed resistances." Most, if not all, observable resistances arise as a defense against some form of patient discomfort, a discomfort that can be called a seed resistance. These seed resistances are none other than the core pains discussed in detail in Chapter 4.

For the purpose of review, these core pains include processes such as the intense pain of isolation, self-loathing, fear of the unknown, fear of an impending loss of internal control, fear of an impending loss of external control, the loss of meaning, or the actual fear of physical pain. An ability to understand and eventually sense the presence of these pains lies at the very root of mastering resistance, because if the interviewer ignores the underlying seeds of resistance, new observable resistances may emerge. This tendency for displacement is not always the case, but it reminds the clinician that one always has the choice of addressing the observable resistance, the seed resistance, or both. As a basic principle, if the clinician finds that resistances repeatedly arise during an interview, then it is often best to consider the notion that underlying seed resistances may be at work. These seed resistances may need to be addressed more directly.

To better understand the concept of seed resistance, an illustration may be useful. In the following example the patient is a young woman in her early twenties. She presents with a sense of agitation, her fingers picking vociferously at each other. She is neatly dressed in a businesslike blouse and skirt. During the interview she seems quite distracted, and at one point asks for an ashtray to be brought to her. Her tone is somewhat demanding. In a few minutes she stands, moving towards the window. Throughout the exchange she has seemed hesitant, resulting in the development of a shut-down interview. After she stands up, the interviewer gently says, "You might find that in the long run you'll feel a little more comfortable sitting." She tersely responds, "I prefer standing."

She continues to appear unsettled and anxious. After a few more terse responses, the interaction continues as follows:

Clin.: What are some of the things that have been concerning you recently?

Pt.: You know, I really need to take a break. I'm going to sit out in the lobby. If you want to continue the interview, there that's fine with me.

Clin.: Before you step out, why don't you and I talk frankly for a moment. I guess that both you and I realize that this is an anxiety-provoking situation. It's difficult sharing important and personal material with a professional, who is also a stranger. I'm wondering what you thought was going to happen today?

Pt.: I don't know, I guess you're going to "shrink my head," isn't that what shrinks do?

Clin.: Well, I guess that depends upon what you mean. In all seriousness, what were you actually expecting today?

Pt.: (said with some exasperation but with less tension) I don't know. I just don't know. I thought I would be layed out on some couch and analyzed. I also thought that some students would probably be brought in to "see the nut."

Clin.: Well, I'm not surprised that you were feeling a little anxious. I can fill you in a little better on what's going to actually happen. Would you like that?

Pt.: I guess so.

Clin.: There is no promise that you'll feel better, but it might help.

Pt.: Sure.

Clin.: First of all, there won't be any such couch or any students. As I said earlier we will talk for about forty more minutes. But we will talk about what you feel is important. If something is too difficult to talk about, I want you to tell me. You don't have to talk about something that is too painful at present. I leave that up to you. We need to move at your pace. Is that all right with you?

Pt.: Yeah, that will be fine.

Clin.: By the way, one thing you said concerned me. You had said that you felt students would be brought in to see "the nut." Are you worried that I'm going to see you as unstable or "nuts," as you said?

Pt.: I must say the thought crossed my mind.

Clin.: What exactly are you worried about?

Pt.: My boyfriend thinks I'm crazy. He's convinced of it, and I'm beginning to wonder myself.

From this point onwards the interview could proceed more smoothly and with a significantly stronger blending. The observable resistance consisted of repeated requests by the patient, eventually highlighted by the request to leave the room, a not so veiled invitation to end the interview itself. The interviewer could have addressed these observable resistances directly and even bluntly denied them. But instead the seed resistances were explored.

This patient appeared to be struggling with both a fear of the unknown and a fear of an impending loss of external control. To counterbalance these fears, she began to "take control" of the interview by making demands upon the interviewer. Her requests were merely manifestations of her seed pains or fears. If the interviewer would have ignored these seeds, perhaps by following the patient out the door, then new observable resistances would most likely have emerged.

At the moment that the patient requested to walk out, the clinician did not address the observable issue of whether the patient should leave or not. Instead, an inquiry was made as to what the patient was feeling about the entire situation. In this fashion the clinician was able to explore some of the seed resistances. Not only did the clinician explore these seed resistances, the clinician relieved them. For instance, concerning the patient's fear of the unknown, the clinician described what would be happening. With regard to the patient's feeling that she had no control in the interview, the clinician literally gave her control with phrases such as, "If something is too difficult to talk about, I want you to tell me."

In this fashion an interview that could have become quite an exercise in antagonism resolved itself. This example illustrates the concept of seed resistances. The interviewer can choose to address either the observable or the seed resistances. Different situations require differing techniques. Generally speaking, as mentioned earlier, if the clinician finds that resistances keep popping up or returning, it is often a good idea to consider the possibility that a seed resistance is not being adequately addressed. For example, this woman may also have been coping with a fear of an impending loss of internal control, as suggested by her statements about going "nuts." The interviewer was wisely beginning to explore this issue, for if it had been left unattended, new resistances may have eventually arisen.

The Direction of Clinician Response to Resistance

This example introduces another basic piece of language concerning resistance. In the handling of any resistance, one can delineate whether the clinician went "with" the resistance or "against" it. Of course, in many instances, the clinician moves somewhere between these two poles. The task consists of determining where on this continuum the clinician acted. In the above example the clinician would have been fully going with the resistance if he had said, "Sure, why don't we both step outside to finish the interview."

The clinician could have directly opposed the resistance by saying, "I'm afraid that it is impossible to go outside, I never interview in public like that. We'll just have to stay here." Both of these responses would also represent attempts to address the observable resistance itself without addressing the seed. In our actual example, the clinician tended to avoid committing himself in either direction, for he chose to address the seed resistance instead. To some degree his willingness to address the patient's concerns probably also supplied an important metacommunication, that he was not strongly opposed to the patient's views in general and was certainly willing to listen. In this sense, he moved subtly with the resistance.

One might ask what is the best track to take, moving with or against the patient's resistance. But this is the wrong question, for no single answer exists. Once again, flexibility remains critical for success. In some instances the clinician must eventually oppose certain resistances. Certainly, in ongoing therapy, specific character types, such as borderlines, benefit from the consistent application of appropriate limits. And in the initial interview, limit setting is sometimes needed. But in general, the more the clinician conveys a willingness to move with the patient, the more likely it is that the resistance will resolve. The more intensely the clinician attacks the requests of the patient, the more likely it is that the patient will "dig in."

Strongly opposing a resistance is asking for a fight from the patient, and the clinician will usually get it, if the clinician authoritatively denies the patient's needs. If a clinician discovers a need to consistently and rapidly oppose patient requests by laying down the law, then the clinician should explore his or her own psychological dynamics. Seed pains are not always found only in patients.

Let us review for a moment (see Figure 12). Thus far we have determined that in any given resistance, one can examine the following points: what was the observable resistance, how was this resistance manifested (was it verbal or nonverbal?), what were the seeds of the resistance, and did the clinician move with or against the resistance? This basic language allows one to discuss and learn from any example of patient resistance. At this point a few more terms will complete the

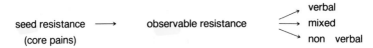

FIGURE 12. Forms of resistance.

tools necessary for understanding resistance. These terms deal directly with techniques of handling resistance.

Specific Approaches for Handling Resistance

Three basic approaches appear most frequently (Figure 13). The clinician can attend to the content of the patient's comment or to the process of the patient-clinician interaction, or the clinician can sidetrack the patient away from the area of resistance. Each technique has its pros and cons.

CONTENT RESPONSES TO RESISTANCE

One of the most common approaches consists of directly responding to the content of the patient's statement. In other words, the clinician answers the question. This approach is common, for it represents the natural manner in which people in an everyday situation respond. If a spouse asks, "Why didn't you tell me we were supposed to be dressed up?" the queried partner generally responds directly to the content of the question. The partner might say, "I'm sorry, I simply forgot." This alibi should probably not be relied upon too frequently, but in a pinch it will do. A clinician is answering the content of a resistance whenever the clinician provides a specific answer to the actual question of the patient. It should be kept in mind that if one responds to the content, then one is automatically placing oneself on the continuum of going with or against the patient's intentions, in which case the patient may either like or dislike the clinician's stance.

For clarification purposes let us take another look at the dialogue used to introduce this chapter, in which the paranoid woman suspected that I was not a doctor, because I had never been possessed. Instead of handling it in the fashion shown, we shall imagine what might have happened if I had attempted to respond solely to the content of the patient's accusation.

> **Clin.:** Mrs. Weston, one thing that you could help me to understand a little better is what it's like to be hit by a demon. I've never had that experience and I'm wondering what it is like.
>
> **Pt.:** You never been hit by a demon? (said with surprised indignation).
>
> **Clin.:** Well . . . I've never had that exact experience.

Pt.: Then what are you doing talking to me? (She sits bolt upright, shaking her finger brusquely.) You ought to know all about this stuff, and you're telling me you ain't been hit by a demon. Who are you anyway? You can't be a doctor. I ain't talking to you no more (mumbled angrily beneath her breath).

Clin.: I assure you that I am a doctor. You see, not all doctors are familiar with demons and possession. It depends on what your own beliefs happen to be. One does not have to believe in demons in order to be a good doctor. What remains important is that one cares.

Pt.: Are you telling me that you don't believe in demons?

Clin.: I guess at some level that's true. What I'm trying . . .

Pt.: (patient cuts off clinician) What you're trying to tell me is that you ain't no good Christian. You're with the devil, aren't you?

Clin.: No, I'm not with the devil.

And here we see aptly illustrated one of the main hazards of responding to the content of the patient's resistance. The clinician can rapidly be drawn into a never-ending debate. As the debate thickens, the interviewer may quickly find the patient becoming progressively

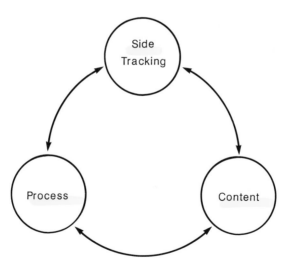

Possible Approaches:

   1) Side-tracking alone
   2) Content alone
   3) Process alone
   4) Combination of two or three of the above

FIGURE 13. Methods of handling resistance.

more hostile. The clinician may find it difficult to know how to respond. It is just this tendency to respond to content that places Alice into such difficult situations in Wonderland, for she frequently responds to the content of what she is asked. This tendency is also extremely common among therapists, for it is a natural response to explain oneself if one feels misunderstood.

One of the other problems with responding to content is the fact that such immediate responses tend to eliminate the chance of learning about the patient's defenses — in short, learning why the patient needed to ask the question in the first place.

On the other hand, in some cases, it may be expedient to directly respond to the patient's content. At times it is the best way to handle a particular situation. Clinicians who develop the rigid habit of always avoiding the content of the patient's inquiries, by addressing the process with questions such as, "What made you ask?" can dig themselves into a deep pit of trouble. With certain patients such process responses may be simply ill-timed and very frustrating.

For example, one can well imagine the response from the psychotic woman just described if the clinician had made a process statement such as, "You seem to be angry that I'm not familiar with demons. I'm wondering why you have such a need to present yourself so hostilely?" If the clinician is lucky, the patient will not have any idea what he just said so obtusely. If unlucky, and the point strikes home, then one hopes this clinician has his running shoes on. A rigid need to never answer questions directly probably represents an error in training and/or a need for control on the part of the clinician. Later we shall see examples in which content responses seem quite effective.

PROCESS RESPONSES TO RESISTANCE

We have already hinted at the basic mechanics of the second major method of handling resistance, namely to address the process of why the question is being asked. This is not the manner in which one is raised in our culture to respond to questions. As an adolescent one does not turn to the school principal and ask, "Gee Mr. Claybourne, I'm wondering why you have such an urgent need to know why I was smoking in the bathroom, and I might add that you are wearing a very handsome suit today." An obsequious Eddie Haskell from the "Leave It To Beaver" show might have said something like this, but few principals would be impressed. The point of this excursion remains the fact that because process responses are not natural, their effective utilization can be difficult to learn.

And what a shame it would be not to learn the nuances of such a powerful technique. In the long run, effective process responses are essential elements of intensive psychotherapy, and they also can guide the clinician out of many a jam in the initial interview.

In an operational sense, process is addressed whenever the clinician asks the patient to reflect upon what is happening in the interview itself, within the patient, or within the clinician. The clinician does not attempt to directly answer the specific question of the patient, but rather attempts to shift the focus of the patient to the actual process of the interaction itself, the feelings generated by the interview, or the thoughts that led to the patient's question in the first place. A variety of methods of attending to process are available to the clinician. Let us make a quick review of some of these techniques, which we shall see in more detail in the second part of this chapter. It is valuable to be familiar with all of these techniques, while discovering new ones from experience.

To begin the survey, one of the most basic methods of focusing on process consists of pointing out to patients their own behaviors. For instance, the interviewer may notice that an interview is becoming shut down after an animated beginning. The clinician could turn to such a patient and say, "You know, during the last couple of minutes I've noticed that you've become pretty quiet. I'm wondering what you are feeling."

At times the interviewer may choose to be more specific about the exact change in behavior. A patient may begin asking a variety of questions as the interview proceeds such as, "What do you think I ought to do?" At such a point the clinician may ask, "In the past couple of minutes you've asked a lot of questions. You weren't asking many questions earlier. I'm wondering what has changed so that now you seem to want some answers from me?"

The interviewer could also explore process by directing attention to the immediate effect of one's actions upon the patient. For instance, with the previous example one could say, "I guess you've noticed that I'm not directly answering many of your questions. I'm interested in how you're feeling about my apparent reluctance to answer directly." A response to this question may reveal some important traits in the patient, such as an ability or inability to be appropriately assertive. By way of example, a patient exhibiting many dependent traits may feel quite awkward at this point, saying, "Oh don't worry about it, I guess that's just your job." A person with narcissistic traits, on the other hand, may snarl a sarcasm such as, "Shrinks are too afraid to deal with people like people, isn't that right?" In any case the process question has provided significant material for exploration.

In other instances, the clinician may choose to address the patient's affect as opposed to the patient's behavior per se. A patient may begin to appear sad. The clinician may directly point out the affect with, "You're looking sort of sad right now, what's going on?" Or the interviewer may inquire at a more general level such as, "I was wondering what you were feeling just a moment ago, when you spoke about your Dad?"

In a somewhat similar vein, if the clinician senses a growing hostility from the patient, the clinician may choose to note the affect itself. "Mr. Jason, it looks like you're feeling a little angry, what's going on?" In some instances, the clinician can directly point out the problems arising in the blending process. An angry patient may say, "Look, there's nothing wrong with me that a little time won't cure, get the picture!" To this the clinician may respond, "I'm sorry if you are starting to feel some anger, let's see what's happening here. It looks like some of my questions are irritating. What am I asking that seems uncalled for?"

At this point one of the characteristics of process interactions seems more apparent. Specifically, when addressing process, the clinician cannot afford to be afraid of exploring the resistance itself, no matter what emotions are being aroused. Instead, the clinician moves into the "eye of the storm," while carefully trying to understand what is actually being experienced by the patient. Many times patients appreciate this honest attempt of the clinician to "uncover the real problem here."

In an interview in which a patient is becoming more distant, but is unable to verbalize anger, the logjam can sometimes be broken by personalizing the interaction, as with, "Mr. Wilkins, are you feeling a little angry with me?" Once the patient becomes engaged in talking about his or her own anger, some of the anger may actually dissipate. It is somehow harder for patients to be angry with someone who can openly acknowledge true feelings. At such moments the interviewer seems more human and less like a sterile clinician. In general, one of the best manners with which to make covert resistance less obstructive is simply to make it overt, put the cards on the table so to speak.

Another fruitful method of addressing the process consists of asking patients what answer they are expecting. The patient may ask, "Do you believe in God?" The clinician may respond, "That's a tough question, John. What kind of difference would it make to you if I said yes or no?" In this fashion the clinician may get a good warning as to what results may follow if the clinician would choose to respond to the actual content of the question. But in many cases, once the patient begins answering what difference it would make, the original question never returns.

Herein lies another hallmark of process responses in general. Process responses provide clinicians with time to think and re-collect themselves. They are punts of a sort, which clearly put the ball back in the patient's hands. During the time in which the patient must come up with a response, the clinician can get a better idea of how to ultimately respond to the resistance in question.

In a behavioral sense, process comments may also serve as punishing reinforcers to patients who are simply trying to needle the clinician with tricky questions. Each time these patients ask a bothersome question, the process comment turns the focus back upon themselves. Soon enough they tire of being put on the spot. By way of example, one might say to such a patient, "You seem to get a charge of putting me on the spot. Any ideas why you like to do that?" If the patient persists, the clinician can continue to pursue the point, "There's another one of those pointed questions. What are you feeling when you ask questions like that?" Done with a calm and nonvindictive tone of voice, these questions serve the dual purpose of helping the patient to look at himself, while simultaneously decreasing the frequency of such barbed questions.

A final process technique, which we have not yet discussed, is the judicious use of self-disclosure. If one feels frustrated by the appearance of repeated resistance, one may turn to the patient saying, "You know, I'm feeling a little puzzled right now. We don't seem to be getting anywhere. Do you have any ideas about what is going on between us?" A more interpretive variant of such a response may be, "Do you have any ideas why we are getting into a debate here? Is this the same type of argument that you find yourself in with your wife, or with your boss?"

As a final example, one of the most common process techniques is to respond to a patient's question with a simple, "Why do you ask?" To me this question is occasionally useful, but, in actuality, it is often not fully understood by the patient in an initial interview, for these patients are not yet trained to understand process as opposed to content. In short, they wonder, "What does he mean, why do I ask?" Moreover, I have noticed that many supervisees automatically snap off this response any time a patient asks a question. More often than not, the accompanying tone of the clinician's voice has a defensive quality to it. Utilized in this fashion, this question can be malproductive. If the clinician keeps these potential problems in mind, this standard example of a process response remains a viable option.

Now that we have delineated various methods of responding to process as opposed to the content of the patient's statements, the question becomes one of uncovering the possible advantages of such process responses. Several advantages come to mind. Process statements and questions provide time in which the clinician can reorganize, as stated earlier. They also push the patient to begin a self-exploration, which will hopefully continue if the patient proceeds into psychotherapy. Moreover, as the patient responds, the clinician gains a chance to understand the patient's defenses, fantasies, and interpersonal style. If a question is answered on a content level by the clinician, much of this opportunity may be lost. Finally, when clinicians respond to process as opposed to content, the issue of going against the resistance is somewhat muted, for no opinion has actually been offered. Consequently it becomes less likely that the clinician will put his or her foot in his or her mouth.

All in all, process comments and questions appear to have many advantages. It is probably not too risky to state that process responses are generally better than content responses. But there are times when content responses may be superior, and one should be familiar with both methods. Another very important point remains the fact that the clinician may frequently find it useful to combine process and content techniques.

Let us take a look at some process maneuvers in an actual clinical situation. Although this particular dialogue was not in an initial interview, it illustrates the advantages of a process approach when it hits its mark. The patient was a young man, whom we have discussed before. He had a long history of a compulsive drive for success, which had brought him many societal rewards but left him feeling empty and unloved. He appeared to benefit significantly from psychotherapy as well as the interim use of a tricyclic antidepressant.

In the termination phase of his psychotherapy the following exchange occurred generally as follows. In it we shall see the patient ask a specific content-oriented question. Rather than respond to the content of the question, a series of process questions provided an entrance into a wealth of psychodynamic material.

Clin.: What was the last session like for you?
Pt.: It was uh, pretty upsetting. I don't like thinking about the death of my parents. And I was a little surprised at how upset I was feeling. I've been thinking about the ending of the therapy a lot. I think I'm ready, but uh, it's, it's a little scary . . . I don't like saying good-bye and you had asked what I'd do if my father was dying . . . I really don't know. But there has to be something more than death. There has to be a life after death or else all this would be so senseless . . . What do you think, do you think there is life after death?
Clin.: When you ask that question, what do you picture me answering?
Pt.: Oh I don't really know. I guess I hope you'll say yes, because, because that's what I think too.
Clin.: Well what would it mean to you, and this isn't necessarily my answer, but what would it mean to you if I said, "No"?

Pt.: Uh, hmm, I think that would upset me.

Clin.: In what way?

Pt.: Because it would mean that you disagreed with me and I wouldn't like that. That would bother me, that would bother me a lot.

Clin.: Why?

Pt.: I don't know. I, I, guess it's important to me what you think of me.

Clin.: So let's get back to your question, because what seems important about it is the fact that you are hunting for me to agree with you, as if you need my approval to be "good." What do you make of that? *think @ your beh.*

Pt.: (slight smile) It reminds me of earlier in the therapy, when I needed you to praise me in order to feel good. Like when I got mad at you because you hadn't read the newspaper articles about my ball games. That upset me, it was like I needed your approval to be O.K. And I know that I've felt that need about my father for years. He was the reason I played ball . . . I felt I had to play ball or he wouldn't love me. But I thought I got over that need.

Clin.: I guess not entirely. You did it just now with me again. You wanted my approval of your answer. But the point is that you don't need an answer from me. You don't need my approval. It would be fine for us to disagree. You won't be destroyed. Our relationship will not end simply because we disagree or because I wouldn't approve of one of your beliefs.

Pt.: I know that, but sometimes I have a hard time feeling it. I thought I was totally over that feeling, but I guess there is a part of me that still demands approval, perhaps too strongly. (pause) I was very upset with something my sister said to me a couple of days ago. She told me that I'd better stay in therapy a little longer, two years wasn't enough. And that really bothered me . . . but I eventually realized that it didn't really matter what she thought. I know that I've made a lot of progress. And I may not be perfect, but I'm not so bad either. And she doesn't really know me. I am cautiously optimistic about the future. I really think that I am ready to end therapy. It won't be easy, but I don't think it ever would be.

In this excerpt, the focus was turned back upon the reason why the patient asked the question. No effort was made to actually answer his question directly on a content level. The approach, via process, led the patient into a rich area of reflection, which cut directly to one of the main themes of the therapy as it related to the issue of termination. Eventually the patient achieved a deeper understanding of why he "needed" an answer, a need that was gradually decreasing as his sense of self-esteem improved. To have responded with a content approach would have completely short-circuited this powerful therapeutic interlude.

We can see the power inherent in responding to the process as opposed to the content. When done effectively, the patient and the clinician are often moved inward. Although this excerpt originated from an exchange during the termination phase of therapy, it nicely illustrates the basic principles and strengths of a process-oriented technique.

At this juncture, one might argue that if process responses can provide such insight, then why would a clinician ever use anything but a process-oriented approach. And here lies an important but often underplayed point. The immediate goal of the clinician, when handling a resistance, is not necessarily to provide insight. Let us backtrack for a moment in order to explore this issue in more detail.

When working with resistance, the clinician may choose to achieve any of the following three tasks: (1) to decrease the resistance itself, so that communication is improved in the setting of a strengthened engagement process, (2) to learn about the patient's defenses, while uncovering the anxieties that stirred these defenses, and (3) to help the patient learn a method with which to explore the patient's own dynamics. Each of these goals is important. But the emphasis placed on each goal by the clinician may vary considerably, depending upon the stage of therapy. Once again, as with the interview itself, goals and tasks change with each phase of the therapeutic encounter.

In the above excerpt the patient was in the closing phases of a long-term, dynamically oriented therapy. At this stage of therapy the alliance is generally extremely strong. Consequently, the first task listed above is of little relevance, the alliance having been secured much earlier in the process. Indeed, during this stage of therapy, I was able to be fairly confrontational with this patient without endangering my alliance with him. On the other hand, while in the termination phase of therapy, both participants should be concerned with recognizing and understanding the patient's anxieties and defenses. If the therapy has proceeded well, the patient should be nearing a phase in which he progressively functions as his own therapist. The last two tasks mentioned above are of prime importance. Process questions and interpretations remain the best method of accomplishing these tasks.

Let us look at the needs associated with an initial interview as compared with later stages of therapy. The main goal is not to uncover defenses in detail or to help the patient gain insight. Instead the most important task is the establishment of a sound alliance, while gathering the most valid information available in order to determine the treatment options available for the patient. Patients may gain psychotherapeutic insight in the process, but there will be plenty of time in the subsequent therapy for a focus upon the acquisition of insight.

In this light, it becomes apparent that the last two potential tasks associated with handling resistance, mentioned above, are not of major importance in the initial interview. The first task of decreasing the resistance in order to allow the gathering of further data becomes paramount. In this sense process maneuvers are frequently valuable, but other methods of handling resistance may also be valuable, and in some cases more useful for the task at hand. This is why we mentioned earlier that content responses to resistance have a real place in the initial interview, for the task of the initial interview is a unique one. This distinction between the goals of the initial interview as opposed to ongoing therapy is further highlighted if the initial interviewer is functioning as a consultant or triage agent, who may never see the patient again.

SIDETRACKING RESISTANCE

While considering the above line of thinking, it is worth mentioning another method of handling resistance besides the previously described techniques of addressing content or process. This other technique is much more commonly utilized during initial interviews rather than in ongoing therapy, for it certainly provides no insight for either the patient or the clinician. Yet it can work surprisingly well in breaking up a logjam of resistance. The technique is called sidetracking the patient, which in less euphemistic terms one might call ignoring the resistance.

At first glance this sounds like an unsavory undertaking. But let us see it in action before passing judgment. Imagine a mildly angry man of about thirty, brought in for an evaluation, somewhat against his will. His family describes symptoms suggestive of incipient mania, and he indeed displays both a pressured speech and a flight of ideas. We will pick up the interview somewhere in the opening phase.

> *Clin.:* Mr. Preston, a little earlier you had mentioned that you had been thinking of hurting yourself . . . (patient cuts off clinician).
>
> *Pt.:* What is it with you shrinks, you're always talking about people killing themselves, can't a man kill himself if he wants to? Can't a man control his own destiny?
>
> *Clin.:* Who else has been trying to control your life?   *not me*

> *Pt.:* Who hasn't! You name them, the President, the Pope, and all the saints in heaven. My wife is the big know-it-all. She's the boss. To her everything makes sense but me. But she don't know it all, trust me.
>
> *Clin.:* Besides feeling angry with some of these people, have you been feeling sad at all?
>
> *Pt.:* You know it's the strangest thing but I do get sad some-times real sudden-like.

This example nicely illustrates the successful use of a sidetrack. The patient's anger at the clinician has subsided, and the interview is proceeding into a data gathering phase. But the patient's questions concerning "shrinks" and their generic interest in suicide has been side-stepped. The clinician will reapproach suicidal ideation at a later point in the interview, but for now the flow of the interview has been restored. An attempt to respond either to the process or the content of the patient's question may have been considerably less productive in moving through this resistance.

Sidetracking is frequently useful with hypomanic or manic patients, for it takes advantage of the patient's inherent tendency to jump from topic to topic. A few other points concerning sidetracking are relevant. If the clinician uses a sidetrack, the clinician needs to carefully watch the patient's response. If successful, the patient will quickly follow up on the new topic. If the patient returns to the patient's original question, then sidetracking is probably not going to work and a content or process response will be needed. It is generally not wise to continue sidetracking an issue, for such persistence is often irritating and rightfully so to a patient. If a sidetrack fails, try a different technique.

Another point to keep in mind is that sidetracking frequently works best when the interviewer changes the topic to an area of high importance or affect for the patient, as was demonstrated in the excerpt above. It is also useful to sidetrack the topic away from oneself if the patient is expressing anger towards the clinician.

A Direct Application of the Language of Resistance

Thus far we have discussed three methods of handling resistance: addressing the content, addressing the process, and sidetracking. These techniques complement each other and may be used singly or in conjunction with each other. We have also seen that depending upon the phase of therapy and/or the patient's clinical state, different techniques may be more or less useful. Combined with the concepts of observable resistance, seed resistance, and direction of clinician response (either with or against the resistance), we have developed a language that can allow us to explore essentially any example of resistance encountered in clinical work.

For instance, these terms can be readily applied to the striking piece of resistance illustrated in the beginning of this chapter. It may be of value to review this piece of dialogue as viewed with the concepts delineated above. The patient was the thirty-year-old woman escorted by the police into the emergency room on an involuntary commitment after she had been found destroying her "demon-possessed" furniture. The dialogue had proceeded as follows:

Clin.: Mrs. Weston, one thing that you could help me to understand a little better is what it's like to be hit by a demon. I've never had that experience and I'm wondering what it feels like to you.

Pt.: You never been hit by a demon? (said with surprised indignation).

Clin.: Well . . . I've never had that exact experience.

Pt.: Then what are you doing talking to me! (She sits bolt upright, shaking her finger brusquely.) You ought to know all about this stuff and you're telling me you ain't been hit by a demon. Who are you anyway? I ain't talking to you no more (mumbled angrily beneath her breath).

It is rather easy to pick out the observable resistance at this point, as mentioned earlier. On a verbal level the observable resistance begins with the accusatory question, "You never been hit by a demon?" This is quickly followed by a deeper pit of resistant statements, culminating in a refusal to talk anymore.

All of these verbal antagonisms were accompanied by many observable signs of nonverbal resistance. Her tone of voice became acrid, accompanied by an angry stare. The stare itself was waved in by a hostile wagging of her finger. In short, the observable resistances, on both a verbal and nonverbal level, were openly displayed.

But what of the potential seed resistances? Which core pains may have been at work with this particular woman? One must remain somewhat speculative in this regard. And yet the seeds of her resistance seemed fairly apparent. In the first place, the situation itself, of being brought in by the police involuntarily, suggests the likelihood of a great deal of fear and anger concerning the issue of a loss of external control. Earlier in the interview she had animatedly discussed the need for all people to convert to her religious beliefs. Beneath her intensity one could sense a feeling of inferiority, which she guarded by putting all other faiths down. In this sense another possible seed resistance was a feeling of low self-esteem. These two core pains seemed most acutely active, but other tensions such as a fear of the unknown or a fear of a loss of internal control (ergo violence) may also have been at work.

It appears that the actual resistances, both overt and covert, can be categorized nicely by the language developed so far. The next question becomes one of delineating the actual attempt to resolve the resistance, for this interview had potentially reached a dead-end.

In the first place, the resistance is addressed by my immediate reply, "Mrs. Weston, it looks like you're concerned about my lack of knowledge about being hit by demons." This statement represents a process response, in which the patient's affect is being acknowledged. This pathway is furthered by my next question. "What specifically about that is upsetting you?" Once again this statement focuses upon the process of what is disturbing to Mrs. Weston. It acknowledges her right to be angry, and it suggests a willingness on the part of the clinician to find out how he is upsetting her. The metacommunication is clear and reassuring to the patient: "I would like to find out what I'm doing to upset you, and I may be able to change it."

The tone of voice used was a gentle one. In this regard a nonverbal as well as a verbal medium was utilized to respond to the patient's resistance. Both the verbal and the nonverbal response were nondefensive. They represent a moving with the resistance. No attempt is made to contradict or block the patient's anger, as would have been displayed with a clinician response such as, "Now there's no need to be angry here" or "You're going to have to talk to me so that this can be straightened out." Both of these statements represent content responses, for they immediately address the patient's stated demands. Such statements would probably have served to anger this patient even more, for in essence they strip her of even more control.

The process techniques actually used began to soften the patient's resistance, as shown below.

> ***Pt.:*** It would mean you ain't no doctor, that's what it would mean.
>
> ***Clin.:*** And how would it mean that I wasn't a doctor?
>
> ***Pt.:*** Because to be a doctor you got to deal with demons all the time, any idiot knows that . . . I just don't know what is going on here, I just want help with these demons and they send me to a moron.

Clearly the patient remains hostile, but her admission of feeling confused is suggestive that the hostility is residing. One may be able to reach her on a more cooperative level. In general, once a clinician acknowledges a patient's anger in a nondefensive fashion, it is not unusual to see the beginning of a de-escalation of affect.

In the next few statements I employed a slightly different tack with, "I'm going to be very honest with you because I think that is very important. I must admit I may not know everything about things that are important to you, but I am honestly trying to understand better, and you can help me to do that." This represents a content response, which directly acknowledges the patient's statement that I essentially do not know what I am doing. There is a toned down admission that the clinician is "guilty as charged," but this is turned to advantage by asking for the patient's help. Here we see a seed resistance being addressed. The patient has a need to feel superior, and the clinician responds to this need by taking a one-down position.

The next two statements, "And I didn't mean to upset you. If other things I say upset you, please let me know," address the other seed resistance discussed earlier. More specifically, these statements give some control to the patient, thus decreasing the tensions surrounding her fear of a loss of external control while conveying a sense of respect.

Directly on top of these efforts to decrease the patient's core pains, a sidetracking technique was employed. The patient was asked, "I'm wondering if the demons have tried to hurt or enter your daughter?" As mentioned earlier, an effective side-track tends to move the patient into an area of high affect or interest. In this case the area involved the patient's daughter and completely moves the discussion away from the immediate interviewing situation. Fortunately the patient accepted this sidetrack, probably because her anger towards the clinician was resolving. It is frequently useful to piggyback sidetracking statements onto other techniques as shown above. The trick is to quickly move the topic of discussion, thus decreasing the likelihood of the patient's anger rekindling.

At this point a series of close-ended questions was used to keep the patient in the new area of discussion, thus cementing the sidetrack. A decision was then made to continue using the daughter as a focus of discussion, for the patient seemed to increase her blending around this topic. Eventually the further expansion of the psychotic region and the lethality region was accomplished utilizing this new focus of discussion. The interview proceeded more smoothly, the resistance having fallen away.

By examining this particular resistance in detail, it is apparent that we have indeed developed a language with which to explore the subtle nuances of the complex phenomenon known as resistance. In the next section, this language will allow us to directly address specific resistances commonly encountered during the initial interview.

PART II: HANDLING COMMON RESISTANCES

That the yielding conquers the resistant and the soft the hard is a fact known by all men, yet utilized by none . . .

Lao Tzu (Chinese Sage)

Resistances Concerned with Clinician Competence

Certainly one of the more common forms of resistance is illustrated by questions such as, "What type of training have you had?" or "Are you a student?" Patients may be concerned about a variety of issues such as training, professional affiliation, age, sex, and race. The issue becomes one of to what degree should the clinician directly respond, and whether the response should be on a content or process level. As one would expect, there exist no pat answers, but some guiding principles can be discerned.

In the first place, these types of questions commonly stem from a single seed resistance, the fear of the unknown. In this case the specific fear can be succinctly stated as, "Can this particular clinician help me?" With this idea in mind, the goal becomes one of helping the patient to recognize the nature of the question actually being asked, to help the patient see where such a question may be coming from in a psychological sense, and to decrease the patient's anxiety.

It is also relevant to realize that such questions may not actually always represent resistance. They may represent intelligence. It is not inappropriate, when seeking a professional, to want to know if the supposed professional is any good. Many patients have no way of prescreening and simply end up choosing a number from the telephone book or receiving a referral to their local mental health center.

Around this issue of whether these requests represent resistance or not, two schools of thought have evolved. For those who view it as a form of resistance, an argument is generally advanced that only a process response is appropriate from the clinician. According to this school of thought, the clinician should find out why the question is being asked. To answer directly will short-circuit the opportunity to uncover important psychodynamic information. The clinician also runs the risk of providing an answer that will unsettle the patient. For example, the clinician might quickly respond that the clinician's training has been in behavioral techniques. If the clinician is unlucky, the patient may possess all sorts of distorted views about behaviorism, resulting in an immediate wariness of the clinician.

The second school views these questions as a legitimate aspect of the contract and leans towards answering them directly, utilizing a content-oriented response. One does not go to a surgeon without finding out whether the surgeon is skilled. With something as sensitive as one's personal memories, it makes sense to find out if the clinician is talented and trustworthy. This argument is strengthened by the fact that many unskilled and poorly trained people can label themselves as therapists without ever having spent a single day in a legitimate school of counseling.

Both of these arguments seem to hold water as one reads them. This somewhat contradictory situation arises because both of these arguments are, in reality, quite legitimate. The wisest resolution may be to incorporate both arguments, utilizing both a process and a content response. For instance, the clinician may respond as follows, "I think your question about my training is a very good one. In just a little while, I'll answer any basic questions you have about my training, but first I'd like to get an idea of what some of your concerns may be. For instance, what type of clinician were you hoping to find here today?" As the patient begins to describe specific concerns, a variety of follow-up questions can be asked, including the following:

a. What was it like coming here today?
b. What types of concerns did you have about coming to the appointment today?
c. What had you imagined it would be like talking with a psychiatrist?
d. What are some of your specific fears about my training or background?
e. Did you have any dreams or fantasies about coming to see a psychologist?
f. What have you heard about social workers or other mental health professionals?
g. What does seeing a psychiatrist mean to you?

All of these questions are process oriented in nature, allowing ample room for the clinician to explore some of the dynamic issues behind the original question. The information provided by the patient may also help the clinician to choose a better method of responding on a content level. For instance, if the patient relates distorted information about therapy in general or specifically, then the clinician can gracefully acknowledge the patient's anxiety, while hopefully decreasing it through appropriate education. The clinician may say something such as "I can understand why you would have concerns about behavioral therapy. Let me clarify some issues, and I think you'll find that the therapy we are discussing, although behavioral in nature, is quite different from what you've heard."

Other methods of returning to the content response, which was promised to the patient, may be as simple as saying, "I appreciate your sharing some of your concerns, let me tell you a little about my background as I said I would." Besides providing appreciated information, this comment conveys the metacommunication that "this clinician keeps his or her word" and respects the needs of the patient.

To me, the combined process/content technique described above allows the clinician to gather a substantial amount of pertinent information, while also answering the legitimate questions of the patient. Once again, in an initial interview, as opposed to ongoing therapy, the premium is upon engaging the patient, not upon providing insight. The above technique is strongly engaging while providing an appropriate degree of dynamic exploration.

With regard to issues such as sex, age, and race, a similar approach may be taken. The trick is not to become defensive. The clinician attempts to provide a safe milieu within which the patient can discuss concerns. The clinician might ask, "I noticed that you mentioned that I seem young, I'm wondering what some of your concerns are about my youth." The nondefensiveness of such a response probably conveys more professionalism than a string of diplomas hanging on the office wall.

After hearing the patient's concerns, the clinician will have a better idea of where to move next and whether to directly respond to the content of the patient's questions. Once again, content responses can be valuable. In the next illustration the clinician will follow a process response with a content-oriented technique, in which an attempt is made to acknowledge the inherent differences between the patient and the clinician, raised by the patient herself.

    Clin.:   What I'd like to do today is spend the next forty or so minutes trying to gather from you what you see as the major problems. Perhaps we could start with what brought you here today.

    Pt.:   You know, before we start I need to say something.

    Clin.:   Sure, what did you want to say?

    Pt.:   Well, I don't know how to put this, uh, well, I might as well just say it. I really would strongly prefer talking with another woman. I don't feel comfortable talking to a man. You know, I had requested a woman as a therapist.

    Clin.:   I must have been quite a shock (smiles gently).

    Pt.:   No kidding! But you, you seem nice and all that, but I really would prefer talking with a woman.

    Clin.:   Sometimes that can be important. Before we decide what to do, tell me a little bit about what your concerns are about talking with a man, in this case me.

    Pt.:   Well, there is no way that a man can know what I've been through. A lot of my problems have to do with guys and some of the sexist things they do. Every man I meet seems to want something from me and I resent that. And so, well, I need a woman who will understand, because she has experienced the same things as I have.

Clin.: Hmmm, I see what you mean. First let me state that I agree that I can't know exactly what you are feeling. Only a woman can know exactly what it is like to be a woman. Moreover, even if I was a woman, I couldn't know exactly what you are feeling, because each person's feelings are unique. But in therapy the goal is not for me to know exactly what you are thinking, but to help you to explore your own thoughts and feelings. And I have had considerable experience with people of both sexes who have felt put down and abused. For each person I've worked with, I've learned something, and some of the things I've learned may be helpful to your own understanding.

Pt.: I understand what you're saying and actually it makes sense, but somehow I think I would feel more comfortable with a woman.

Clin.: Well that brings up another important point.

Pt.: What's that?

Clin.: Perhaps you'll miss an opportunity if you avoid a male clinician.

Pt.: In what sense?

Clin.: The very thing you want to learn about is how you react and respond to men. With a male therapist you may have a better chance to see what your natural responses, fears, and expectations are like. Does that make any sense?

Pt.: Yes it does, and I never thought of it that way.

Clin.: I'll tell you what. Let's try to work together and if problems arise I want you to tell me immediately. O.K.?

Pt.: O.K., you got yourself a deal.

In this example the clinician discussed in a matter of fact manner the specific resistance voiced by the patient. The resistance was, at that moment, dealt with on a content level. The patient was convinced of the usefulness of at least trying to work with the male clinician. The clinician also tended to move with the patient's resistance by acknowledging that he could not know exactly what she was feeling. To move against the resistance, with a statement such as, "Even though I'm a man I think I have a good idea of what you are feeling" would probably have disengaged the patient. In response, she might have proceeded to further argue her point.

With the phrase, "I must have been quite a shock" the clinician utilized humor effectively to break the tension. Well-timed humor can be very effective in this regard. The clinician also utilized another sound technique, a trial agreement when he said, "Let's try to work together and if problems arise I want you to tell me immediately. O.K.?" This concept decathected the situation by not forcing the patient to make an immediate decision.

Perhaps more than the issue of sex, the inexperienced mental health professional is in fear of questions such as, "Are you a student?" Most students are naturally sensitive to their lack of experience. At some level this is an appropriate realization. But a lack of experience does not imply incompetence. To the contrary, if the clinician listens carefully, the interview will probably proceed well, resulting in the collection of a useful data base from which to help the patient. An interview can be very useful without being perfect. There exists no need for a young clinician to become defensive over such a question. The very act of calmly responding to such challenges often conveys a reassuring sense of competence to the anxious patient, as shown in the following:

Pt.:   You know, just looking at you, I'm getting a little concerned, I mean are you a student or what?

Clin.:   Yes, I am a student, I'm in my second year of graduate training. You look like it is a little unsettling to be working with a student. What are some of your concerns?

Pt.:   Oh, I, I, well, I just think that someone with more experience might be more able to understand what is going on here. I mean this is pretty complicated.

Clin.:   It certainly seems to be very complicated. And if I were you I might also be concerned about my age, but I'll tell you what, the most important thing for a clinician to do is to listen carefully and with a sensitive ear. And that is something that I do well, in fact it is one of the main reasons that I entered this field. And I'd like to try to help you today. If there are specific problems that arise as we go along just let me know. We'll get an idea soon enough whether we will work well together or not. Let's start with why your wife sent you here. Do you agree with her views on the problem?

Pt.:   No. She's got it backwards. I haven't been depressed, I've been angry and she should know that.

Clin.:   And how should she know that?

Pt.:   Because she's the one who is causing all the friction, what with her stupid meddling into my business affairs. She should know better. I know what I'm doing, I don't need her eight-foot nose in my way, sniffing around my office.

In this example the clinician has used both process and content techniques to move through the resistance. Without appearing defensive the clinician has reassured the patient that the clinician himself feels confident in a realistic fashion. A sidetracking technique was then utilized to get the conversation moving.

Along these lines, the clinician should feel perfectly safe mentioning the fact that supervision is also going to be utilized. These statements may actually calm the patient. By way of example, the clinician may say something like, "Your point is a good one, which is one of the reasons that we are always closely supervised in our work. In fact as soon as we are done talking I will be discussing what we learned with a very talented supervisor, Dr. Jones. We work well as a team. So let's try to get at least a start in understanding what is going on here. Now what was it your husband said he didn't like about the way you handled your son?" Once again the trick is in not becoming defensive. In the last analysis, the enthusiasm and willingness to listen carefully, which is so common in the young clinician, sometimes counterbalances the lack of experience that comes with the turf of being a trainee.

Before leaving the topic of challenges to the clinician's competence, another point is worth mentioning. In situations in which race may be an issue, it is wise to carefully attend to nonverbal as well as verbal clues that the patient is ill-at-ease. Unlike the woman above, some patients will not spontaneously bring up their discomfort. But if it is not addressed, the patient may never reappear for a second appointment. If I feel that a patient of a different race or culture is looking uncomfortable, I may raise the issue myself in a gentle fashion with phrases such as, "Mr. Macken, one thing I'm wondering about is what it's like for you to be working with a white clinician?" This may bring the covert resistance to the surface where it can be examined and hopefully worked through.

Many of the above ideas concerning challenges to the clinician's competence are excellently discussed by Anderson and Stewart, two family therapists who have carefully examined the entire range of resistance behaviors. Their book stands as an outstanding introduction to the issues of resistance in various aspects of therapy.[2]

Attempts to Gain Personal Information About the Clinician

This type of situation represents a more invasive extension of the issues just discussed. Instead of wanting to know appropriate information about the clinician's background, the patient wants the scoop or low-down on the clinician. This type of situation can be truly more threatening. Probably because of this threat, clinicians frequently over-react by abruptly going against the resistance with phrases such as, "I'm afraid that is not what is important here, we are here to talk about you, not me." This curt oppositional approach may lead to problems, as shown in the following:

> **Pt.:** Yeah, so I've been out of sorts since I began having this affair, you know how it is, you've had an affair haven't you?
>
> **Clin.:** Mr. Raphael, I fail to see how that is relevant. Let's get back to your problems.
>
> **Pt.:** But it is important, if you haven't had an affair how are you going to know what I'm talking about?
>
> **Clin.:** Well, I guess you'll just have to deal with that, because psychiatrists don't discuss their personal lives with patients.
>
> **Pt.:** I guess that settles that.
>
> **Clin.:** I guess so.

With such an antagonistic exchange, there exists a very good chance that the rest of this interview will be of little consequence. An initial attempt, utilizing a process response, may have been more rewarding, as demonstrated in the following:

> **Pt.:** You've had an affair, haven't you?
>
> **Clin.:** You make it sound like it would be odd if I said I had never had an affair.
>
> **Pt.:** I think that would be sort of odd, I thought all men had affairs at some point or another.
>
> **Clin.:** Do you think that you make a lot of assumptions about what the people around you are thinking, for instance what you think your wife is feeling?
>
> **Pt.:** That's hard to say. I never really gave it much thought.
>
> **Clin.:** Suppose for a moment that I told you that I had never had an affair. How would that affect you?
>
> **Pt.:** Uh, it would make me think that we were pretty different people, and I don't know how comfortable I'd be.
>
> **Clin.:** So then you feel uncomfortable if someone seems different from you?
>
> **Pt.:** I suppose that at some level, I do.
>
> **Clin.:** In what sort of ways?

In this example the clinician has moved around the resistance, and the process questions serve to guide the patient toward self-reflection. But what if the patient were more stubborn? How might one proceed?

>   **Pt.:**   You've had an affair, haven't you?
> **Clin.:**   What makes you ask?
>   **Pt.:**   That's for me to know and you to guess (patient smiles);
>   you're a doctor, surely you've had an affair?
> **Clin.:**   Looks like you're going to keep at it until you get an
>   answer of some sort.
>   **Pt.:**   That's right.
> **Clin.:**   Well, I'll be honest with you. In the past I've found that
>   my sharing of personal information always gets the ther-
>   apy into trouble. And if you wish, I can go into detail later
>   about how such information hurts the therapy itself. But
>   in any case I won't be supplying those types of answers.
>   On the other hand something has just happened that is of
>   interest. Do you know what it is?
>   **Pt.:**   No, I don't think so.
> **Clin.:**   Well, I was feeling put on the spot by you. And while you
>   did it, you were smiling to yourself, it seemed sort of
>   pleasurable for you. Are there other instances in your life
>   where you purposely put people on the spot?
>   **Pt.:**   I got to admit, I've been known to do that on occasion.
>   Like, it's just sort of a way to tease, you know what I mean
>   (smiles).

This example illustrates that at times the clinician must set limits. But limit setting is not the immediate response of this clinician, nor his only response. Also of interest is the fact that the reason for the limit was conveyed. The clinician did not merely pass on an authoritative proclamation to the patient.

Patients may make inquiries concerning a broad range of areas, including marriage, dating patterns, sexual activity, children, financial situation, religion, and many others. The clinician must decide what type of information is appropriate to disclose. Clinicians will vary on this issue, but I think that most clinicians would state that in an initial interview little if any background personal information should be disclosed. Many clinicians disclose little personal information even later in therapy. Such self-disclosure opens the clinician up to personal attack and loss of respect from the patient, and also short-circuits the projection of the patient's issues onto the clinician.

Another point is of interest here that can affect the manner in which the clinician chooses to respond to such personal inquiries. The seed resistance represented by such inquiries tends to fall into two different camps. In one camp these personal inquiries represent yet another fear that the clinician will not be able to help. For instance, a patient may ask whether the clinician has children or not. This request may stem from the patient's fear that a childless clinician could not possibly understand. In these instances, as shown before, the clinician will want to help the patient to bring this fear into the open.

But the patient above, who kept pushing the clinician to talk about affairs, represents a different camp. This hounding of the clinician probably represents a characterological display of sorts, like a peacock fanning its plumage. In the case just shown, the patient demonstrated a rather curious pleasure in watching the clinician squirm. Perhaps his mild sadism represents a counterreaction to some deep-seated core pains, such as feelings of inferiority. The clinician can file this information away, while later stroking the patient, so as to decrease the patient's need to attack. On a more immediate level, these characterological patients may need limits set, while being helped to look at the reasons that limit setting was needed. This type of reflection must be done in a noncritical fashion and without any angry countertransference response. When done well, the patient does not feel confronted. Once again the technique is flexibly matched to the needs of the patient and of the clinician.

Resistance in the Form of Patient Requests

It is not uncommon, during an initial interview, for a patient to make a request of the clinician. These requests can range from innocuous issues such as wanting a glass of water to more extravagant requests such as wanting a date. Once again the key lies in attempting to understand the reasons behind the requests. Does the request for water represent a need to control the interview, a manifestation of oral needs, or simply a thirsty patient? In a similar fashion, is the request for a date a defensive posturing or the workings of a manic process?

If a request is made for a simple physical issue such as a glass of water or a trip to the restroom, it can often be accommodated by the clinician. Unfortunately, especially if repeated, these requests may, if granted, use up valuable and limited clinical time. In such instances, I have found that a simple explanation of the situation will often satisfy the patient. One might say, "Mr. Miller we've got a little bit of a problem with time. Let's try to go on with the interview without any breaks, because you're bringing up a lot of important information that I need to hear. If you feel later that you must get another drink of water, please mention it again."

Probably a more frequent request, as opposed to asking for an activity or an object, is an attempt to procure an opinion from the clinician on a topic on which the clinician should not be offering his or her two bits.

> *Pt.:* The bottom line of all this remains the fact that I'm a hard-working single mother. Trust me, it isn't easy and my sister thinks that I should also be taking care of my sick father. Now you're a professional, what do you think of that?
>
> *Clin.:* I think that it upsets you a lot. What do you say to your sister when she brings up the topic?
>
> *Pt.:* I tell her to forget it; sometimes, sometimes I, I would just like to belt her!
>
> *Clin.:* What do you do with your anger?
>
> *Pt.:* I let it out, and I've got a right to let it out. She's lucky I just don't burn her house down.

In this example the clinician moves past the resistance by offering an opinion, not on the patient's question, but on what the question signifies about the patient. In essence, this is a variant of sidetracking.

At times patients may be a bit more persistent.

> *Pt.:* Then my mother had to put her two cents in. Nothing new about that. Believe it or not she had my phone tapped. Now tell me the truth, she's way out of line, right?
>
> *Clin.:* Well she certainly has made you very angry.
>
> *Pt.:* No joke! But seriously, don't you think she's way out of bounds?
>
> *Clin.:* What would you like me to say?
>
> *Pt.:* I don't know . . . agree with me I guess.
>
> *Clin.:* I don't think that my agreeing would do that much for you, but have you found much support among your friends or family?
>
> *Pt.:* I haven't found much support from anyone at any time. Everyone views me as a loser.

Here the clinician first tried the sidetrack previously demonstrated, but this time the patient persisted. Then the clinician used a process question that bought some time and resulted in a new line of response. The patient was successfully sidetracked using this new avenue. Flexibility remains critical for success.

Awkward Situations Encountered with Psychotic Patients

There are many unusual situations that can arise for the clinician when dealing with psychotic patients. But two stick out as occurring fairly frequently. Both interactions once again involve patient requests for the clinician's opinion. The first occurs when a delusional patient asks a clinician whether the clinician believes in the patient's delusion. The second potentially awkward moment arises when a psychotic patient asks whether he or she is crazy. The frankness of this question frequently catches interviewers off-guard. Let us begin with the first situation.

It is not unusual for a delusional patient to wonder whether the clinician believes the patient's story. In one sense this represents a healthy attempt by the patient to check with reality. It also places the clinician in a rather unsettling spot. If the clinician goes along with the patient, then the patient is being given a false verification of delusional material. On the other hand, if the clinician flatly disagrees with the patient, then the patient has only one of two conclusions to reach. First, the patient can feel that the clinician believes the patient is lying. Second, the patient can feel that the clinician believes that the patient is insane. Needless to say, neither of these perceptions by the patient is likely to increase blending.

In general, I feel that it is seldom appropriate to agree with the patient's delusional system. There may be exceptions, which will be discussed below. To agree with the delusional material is risky business. By way of illustration, if the clinician would agree with a paranoid patient that someone is "out to get the patient," there is always the risk that the clinician will eventually be included as one of the persecutors in the evolving delusional system. At such a point the clinician, who is now being accused by the patient, cannot suddenly change his opinion, telling the patient that he was kidding earlier. Furthermore, it can make it very difficult for the subsequent treatment team if the patient keeps saying, "But Dr. Blake believed me, why don't you?" Dr. Blake will not be popular with his fellow mental health workers.

To me, the best method of handling such a situation so that one does not antagonize the patient is an honest approach, coupled with a suspended judgment, as illustrated in the following:

Pt.: The entire string of circumstances terrifies me. I am convinced that my husband has been contacted by aliens.

Clin.: And how do you know that?

Pt.: Oh, I've been keeping tabs on him for months. Every night when he comes home he has a funny smell to him. It's the smell of aliens. And, I have seen him sneaking out at night. I believe he is planning to give our boy to the aliens for experimental reasons. Oh you've got to believe me, tell me you believe me and will help me.

Clin.: Mrs. Jason, I'm not at all surprised at your concern. I'll be very honest with you, as I'm sure you are aware, what you are saying is so unusual that it is hard to believe. But I want to learn more. When do you think he made contact with the aliens?

Pt.: I'm not certain, but I think it was at least a month ago. It is also possible that he intends to get rid of me.

Clin.: Have you done anything to protect your son and yourself against him?

Pt.: . . . Yes . . . yes, I have gotten the gun out of the attic. And I bought some new bullets for it; oh I can't believe this is happening.

The approach taken by this clinician has conveyed a feeling of unconditional positive regard, while indicating that the clinician has some doubts about the validity of the story. Despite these doubts, the clinician conveys an active interest in hearing more. This clinician interest frequently appeals to delusional patients, who seldom find anyone who will listen to their story attentively. The clinician caps off the movement through this resistance point by quickly sidetracking the patient with a specific question.

In the initial interview the goal is to build an alliance strong enough that important information will be conveyed to the clinician. To have told this woman that her story makes no sense or as some clinicians phrase it, "I can see that you believe your story, and that's what counts" runs the risk of jeopardizing the tenuous blending so characteristic of paranoia. At an early stage of the interview, there is seldom a need to tell the patient point blank that you do not believe the patient's story.

This excerpt demonstrates the need to continue the interview in an effort to determine the potential dangerousness of the patient. This particular woman has already taken a striking action towards violence. If she reaches a point in which she truly feels that her husband is about to harm her child, a shooting would not be out of the question. If she had felt disbelief from the clinician, this critical material may never have been shared.

In the closing phase of the interview, clinicians can more appropriately bring up their feelings of disbelief in a fashion that is not overly confrontational such as, "Mrs. Jason it is a very frightening story. Once again, I'm going to be very open with you. It's still very difficult to believe, but I realize that it is very real in your opinion. Sometimes, and I'm not necessarily saying that this is the case, but sometimes one's mind can perceive reality in a slightly distorted fashion, for instance when a person clearly sees water in a desert when no water is around. Do you think that this might be the case with you?"

If the delusion is fixed, the patient will probably say something like, "No way, this is not a trick of my mind." With a less fixed delusion the patient may be more open to considering the possibility. But, in any case, by this time the clinician has gathered the critical information needed for triage, while still providing some reality contact for the patient.

Earlier I stated that on rare instances it may be appropriate to go along with the patient's delusion temporarily. This may be the case if the patient is rapidly escalating towards violence and any antagonism from the clinician could set him or her off. I am reminded of a humorous example of this process.

A young and agitated woman of about thirty was brought into the emergency room on an involuntary commitment. She was terrified that "the lesbians are all around me. They want to kill me, they want to kill me!" She had already attacked one person, and it was soon clear that she would need admission. Unfortunately, a former male partner of hers had been brought into the emergency room, close to the same time, also on an involuntary commitment. The charge nurse felt that he was "ready to blow." He also happened to be acutely intoxicated. Needless to say the charge nurse thought that it would be a very bad idea for the two patients to meet.

As the fates would have it, the first patient decided that now was the time to escape, and she headed for the door leading to the receiving area, where her past partner was stomping about. Not feeling that it was safe to try to physically stop her by myself, I stood aside. But for whatever it was worth, an idea crossed my mind, and I told her, "I wouldn't go out in that waiting room if I were you, it's packed with women." I don't think her eyes could have gotten much wider. It took her about two seconds to run back into the safety of the interviewing room.

The other problem mentioned earlier arises when the patient pointedly asks for a judgment on his or her sanity. Early in an interview a patient may ask, "Look, I need to know, am I nuts?" If the patient has been animatedly discussing a recent lunch with Neptunians, the clinician may have a perverse desire to say something like, "You're not nuts, you're very nuts." Clearly this is totally inappropriate, and it must be locked away in the recesses of the clinician's id. But all humor aside, what can the clinician say?

Probably a variety of techniques are useful. I tend to reframe what the important point is while proceeding with a rapid sidetrack to this new point, as shown in the following:

> **Pt.:** I just don't know what to do. I honestly think I'm losing my mind. Am I crazy?
>
> **Clin.:** Mr. Bach, I'm not really certain what people mean by

that term. And I don't think that's the major issue for us. Rather it is obvious to both of us that you are not feeling yourself, and that's what we need to look at.//How long have you been feeling depressed?"

Pt.: Oh about three or four months. I know that, because four months ago I visited my son and his family, that's when the trouble began.

The clinician can also tell the patient about misgivings concerning such a term as "nuts" or "crazy." Or the interviewer can utilize a process maneuver by asking the patient questions such as, "Have you been thinking that you are crazy?" or "What exactly have you been worried is happening to you?" Naturally, if the clinician has gathered enough data in order to feel comfortable that the patient is not psychotic, then one can share this opinion with the patient. This simple gesture can be remarkably calming for some neurotic patients who were becoming convinced that they were really going insane. Some patients, on the other hand, have not come for an opinion. In fact, they wish that they had not come at all, as the next section illustrates.

Situational Resistance: The Unwilling Patient

There are probably at least three different types of patients who could be considered unwilling: (1) a patient who is self-referred but feels extremely ill at ease, (2) a patient who came only at the insistence of another person, and (3) an involuntary patient on a commitment. The seed resistances may be significantly different with each type, resulting in differing possibilities for resolving the observable resistance of a shut-down interview.

In the first instance, a patient who feels tenuous about the whole idea of seeing a therapist, the seed resistances may be manifold. The patient may have low self-esteem and consequently be frightened of rejection by the clinician or of being "found out" as a weak person. A fear of the unknown may be actively at work, as the patient imagines all sorts of nasty things that a psychiatrist might do. Frequently, patients are concerned that somehow or other, they will not be in control of what they say, suggesting another possible core pain, the fear of a loss of internal control. The list could go on and on. But the important point remains the fact that there is a reason behind the patient's reticence.

If a patient continues to remain shut-down, despite the use of the many techniques described earlier for opening up such interviews, then the clinician should probably attempt to make the covert resistance overt. In a gentle tone, the clinician may simply say, "Mrs. Ford, I know that it's difficult to talk at first. I'm wondering what some of your concerns are about being here today?" A different tack may be to demonstrate a willingness to help relieve the tension with a statement such as, "Mrs. Ford, it can be hard to talk about personal matters, it certainly is for me. What can I do to make things easier?"

If the clinician obtains a better idea of what the seed resistance is, it can be addressed even more directly. For example, suppose the clinician suspects that the patient is afraid of saying something self-incriminating. The clinician might say, "It's tough to begin talking with a stranger, and it may take time for you to trust me. That's natural, and I don't want you to say anything that you feel uncomfortable with until you're ready."

The above example also brings up the issue of using paradox, in short, telling the patient not to talk, with the hope that this will trigger a desire to continue. When done gently, this technique can be strikingly effective, as was the case with a young man sent by the Army after trying to hang himself. He gave a long history of impulsive behavior and seemed concerned about his tendency for violence. When probed, he began to be resistant, but a gentle paradox quickly resolved the tension.

> **Pt.:** I have had problems with my temper in the past, and I'm afraid of what it all means.
>
> **Clin.:** What exactly are you afraid of?
>
> **Pt.:** I've been in some pretty bad fights, uh, I guess that's what bothers me.
>
> **Clin.:** Have you ever been hurt in one of the fights?
>
> **Pt.:** Not really, a few stitches here and there, nothing to brag about.
>
> **Clin.:** What about the other guy, did you ever hurt one of them pretty badly?
>
> **Pt.:** Yeah, pretty bad, I had a knife on me and it caused some problems.
>
> **Clin.:** Did you actually knife him?
>
> **Pt.:** (The patient began moving around in his seat and put his head down.) I, I don't want to talk about it, I don't even want to think about it right now.
>
> **Clin.:** That's all right. There's no need to go into that right now. It may be of value in the future to talk about it. It might help you to feel a lot better.
>
> **Pt.:** Yeah, I know that. The funny thing was I didn't really want to hurt him, but when he came at me, I just stuck it

> in him. I think I might still do the same thing, it really was, uh, self-defense. You see, we was out looking for some action and I was a little drunked up.

In this instance the patient apparently felt a need to talk, although guilt was blocking the way. Paradoxically, when assured he did not have to talk, he proceeded to tell his story in great detail.

Usually the above types of techniques help to resolve the resistance. Just the process of talking about the resistance frequently increases the patient's duration of utterance and gets the ball rolling. Things can be a little more difficult with a patient who is in the office at the request of someone else and who, unlike the Army recruit, does not want help.

Patients may find themselves in a "shrink's office" at the order of their bosses, friends, or family. It is not uncommon for a spouse to threaten divorce unless the patient seeks help. Clearly this is an awkward situation for both the patient and the therapist. To handle it, Herbert Strean provides some excellent guidelines in his book *Resolving Resistances in Psychotherapy.*[3]

He emphasizes several points. These patients, who are essentially psychologically hand-cuffed, frequently are very angry. They may need a chance to ventilate some of their frustration before proceeding into the body of the interview. They may also view the clinician as somehow "in on it." Consequently, it becomes important to help the patient differentiate between the clinician and the person who pressured the patient to seek help. An open acknowledgment of the situation can help break the logjam, as follows: "Mr. Sanders, it looks like we both feel some tension here. I realize that you don't want to be here, and I respect that. I guess we are both in an awkward position. Let's try to find out if there is anything that you can gain from our talking, and let's leave your wife's desires out of it for a while. Tell me a little more about what your relationship was like at the beginning."

In this fashion the clinician is actually addressing the seed resistance, for the patient is experiencing a loss of external control. With the words "and let's leave your wife's desires out of it for a while," the clinician has effectively released the hand-cuffs. The patient is being given a chance to create his own agenda. At the tail-end of the statement, the clinician is sidetracking the patient toward an affectively charged topic.

Of course, some patients present with real hand-cuffs, representing the third category of unwilling patient, those patients who are involuntarily committed. This situation is obviously not ideal for interviewing. One of the keys to successfully navigating it consists of realizing that both the patient and the clinician are uncomfortable. In essence, there is a common enemy, the situation itself. If the patient refuses to talk, it often pays to point out this common enemy, while matter of factly describing the situation more clearly, as depicted in the following:

> **Pt.:** Look we've been talking for ten minutes and I don't want to talk anymore, period. Got it?
>
> **Clin.:** Mr. Phillips, I'd be upset if I was in your spot too. In fact, I'm not particularly at ease with this situation to begin with. It's awkward for both of us, but here's the bottom line. I know that you want to get out of here. By law, I'm supposed to determine whether you need to be here or not. If I can't talk with you and get more information, I'll have to act cautiously and consequently continue the commitment, because I can't risk letting you hurt yourself. The only way for me to decide whether you can leave is to talk with you. And I'm not pulling any punches here, I'm not saying that if you talk I'll let you go. I'm just saying that if you don't talk you'll definitely have to stay.
>
> **Pt.:** Well, what do you want me to talk about?
>
> **Clin.:** Let's start with your side of the story. What actually happened last night?
>
> **Pt.:** What happened was that I found out that little innocent Susan wasn't so innocent. She was out getting some action. I loved her and she kicked my face in!
>
> **Clin.:** Any ideas why she did it?
>
> **Pt.:** That's what I don't understand, I just don't understand it!
>
> **Clin.:** What happened after you found out?

In this excerpt the clinician also asks the patient for his opinion on what happened. Most committed patients feel that no one is seeing their side of things. If given an opportunity to tell their story, they often will eagerly accept that opportunity. Of course, all of the previously described principles for resolving resistance are equally applicable to the committed patient as well.

The main point is to avoid a battle for control as instigated by statements like, "You have to talk with me and that's that." With these patients the core resistance is frequently a fear of a loss of external control, which for the most part has been stripped away from them. It is indeed a terrifying feeling. The more that the clinician can offer some semblance of control to the patient, while establishing a common agenda, the more likely that the resistance will settle.

Resistance in the Form of Anger

During the initial interview, anger may stem from a variety of causes. In the patients discussed above, the anger was primarily situational in nature. At other times the anger may stem from character pathology, as seen with the primitive rage of borderline and narcissistic personality disorders. In other instances, the clinician may not find the anger coming from the patient. Instead, the clinician faces the brewing anger of irate family members.

One of the first steps necessary in handling angry patients well has nothing to do with the interview itself. It has to do with the clinician's realization that the patient's anger should not be taken personally. No one likes to have people angry at them, but all clinicians will sooner or later have patients who are inappropriately hostile.

One method of placing the patient's anger in perspective is to view the anger as a reflection of pain. Narcissistic rage is often the end result of intense feelings of inferiority. In a similar light the borderline patient's anger may be an artifact whose roots lie in fears of annihilation or abandonment.

Keeping these ideas in mind, certain principles in handling angry patients (and I am not referring to violent or psychotic patients here) are worth examining in more detail. In the first place, one often needs to offer the angry person a chance to ventilate appropriately. In a curious sense, one could say that the clinician attempts to provide the patient with a safe environment in which to be angry. This safety arises from the fact that the clinician will not counterattack, matching force with force. The interviewer steps out of the way of the patient's anger by not providing opposition. The patient cannot resist if there is nothing to resist against.

The clinician should calmly try to determine what exactly is angering the patient. Patients tend to appreciate an honest effort to sort things out. More importantly, if the clinician can decipher which seed resistances are driving the rage, then these core pains can be assuaged more directly. Perhaps the key point consists of conveying to the angry patient that the clinician is listening carefully. The interviewer listens to the patient's demands calmly and with fairness. Patients who become progressively angrier almost invariably feel that their needs are being ignored. Such an escalation in hostility can frequently be prevented by attentive listening.

In the following scenario, the father of an anorexic girl is throwing a fit in the emergency room waiting area. His family has been waiting for about an hour to see the initial interviewer. When the father discovers that the clinician is a psychiatric nurse, the father becomes livid, even though he has been told that a doctor will also see his daughter.

Fath.:   Just what is going on here?! My daughter is not talking with a nurse. We did not drive one hundred miles to see a nurse.

Nurse: Mr. Landis, I'm sorry that this has caused you to get so angry. That concerns me and I need to find out more about what it is about my seeing your daughter that is so upsetting. By the way, I understand that you've been waiting quite some time. We appreciate your patience; as you can see, things are very busy here today. I apologize for the delay and will try to move things along for both you and your family. But first, what are your specific concerns about my seeing your daughter?

Fath.:   I don't think that a nurse is qualified to see my daughter. The problem is far too complex. It's nothing personal, we just don't want a nurse.

Nurse: I see. Just to give me a little background, what are some of the main problems that your daughter is having?

Fath.:   She's got this thing called anorexia nervosa, and it's driving us all mad. The last clinician, a psychologist, didn't do beans for her. And the shrink before him didn't have a clue as to what is going on with her. And we heard that Dr. Wilson here is an expert so we set up an intake appointment.

Nurse: I see. Well, it certainly does seem like a complicated problem, and I also see why you were upset when you saw me coming. Clearly you were expecting a physician. And I certainly agree that Annie needs to see a physician. If you could give me just a moment of your time, I'll try to clarify things and once again get things moving so that Annie can see the doctor. The way Dr. Wilson likes to handle all new referrals is through us. He always has a team approach, because he feels that, especially with eating disorders, it is valuable to get several clinicians thinking about the case. I always see the patient first to scout out the information. After I speak with Dr. Wilson he will want to talk with all of you in some detail. Are there any questions so far from any of you?

Fath.:   So she is definitely going to see the doctor?

Nurse: Absolutely, we wouldn't have it any other way. And the sooner that Annie and I get talking the sooner she'll see the doctor.

Fath.:   O.K., let's get rolling then.

Nurse: By the way, while I'm talking with Annie be sure to organize and prepare any questions you may have for

the doctor. He'll want to hear them all. It is very important for us to hear your opinions on what is going on.
We'll try to make this long trip a worthwhile one for
everyone.

Fath.: Well, it will be if my little girl gets some help.

What could have been a real mess has been resolved gracefully.
This clinician earned her pay and then some. By remaining poised and
nondefensive, she was able to put her ego aside as she dealt with the
bruised ego standing before her. Core pains were quickly addressed,
and the clinician gained ground by giving ground. How differently this
interview might have gone if the clinician had made content responses
such as, "Mr. Landis, you'll have to realize that I am extremely well
trained and am more than well qualified to see your daughter" or,
"Listen, you're going to have to wait just like everybody else here, I
don't care how far you came." Meeting angry statements with more
anger is seldom productive.

The clinician also demonstrated several other subtle yet effective
techniques. Her opening two statements were as follows, "Mr. Landis,
I'm sorry that this has caused you to get so angry. That concerns me
and I need to find out more about what it is about my seeing your
daughter that is so upsetting." Although a bit convoluted, the statements have personalized the conversation with the use of the word
"my." It may be harder for Mr. Landis to be mad at this specific person
as opposed to nurses in general. Indeed the desired effect appeared to
occur, for Mr. Landis literally made a subsequent point of saying that
his concerns were not personal in nature. At this early stage, the
resistance had already begun to soften.

Once the clinician realized the father's strong commitment to Dr.
Wilson, she took advantage of this fact by aligning herself with the
physician. This was accomplished by emphasizing the team approach
and by using the word "we." Furthermore, she deflected responsibility
for the situational circumstances irritating the father by stating, "The
way that Dr. Wilson likes to handle all new referrals is . . . " but of
even more significance, she made the father feel important, while
listening carefully to both his conscious and unconscious needs. In
essence, the clinician does not want to reflect the patient's anger, the
clinician wants to absorb it. This process is difficult at times, especially
for trainees, but the payoffs are immense.

It seems appropriate to be concluding this chapter by discussing
the approach to angry patients, for all of the principles concerning
resistance are brought to the forefront in such situations. It also serves
to highlight the point, mentioned earlier, that the real goal is not to
oppose resistance but to understand it, learn its directions, and move

with its tensions. This skill is not always easy to master, but few skills yield more positive rewards.

In putting the final touches to this chapter, dear old Alice comes back to mind. Hopefully our work with patients is a good deal less confusing than Alice's interactions in Wonderland. But who knows? Perhaps even in Wonderland, the principles discussed here would have been of service. It probably would not have taken long to intuit the core pains behind a figure as fragile as Humpty Dumpty. And once Alice understood his needs, perhaps she would not have found herself quite so speechless.

References

1. Brower, D. (editor): *Of all things most yielding.* San Francisco, Ballantine Books, date of publication unlisted, p.18.
2. Anderson, C., and Stewart, S.: *Mastering Resistance, A Practical Guide to Family Therapy.* New York, The Guilford Press, 1983, pp.120–150.
3. Strean, H.: *Resolving Resistances in Psychotherapy.* New York, John Wiley & Sons, 1985, pp.120–148.

Supervision Utilizing Facilic Analysis

Helping trainees to understand the nuances of structuring the interview, while actively attending to engagement, represents a challenging task for the supervisor. The concepts of facilic analysis can be graphically employed in a fashion that brings the interview to life for the trainee while presenting an easily understood description of what actually took place. In this Appendix a brief description of this graphic system is presented. It is not meant to fully describe the system but to provide an introduction. This system of "shorthand" can be utilized in direct supervision, class discussion, and videotape supervision.

The system grew out of the observation that modern dancers have developed simple systems of representing their complex movements and choreography. It was felt that the structural choreography of the initial interview may also be amenable to symbolic representation. Two complementary analyses are available. In a longitudinal facilic analysis, the interview and its transition are followed from front to back chronologically. In a cross-sectional facilic analysis, a pie diagram allows the clinician to observe the overall structuring process.

Content regions are depicted as rectangles, with the subject matter abbreviated within the rectangle. The degree of thoroughness in expanding any given content region is depicted by slash marks at the corners of the rectangle. One slash represents 25 percent of the needed information, two slashes represent 50 percent, three slashes represent 75 percent, and four slashes represent a completely expanded region. Process areas such as psychodynamic inquiries are represented by circles. The scouting phase is indicated by a combination of both a rectangle and circle. All transitional gates are depicted as follows:

Spontaneous Gates	~~→	Introduced Gates	—□→
Natural Gates	⟹	Phantom Gates	—⊠—
Referred Gates	----→	Manufactured Gates	—o—o→
Implied Gates	↓__→		

With videotape supervision, the supervisor first watches the tape alone and subsequently reviews it with the trainee. When first watching the tape, the supervisor uses the facilic schematic system to note the flow of the interview as well as adding comments concerning any other technical aspects of the interview such as engagement techniques and psychodynamic concerns. The time of the interview in minutes as well as the videotape counter number are noted periodically, allowing the supervisor to quickly turn to illustrative videotape excerpts. The system also provides a permanent outline of the supervision hour, which can be referred to in future sessions of supervision by both the supervisor and trainee. An example of a longitudinal analysis is shown below:

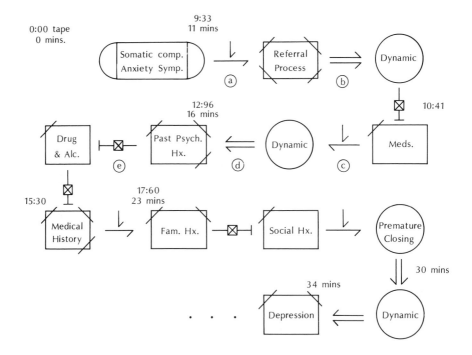

Counter
Settings

I. Transitions (Gates)
ⓐ What made you come to our clinic today?
ⓑ What were some of your feelings about coming here today?

                 ⓒ What role do you think your actions play in some of these problems?

                 ⓓ Have you ever seen a psychiatrist before?

13:10   *   ⓔ Are you a problem drinker?

II. Teaching Points

8:00   1. Scouting phase is appropriately unstructured and free-floating but is too long.

9:50   2. Too much detail and time spent in the referral process region.

10:10   *   3. Good psychodynamic questioning.

10:41   *   4. Decrease use of phantom gates (ask clinician what he was feeling at this point of the interview).

12:96   *   5. Explore use of chronology as a reference framework.

13:00   6. Good use of empathy: "Sounds like the world was caving in on you back then."

14:00   *   7. Use behavioral incidents when delineating the drug and alcohol history. I think this patient was providing invalid information. (Also comment on note taking — too much.)

18:00   *   8. Here's a series of Type A validity errors including multiple questions and negative questions.

The asterisks represents areas of videotape that may be useful to view with the trainee. It can also be seen that this clinician tends to overuse abrupt transitions and to leave content regions prematurely. These errors may result in a weakening of the thoroughness of the data base needed in this particular style of intake assessment, in which a complex triage was to be determined and a full diagnostic evaluation was requested. Numerous positive comments were also made in the actual supervision, highlighting the skills of the clinician.

The facilic analysis merely provides a framework for discussion. The actual supervision itself is characterized by spontaneity, humor, and discussions of both dynamic and personal feelings related to the interview. The trainee may request certain areas of the tape to be viewed. Emphasis is also placed upon nonverbal interaction.

A second type of facilic analysis, a cross-sectional view, provides an illuminating view of the actual use of time in the interview. Thirty minutes of a cross-sectional analysis are shown on the following page.

In the videotape supervision, a record is also kept of the types of questions asked (e.g., swing questions, open-ended questions, statements of empathy), as used in the opening fifteen minutes.

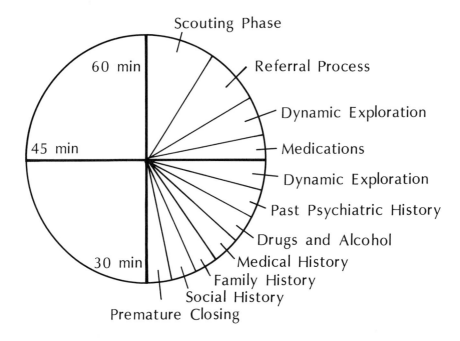

These facilic schematics help to make concrete and manageable some of the interviewing skills that appear nebulous and confusing at first glance. From this common framework of understanding between the supervisor and the trainee, the possibility of actual changes in interviewer behavior arises, leading to both improved skills and a renewed fascination with the interview process itself.

Glossary of Interview Supervision Terms

Blending

Blending is the subjective and objective evidence, collected from the interview, which suggests that the engagement process is going well. For group discussion and supervision purposes, it is useful to rate blending on a scale from zero (patient is hostile toward clinician) to ten (patient and clinician appear extremely natural together). The degree of blending can be determined from three complementary perspectives: (1) the clinician's subjective feelings, (2) objective evidence from the patient's behavior (such as increased eye contact or smiling), and (3) self-report from the patient. The degree of blending depends on two major elements, the clinician's skill and the patient's defenses and psychopathology. Consequently, low blending is not necessarily a sign of poor clinician performance. For instance, a skilled clinician may only achieve a blending of three with a patient who displays active paranoid process.

Closed-Ended Questions

Closed-ended questions are those questions that are extremely easy for a moderately guarded or moderately resistant patient to answer with one word, a short phrase, or a simple "yes" or "no." All inquiries that provide or imply a specific list of answers or ask for specific items, places, dates, numbers, or names are viewed as closed-ended. In patients who are easily engaged, these questions may also tend to decrease interviewee response length, for in many instances the socially appropriate answer is only one word, a short phrase, or a simple "yes" or "no."

Content Region

An area of dialogue in which a specific topic becomes the center of focus. Typical content regions include diagnostic regions, history of the present illness, social history, family history, and the lethality assessment.

547

Engagement Process

The verbal and nonverbal behaviors demonstrated by the interviewer that create an atmosphere of increasing trust, safety, and calmness in the interviewee.

Facilics

Facilics is the study of the flow and structuring of the interviewing process. In its applied format it includes the study of the methods utilized by clinicians to explore specific topics and processes (delineated as "regions") as well as the study of transitions (delineated as "gates") between these regions. A method of diagramming the various regions and transitions has been developed and is currently utilized as both a supervision and research tool. In a pure research form, facilic analysis can be applied to any dialogue, whether an everyday conversation or a television interview.

Gentle Assumption

A technique for increasing the likelihood that sensitive material will be discussed more openly. The clinician assumes that the suspected behavior is occurring and frames a question based on this assumption. Thus, the clinician does not ask, "Do you masturbate?" but "How frequently do you masturbate during a typical week?"

Gentle Commands

Gentle commands represent one of the two most powerful open-ended techniques (open-ended questions being the other). They begin with phrases such as "Tell me about your . . ." or "Say something about . . .", which gently direct the patient to discuss a topic. The tone of voice is gentle and nonthreatening. An example of such a statement is "Tell me something about your stress on the job."

Implied Gate

A relatively smooth transition initiated by the clinician, who leaves one topic by discussing a closely related topic that seems to follow the conversation. It does not (as in the case of the natural gate) take its cue from the immediately preceding patient response.

Introduced Gate

These gates do not naturally follow the flow of conversation, but they are relatively smooth, for the clinician verbally notes that a transition is under way. An example is as follows: "For a moment let's change topics to how your mood has been recently."

Manufactured Gate

A technique for setting up a natural transition by bringing up a bridging topic. For instance, if the clinician wants to bring up alcoholism, he or she first inquires about family history. After asking about a family history of drinking, the clinician then smoothly cues off this material into the patient's own drinking history.

Natural Expansion

An exploration of a given topic in which the clinician's questions seem to follow naturally and convey an almost conversational feeling to the interview.

Natural Gate

A smooth transition from one topic to a new topic initiated by the clinician. In a natural gate the clinician cues directly off the patient's immediately preceding statement.

Open-Ended Questions

Open-ended questions are difficult to answer with one word or a short phrase, even if the interviewee is moderately guarded or moderately resistant. It is virtually impossible to respond to these questions with a simple "yes" or "no." Questions that provide or imply possible answers, or ask for specific items, places, dates, numbers, or names, are never viewed as open-ended, for they limit the freedom of answer choice. In patients who are easily engaged, open-ended questions should tend to produce relatively large quantities of speech.

PACE

An acronym representing the four major assessments made by a clinician during the scouting period:

P = Patient's perspective and conscious agenda

A = Assessment of the patient's mental status on an informal basis

C = Clinician's perception of the patient's problems and unconscious agenda

E = Evaluation of the interview process itself (e.g., is the interview shut down, wandering, or rehearsed?).

Phantom Gate

This relatively weak transition occurs when a new topic is introduced with an abrupt entrance that seems to come from nowhere. Such gates may convey a sense of awkwardness or disinterest on the part of the clinician, especially if his or her style is frequently characterized by such blunt transitions.

Pivot Points

A pivot point occurs when a patient spontaneously changes topics. If the clinician is consciously aware of a pivot point, then a decision can be made regarding the wisdom of following or gently refocusing the patient. Uncontrolled wandering interviews frequently result when clinicians miss pivot points and consequently never appropriately focus the patient.

Process Regions

An area of dialogue in which the focus is on the manner in which the patient answers, not the content of what is said. Classic process regions include facilatory regions, psychodynamic regions, and regions in which specific types of resistance are addressed. Other process regions include phenomenological inquiries and educational regions. Sometimes process regions may also function as content regions, as is the case with phenomenological and educational regions.

Referred Gate

A graceful transition in which a new topic is entered by referring to a previous topic raised earlier in the interview. These transitions convey a sense of careful listening and concern. They frequently begin with phrases such as, "Earlier you had mentioned . . ." or "At one point you had talked about . . .".

Region

A region is a facilic analysis term referring to an area of interview in which a specific topic is being explored or in which the clinician is utilizing a specific interviewing tool focused on the process as opposed to the content of the interview (see Content Region and Process Regions).

Rehearsed Interview

This interview is characterized by a moderate to large production of spontaneous speech that focuses only on topics of interest to the patient. It is a method by which the interview is controlled by the patient.

Responsive Zone (RZ)

The range of distances between the clinician and the patient in which both participants feel comfortable and seem to be aware, at least at an unconscious level, of each other's movements. Once within the RZ, nonverbal behaviors of the clinician have the potential to effectively impact upon the patient. Inside the RZ, nonverbal behaviors may be intimidating or overwhelming. Outside the RZ, nonverbal behaviors may seem insignificant and noneffective.

Scouting Period

Generally the first five to seven minutes of a fifty to sixty minute interview. This period is composed of both the introduction and the opening phase of the interview. Open-ended verbalizations tend to predominate, for the main goal of the clinician is the development of a sound engagement with the patient. One or two empathic statements are frequently useful.

Shame Reversal

A technique for increasing the validity of the patient's response by maintaining a nonthreatening stance. The question tends to be phrased in such a fashion that a positive reply does not feel incriminating to the patient but suggests a specific problem to the clinician. A classic example would be the question, "Do you find that other men pick fights with you when you're trying to enjoy a drink at the bar?" If the patient answers yes, it is easy to discover the number of fights and whether the patient actually plays a role in their initiation, as seen in sociopathy.

Shut-Down Interview

In this type of interview, the patient answers tensely and shows little spontaneity or interest in engagement. Eye contact is frequently poor, and gesturing is at a minimum. A variant of this style is the hostile interview, in which the patient's tone of voice may be angry and the content of the patient's responses may be sharp or antagonistic. In the hostile interview, eye contact may be prolonged and glaring.

Side-Tracking

Side-tracking is a method of handling resistance in which the clinician switches topics away from the issue raised by the patient. It can be very effective with tangential patients, especially if the clinician chooses a topic about which the patient is invested in talking. If the patient returns to the original resistance, it suggests that side-tracking will not work.

Spontaneous Gate

A smooth transition from one topic to another that is initiated by the patient. The clinician completes the transition by asking questions of relevance to the new topic.

Statement of Inquiry

These statements follow the declarative pattern of subject/verb. They represent statements, but the tone of voice suggests that they are intended to be inquiries and are followed by a question mark. Two examples are as follows: (1) "You were always late for work?" and (2) "So you were hesitant to go to college?" In shut-down interviews these statements of inquiry can be answered tersely. On a positive side, they may function to effectively clarify questions or to summarize the patient's story. On a negative side, they may represent leading questions.

Stilted Expansion

An exploration of a given topic in which the clinician's questioning seems highly structured and awkward. It is sometimes seen when clinicians utilize a checklist approach to symptoms or when the transitions between questions are repeatedly abrupt or odd. Stilted expansions can create a "Meet the Press" style of interaction.

Swing Questions

Questions that essentially ask the interviewee whether he or she would like to answer or not. They begin with phrases such as, "Could you tell me . . .", "Would you say something about . . .", or "Can you describe . . .". If engagement is high, such swing questions function essentially as open-ended questions. But if engagement is low, they can easily be answered tersely and hence tend to further shut down the interviewee, functioning as closed-ended inquiries.

Symptom Amplification

A technique for increasing the validity of a patient's response by setting the upper limits of a question at such a high level that when the patient downplays the amount, the remaining sum still suggests a problem. For example, "How much liquor can you hold at one time, say a fifth or two?" If the patient responds "Oh no, not that much, maybe a pint, perhaps a pint and a half at most" then the clinician is still aware that a significantly high tolerance is present.

Tracking

The ability of the clinician to sensitively follow the patient's train of thoughts with appropriate clarifying questions. The clinician can track both the affect of the patient and/or the content of the patient's speech.

Unipolar Blending

A specific type of blending that occurs when the patient appears immediately and unusually at ease with the clinician. This "high engagement" is in reality relatively superficial and arises essentially independently of the clinician's engagement techniques. The patient is often talkative and may be dramatic. The presence of unipolar blending frequently suggests underlying psychopathology such as histrionic traits, a hypomanic or manic state, acute intoxication, or extreme anxiety.

Type A Validity Errors

These errors are related to the content of the interviewer's questions and include leading questions, negative questions, multiple questions, and other phrasing errors.

Type B Validity Errors

These errors are related to paralanguage and nonverbal activity. They include processes such as a curt tone of voice, a horizontal head nod while asking a question, or inappropriately cutting patients off.

Wandering Interview

An interview characterized by a patient with verbose speech production and tangential or circumstantial thought. A variant of this interview type is the loquacious interview, in which the patient produces large amounts of speech but the speech stays on the chosen topic. The wandering interview is furthered by poor structuring techniques on the part of the clinician.

Index

Page numbers in *italics* refer to illustrations; page numbers followed by (t) refer to tables.